Feline Practice: Integrating Medicine and Well-Being (Part II)

Editor

MARGIE SCHERK

VETERINARY CLINICS OF NORTH AMERICA: SMALL ANIMAL PRACTICE

www.vetsmall.theclinics.com

September 2020 • Volume 50 • Number 5

ELSEVIER

1600 John F. Kennedy Boulevard • Suite 1800 • Philadelphia, Pennsylvania, 19103-2899
http://www.vetsmall.theclinics.com

VETERINARY CLINICS OF NORTH AMERICA: SMALL ANIMAL PRACTICE Volume 50, Number 5
September 2020 ISSN 0195-5616, ISBN-13: 978-0-323-75442-2

Editor: Stacy Eastman
Developmental Editor: Nicole Congleton

Veterinary Clinics of North America: Small Animal Practice (ISSN 0195-5616) is published bimonthly by Elsevier Inc., 360 Park Avenue South, New York, NY 10010-1710. Months of issue are January, March, May, July, September, and November. Business and Editorial Offices: 1600 John F. Kennedy Blvd., Ste. 1800, Philadelphia, PA 19103-2899. Customer Service Office: 3251 Riverport Lane, Maryland Heights, MO 63043. Periodicals postage paid at New York, NY and additional mailing offices. Subscription prices are $348.00 per year (domestic individuals), $705.00 per year (domestic institutions), $100.00 per year (domestic students/residents), $451.00 per year (Canadian individuals), $876.00 per year (Canadian institutions), $488.00 per year (international individuals), $876.00 per year (international institutions), $100.00 per year (Canadian students/residents), and $220.00 per year (international students/residents). To receive student/resident rate, orders must be accompanied by name of affiliated institution, date of term, and the *signature* of program/residency coordinator on institution letterhead. Orders will be billed at individual rate until proof of status is received. Foreign air speed delivery is included in all *Clinics* subscription prices. All prices are subject to change without notice. **POSTMASTER:** Send address changes to *Veterinary Clinics of North America: Small Animal Practice*, Elsevier Health Sciences Division, Subscription Customer Service, 3251 Riverport Lane, Maryland Heights, MO 63043. Customer Service (orders, claims, online, change of address): Elsevier Periodicals Customer Service, Elsevier Health Sciences Division Subscription **Customer Service 3251 Riverport Lane Maryland Heights, MO 63043. Tel: 1-800-654-2452 (U.S. and Canada); 314-447-8871 (outside U.S. and Canada). Fax: 314-447-8029. E-mail: journalscustomerservice-usa@elsevier.com (for print support); journalsonlinesupport-usa@elsevier.com (for online support).**

Reprints. For copies of 100 or more of articles in this publication, please contact the Commercial Reprints Department, Elsevier Inc., 360 Park Avenue South, New York, NY 10010-1710. Tel.: 212-633-3874; Fax: 212-633-3820; E-mail: reprints@elsevier.com.

Veterinary Clinics of North America: Small Animal Practice is also published in Japanese by Inter Zoo Publishing Co., Ltd., Aoyama Crystal-Bldg 5F, 3-5-12 Kitaaoyama, Minato-ku, Tokyo 107-0061, Japan.

Veterinary Clinics of North America: Small Animal Practice is covered in *Current Contents/Agriculture, Biology and Environmental Sciences, Science Citation Index, ASCA, MEDLINE/PubMed (Index Medicus), Excerpta Medica, and BIOSIS.*

Contributors

EDITOR

MARGIE SCHERK, DVM
Diplomate, American Board of Veterinary Practitioners (Feline Practice); catsINK Feline Consultant, Vancouver, British Columbia, Canada

AUTHORS

BOAZ ARZI, DVM
Department of Surgical and Radiological Sciences, School of Veterinary Medicine, University of California, Davis, Davis, California, USA

JULIEN BAZELLE, DVM, MRCVS
Diplomate, European College of Veterinary Internal Medicine - Companion Animals; Davies Veterinary Specialists, Manor Farm Business Park, Higham Gobion, Hitchin, Hertfordshire, United Kingdom

REUBEN M. BUCKLEY, PhD
Post-doctoral Fellow, Department of Veterinary Medicine and Surgery, College of Veterinary Medicine, University of Missouri, Columbia, Missouri, USA

LETICIA M.S. DANTAS, DVM, MS, PhD
Diplomate, American College of Veterinary Behaviorists; Behavioral Medicine Service, Department of Veterinary Biosciences and Diagnostic Imaging, University of Georgia Veterinary Teaching Hospital, University of Georgia, Athens, Georgia, USA

MIKEL DELGADO, PhD
Department of Medicine and Epidemiology, School of Veterinary Medicine, University of California, Davis, Davis, California, USA

LINDA FLEEMAN, BVSc(Hons), PhD, MANZCVS
Animal Diabetes Australia, Melbourne, Victoria, Australia

REBECCA F. GEDDES, MA, VetMB, MVetMed, PhD, FHEA, MRCVS
Diplomate, American College of Veterinary Internal Medicine; Clinical Scientist Fellow, Queen Mother Hospital for Animals, Royal Veterinary College, North Mymms, Hertfordshire, United Kingdom

RUTH GOSTELOW, BVetMed(Hons), PhD, FHEA, MRCVS
Diplomate, American College of Veterinary Internal Medicine; Diplomate, European College of Veterinary Internal Medicine - Companion Animal; Department of Clinical Science and Services, The Royal Veterinary College, London, United Kingdom

KATRIN HARTMANN, Prof Dr med vet, Dr habil
Diplomate, European College of Veterinary Internal Medicine - Companion Animals; Clinic of Small Animal Medicine, LMU Munich, Munich, Germany

REGINA HOFMANN-LEHMANN, Prof Dr med vet, FVH
Clinical Laboratory, Department for Clinical Diagnostics and Services, Vetsuisse Faculty, University of Zurich, Zurich, Switzerland

ALBERT E. JERGENS, DVM, PhD
Diplomate, American College of Veterinary Internal Medicine; Department of Veterinary Clinical Sciences, College of Veterinary Medicine, Iowa State University, Ames, Iowa, USA

MELISSA A. KENNEDY, DVM, PhD
Diplomate, American College of Veterinary Microbiology; Associate Professor, Department of Biomedical and Diagnostic Sciences, College of Veterinary Medicine, University of Tennessee, Knoxville, Tennessee, USA

HANS S. KOOISTRA, DVM, PhD
Diplomate, European College of Veterinary Internal Medicine - Companion Animals; Department of Clinical Sciences of Companion Animals, Faculty of Veterinary Medicine, Utrecht University, Utrecht, the Netherlands

DOTTIE. P. LaFLAMME, DVM, PhD
Diplomate, American College of Veterinary Nutrition; Consultant, Veterinary Communications, Floyd, Virginia, USA

DA BIN LEE, DVM
Dentistry and Oral Surgery Service, William R. Pritchard Veterinary Medical Teaching Hospital, University of California, Davis, Davis, California, USA

JONATHAN A. LIDBURY, BVMS, MRCVS, PhD
Diplomate, American College of Veterinary Internal Medicine; Diplomate, European College of Veterinary Internal Medicine - Companion Animal; Department of Veterinary Medicine and Biomedical Sciences, Vet Med Small Animal Medicine and Surgery, College of Veterinary Medicine, Texas A&M University, College Station, Texas, USA

LESLIE A. LYONS, PhD
Gilbreath-McLorn Endowed Professor of Comparative Medicine, Department of Veterinary Medicine and Surgery, College of Veterinary Medicine, University of Missouri, Columbia, Missouri, USA

SHANKUMAR MOOYOTTU, DVM, PhD
Diplomate, American College of Veterinary Pathologists; Department of Veterinary Pathology, College of Veterinary Medicine, Iowa State University, Ames, Iowa, USA

MARYANNE MURPHY, DVM, PhD
Diplomate, American College of Veterinary Nutrition; Clinical Assistant Professor of Nutrition, Small Animal Clinical Sciences, The University of Tennessee College of Veterinary Medicine, Knoxville, Tennessee, USA

MARK E. PETERSON, DVM
Diplomate, American College Veterinary Internal Medicine; Animal Endocrine Clinic, New York, New York, USA

CLARE RUSBRIDGE, BVMS, PhD, FRCVS
Diplomate, European College of Veterinary Neurology; Chief of Neurology, Fitzpatrick Referrals, Godalming, Surrey, United Kingdom; Professor of Veterinary Neurology,

School of Veterinary Medicine, Faculty of Health and Medical Sciences, University of Surrey, Guildford, Surrey, United Kingdom

FRANK. J.M. VERSTRAETE, DrMedVet, MMedVet
Dentistry and Oral Surgery Service, William R. Pritchard Veterinary Medical Teaching Hospital, Department of Surgical and Radiological Sciences, School of Veterinary Medicine, University of California, Davis, Davis, California, USA

PENNY WATSON, MA, VetMD, CertVR, DSAM, FRCVS
Diplomate, European College of Veterinary Internal Medicine - Companion Animals; Queen's Veterinary School Hospital, University of Cambridge, Cambridge, United Kingdom

CRAIG B. WEBB, PhD, DVM
Diplomate, American College of Veterinary Internal Medicine; Professor, Clinical Sciences Department, Colorado State University Veterinary Teaching Hospital, Fort Collins, Colorado, USA

TRACY L. WEBB, DVM, PhD
Research Scientist/Clinical Review Board Coordinator, Clinical Sciences/Research Integrity and Compliance Review Office, Colorado State University, Fort Collins, Colorado, USA

ANGELA WITZEL-ROLLINS, DVM, PhD
Diplomate, American College of Veterinary Nutrition; Clinical Associate Professor of Nutrition, Small Animal Clinical Sciences, The University of Tennessee College of Veterinary Medicine, Knoxville, Tennessee, USA

Contents

Feline infectious peritonitis (FIP) is a mysterious and lethal disease of cats. The causative agent, feline coronavirus (FCoV), is ubiquitous in most feline populations, yet the disease is sporadic in nature. Mutations in the infecting virus combined with an inappropriate immune response to the FCoV contribute to the development of FIP. Diagnosis can be challenging because signs may be vague, clinical pathology parameters are nonspecific, and the gold standard for diagnosis is invasive: histopathology of affected tissue. This article discusses the developments in the understanding of this disease as well as the progress in diagnosis and treatment.

Feline leukemia virus (FeLV) is a retrovirus with global impact on the health of domestic cats that causes tumors (mainly lymphoma), bone marrow disorders, and immunosuppression. The importance of FeLV is underestimated due to complacency associated with previous decline in prevalence. However, with this comes lowered vigilance, which, along with potential for regressively infected cats to reactivate viremia and shed the virus or develop clinical signs, can pose a risk to feline health. This article summarizes knowledge on FeLV pathogenesis, courses of infection, and factors affecting prevalance, infection outcome, and development of FeLV-associated diseases, with special focus on regressive FeLV infection.

Hypertension is a common problem, particularly in older cats. Hypertension secondary to a concurrent disease is the most common form of hypertension in cats, particularly in association with chronic kidney disease or hyperthyroidism. However, idiopathic hypertension may account for up to 24% of cases. Any form of persistent hypertension risks target organ damage (TOD), therefore measurement of blood pressure is vital in at-risk cats to identify occult hypertension before TOD occurs. This article addresses when and how to perform blood pressure measurement in cats, TOD that has been documented in this species, and our evidence basis for treating hypertension.

Primary hyperaldosteronism, also known as Conn's syndrome, is the most common adrenocortical disease in cats. As in humans, this disease is underdiagnosed in cats. Cats presenting with systemic arterial hypertension, hypokalemia, or both quite often are only treated symptomatically without further investigations. This practice may potentially exclude a significant number of cats from receiving appropriate treatment. It is therefore important for general practitioners to be aware of the disease. This article describes the (patho)physiology, clinical presentation, diagnostic approach, and treatment options of for feline primary hyperaldosteronism.

In cats, hyperthyroidism can be treated in 4 ways: medical management with methimazole or carbimazole, nutritional management (low-iodine diet), surgical thyroidectomy, and radioactive iodine (^{131}I). Each form of treatment has advantages and disadvantages that should be considered when formulating a treatment plan for the individual hyperthyroid cat. Medical and nutritional managements are considered "reversible" or palliative treatments, whereas surgical thyroidectomy and ^{131}I are "permanent" or curative treatments. The author discusses how each treatment modality could be the optimal choice for a specific cat-owner combination and reviews the advantages and disadvantages of each treatment option.

Flash glucose monitoring is a novel, noninvasive monitoring technique that is increasingly used in the management of small animal diabetes. This article provides guidance on the use of flash glucose monitoring in cats and demonstrates how this technique can be used in a range of feline diabetic cases, including those where management is proving challenging. Other aspects of complicated feline diabetic care are also discussed, including management of the sick diabetic cat, potassium depletion myopathy, and treatment options for cats with hypersomatotropism-associated diabetes mellitus. The use of insulin glargine 300 U/ml as a promising new long-acting insulin for diabetic cats is also discussed.

In recent years, increased awareness of feline pancreatitis by the veterinary profession and improved diagnostic modalities have led to an increased frequency of diagnosis of pancreatitis in this species. Consequently, pancreatic diseases, especially chronic pancreatitis, are considered highly prevalent, even in populations of apparently healthy individuals. This prevalence has led to the suspicion that the condition may be overdiagnosed. This article summarizes the difficulties of diagnosis of acute and chronic pancreatitis, assesses the reasons why this is a challenging disease to recognize, and considers whether these difficulties could result in either overdiagnosis or underdiagnosis.

Cholangitis is a common cause of hepatobiliary disease in the cat. Feline cholangitis is characterized as neutrophilic (acute or chronic), lymphocytic, or caused by liver flukes. The neutrophilic form is caused by bacterial infection of the biliary system, and identification of the specific bacterial agent guides treatment. Bile is the sample of choice for cytology and bacterial culture in these cases, and percutaneous ultrasound-guided cholecystocentesis is used to obtain that sample. This review covers the literature that provides evidence for safety and usefulness of percutaneous ultrasound-guided cholecystocentesis as part of the diagnostic work-up of cats suspected of having hepatobiliary disease.

Clinical findings with triaditis and individual disease components overlap and may include hyporexia, weight loss, lethargy, vomiting, diarrhea, dehydration, icterus, abdominal pain, thickened bowel loops, pyrexia, dyspnea, and shock. A definitive diagnosis of triaditis requires histologic confirmation of inflammation in each organ, but this may not be possible because of financial or patient-related constraints. Evidence-based data indicate that histologic lesions of triaditis are present in 30% to 50% of cats diagnosed with pancreatitis and cholangitis/inflammatory liver disease. Treatment of triaditis is based on the overall health status of the patient and the type and severity of disease in component organs.

 Video content accompanies this article at http://www.vetsmall. theclinics.com.

The corticolimbic system (prefrontal cortices, amygdala, and hippocampus) integrates emotion with cognition and produces a behavioral output that is flexible based on the environmental circumstances. It also modulates pain, being implicated in pathophysiology of maladaptive pain. Because of the anatomic and function overlap between corticolimbic circuitry for pain and emotion, the pathophysiology for maladaptive pain conditions is extremely complex. Addressing environmental needs and underlying triggers is more important than pharmacotherapy when dealing with feline orofacial pain syndrome or feline hyperesthesia syndrome. By contrast, autoimmune limbic encephalitis requires prompt diagnosis and management with immunosuppression and seizure control.

VETERINARY CLINICS OF NORTH AMERICA: SMALL ANIMAL PRACTICE

SERIES OF RELATED INTEREST

Veterinary Clinics of North America: Exotic Animal Practice
https://www.vetexotic.theclinics.com/

THE CLINICS ARE NOW AVAILABLE ONLINE!
Access your subscription at:
www.theclinics.com

Preface

Part 2: Exciting Changes in Feline Medicine

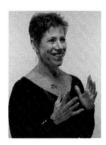

Margie Scherk, DVM
Editor

The previous issue of this 2-part series focused on the role of stress in the development and manifestation of illness in cats. My first love was ethology, understanding who and what a species/creature is by observing their behavior under native environmental situations. As a consequence, I respect them for who and what they are. Over my years in practice and as an educator, this has colored how I see and do things. It has been gratifying to see Cat Friendly and Fear Free movements emerge...as these recognize the stressful and traumatic experience that our patients experience. With the expansion of these programs into the home environment, something that Tony Buffington has championed, we get closer to recognizing who cats are. However, there is still room for this approach when we think about any patient with a medical ailment.

In this issue, more of the medical concerns are addressed. Nutrition is a cornerstone of maintaining health as well as treating disease. In order to attain a good nutritional plane, good oral health is required: an article on oral health addresses the frustrating problem of chronic gingivostomatitis as well as a separate article on the status of stem cell therapies in cats. In that light, there are articles on what the practitioner should know about genetic testing and precision medicine. In-depth updates in feline infectious peritonitis as well as feline leukemia virus are included. Internal medicine topics include hypertension and endocrine diseases, with an article each describing updates in hyperaldosteronism, hyperthyroidism and hypothyroidism, and diabetes. The anterior digestive tract is represented in articles on pancreatitis, ultrasound-guided percutaneous cholecystocentesis, and the complex described as triaditis. The final article is dedicated to newly recognized neurologic entities in cats.

Wherever possible, the role of the whole patient and their relationship to their social/emotional environment are included....easier to accomplish in some articles than in others. It is my sincere hope that this series showcases not only medical advances

Vet Clin Small Anim 50 (2020) xiii–xiv
https://doi.org/10.1016/j.cvsm.2020.06.001
0195-5616/20/© 2020 Published by Elsevier Inc.

but also clinically relevant understanding of how mental/emotional and social factors affect health, disease, and illness.

I have said this previously, but it is no less true for this issue. I am extremely grateful to every author. Thank you for putting up with my nagging, cajoling, and attempts to finetune. Especially, as much of this labor of love has been during the COVID-19 pandemic when every one of you has been stressed to the limit, trying to adapt to the rapidly changing requirements, be it in academia or in private practice. I hope that this pair of issues is greater than the sum of its individual parts. Thank you.

Margie Scherk, DVM
catsINK
Vancouver, Canada

E-mail address:
hypurr@aol.com

Understanding the Nutritional Needs of Healthy Cats and Those with Diet-Sensitive Conditions

Dottie P. Laflamme, DVM, PhD

KEYWORDS

- Obligate carnivore • Protein • Carbohydrate • Lean body mass • Myths
- Diet-sensitive disease sarcopenia • Kidney disease

KEY POINTS

- As carnivores, cats evolved with unique needs. They retain, however, considerable metabolic flexibility.
- Nutritional needs of cats can vary based on age, individual metabolism, and health conditions.
- Sarcopenia, or age-related loss of lean body mass, is common in geriatric cats. Although diet cannot prevent it, certain dietary features, such as increased dietary protein, can slow this loss.
- Although restriction of dietary carbohydrate can be beneficial in the management of feline diabetes, moderate amounts of complex carbohydrates can be beneficial in healthy cats.
- Many of the nutrient modifications thought to be important for the management of chronic kidney disease are not well supported by evidence. Ongoing research likely will identify better diets for cats with kidney disease.

INTRODUCTION

There are 3 main factors in nutritional management of cats, according to the iterative process promoted by the American College of Veterinary Nutrition (www.ACVN.org). These include

- Animal factors, such as species, age, lifestyle, and health
- Food factors, addressing the nutritional content of the food relative to the needs of the animal
- Feeding management, which includes aspects, such as how the animal is fed and how food is consumed

Conflict of Interest: None.
Veterinary Communications, 473 Grandma's Place, Floyd, VA 24091, USA
E-mail address: JunqueDr@yahoo.com

Changes in any 1 of these aspects can have an impact on the other factors, hence the need for iterative re-evaluation. Feeding management is covered in Mikel Delgado and Leticia M. S. Dantas' article, "Feeding Cats for Optimal Mental and Behavioral Well-Being," elsewhere in this issue, so this article focuses on the interface between animal factors and nutritional needs.

This article is divided into 3 sections. Section 1 addresses the dietary needs of healthy cats, including differences among life stages. Section 2 addresses common myths regarding feline nutrition. Section 3 addresses common nutrient-sensitive conditions in cats, including sarcopenia of aging.

SECTION 1: NUTRITION FOR THE HEALTHY CAT

Veterinarians remain the top source of information about pet care and nutrition, although the Internet, social media, and friends and family also are popular sources of information. Unfortunately, some of these sources promote ever-evolving fads and misinformation about nutrition for cats. As such, veterinarians must be confident in their ability to discuss nutrition and dietary management with their clients, which requires a solid understanding about the principles of nutrition. The nutritional adequacy of a diet for an individual cat depends on several factors: the bioavailable nutrient content of the food, the amount of food consumed by the cat, and the actual nutrient requirements of that specific cat.

Nutritional Requirements of Cats

Cats are obligate carnivores. This means that cats have evolved consuming prey-based diets and, as such, require certain nutrients found naturally only in animal tissues (**Table 1**). In addition, compared with dogs, cats require more protein and have uniquely higher requirements for arginine and sulfur-containing amino acids and some B vitamins.[1]

Although wild and feral cats rely on prey as the primary basis of their diets, some intake of plant matter has been noted.[2] The actual prey consumed varies widely based on availability. The prey provides energy and nutrients, just as ingredients in prepared foods provide energy and nutrients. If the available prey provides all the nutrients and energy that the animal needs, it will survive. If not, the individual or the species fails to thrive. The opportunistic consumption of prey-based diets does not mean that cats are biologically limited to such a diet. The same nutrients can be provided from other ingredients, such as those used in either commercial or home-prepared diets.

Food energy is derived from the macronutrients: proteins, fats, and carbohydrates. Most prey contain abundant protein, moderate fat, and limited carbohydrate, although

Table 1	
Unique nutritional requirements of domestic cats that define them as obligate carnivores	
Nutrient	**Why Cats Require These Nutrients Rather than Their Precursors**
Arachidonic acid	Cats lack adequate amounts of the delta-5 and delta-6 desaturation enzymes needed to elongate and convert linoleic acid to arachidonic acid.
Taurine	Cats are able to produce taurine from cysteine but not enough to meet their needs due to low enzyme activity and, to some degree, competition of precursors for production of felinine.
Vitamin A	Cats lack adequate dioxygenase, the enzyme needed to convert beta carotene to vitamin A.

the specific amounts vary and reports suggest variation among different prey animals. Published data suggest average contents of 52% to 63% protein, 25% to 46% fat, and 2% to 12% carbohydrate, all based on percent of energy.[2,3]

Commercial cat foods also vary in their nutrient content, with larger differences between wet foods and dry foods (**Table 2**). Based on modified Atwater values for metabolizable energy (ME), the average distributions of protein, fat, and carbohydrate on an energy basis for dry foods were 32%, 37%, and 31%, respectively, whereas those for wet foods were 41%, 45%, and 14%, respectively, but with considerable variation (Dr Sean Delaney, unpublished 2019).

What Are Essential Nutrients and Minimum Requirements?

Essential nutrients are those needed by the animal and that cannot be synthesized in adequate amounts endogenously so must be provided by the diet. Nonessential nutrients also are required by the animal but are produced within the body in sufficient quantities as long as appropriate precursors are available. Common examples of these nutrients include the nonessential amino acids and glucose. Nonessential amino acids are critical for normal endogenous protein production and many other functions, but are produced by transamination from other amino acids provided in the diet. Likewise, glucose is essential as an energy source for many cells in the body. Although fats and ketones can provide a source of energy for some cells, other cells have an absolute requirement for glucose. Yet, because glucose can be produced endogenously via gluconeogenesis, it is not considered an essential dietary nutrient.

Minimum nutrient requirements are defined as the smallest intake shown to prevent known signs of nutrient deficiencies, to sustain balance in adults, or to support maximum growth in growing animals. Balance studies compare the total intake of the test nutrient to the total loss through feces and urine, with neutral balance at the

Table 2
Nutrient content in typical commercial cat foods available for retail purchase in the United States

Type[a]		Protein	Fat	Crude Fiber	Ash	Nitrogen-free Extract[b]
				Percent of dry matter		
Dry (N = 301)	Mean	36.4	17.4	4.4	7.3	34.7
	SD	5.1	5.2	2.2	0.9	7.9
	Min	14.6	5.6	0.5	3.0	6.7
	Max	57.9	39.2	13.5	11.3	70.2
Soft–Moist	Mean	40.1	14.7	4.6	6.5	34.1
(N = 8)	SD	1.5	1.4	2.1	0.1	0.7
	Min	39.3	13.9	1.1	6.4	32.5
	Max	43.1	17.0	5.7	6.6	34.4
Wet (N = 424)	Mean	46.7	20.9	5.6	10.8	16.0
	SD	8.0	7.9	2.4	3.9	10.2
	Min	25.0	9.1	0.0	3.8	0.0
	Max	79.5	47.4	16.8	20.6	54.2

Abbreviations: Max, maximum value; Min = Minimum value; SD = Standard Deviation.
[a] Nutritionally complete foods grouped based on moisture content: dry foods contain 15% or less moisture; soft–moist foods contain 20% to 65% moisture; and wet foods contain more than 65% moisture.
[b] Nitrogen-free extract is an estimation of the carbohydrate content measured by difference.
Data courtesy of S. Delaney, DVM, MS, DACVN, Davis, CA.

lowest intake taken as the minimum. Such scientific studies are performed mostly with purified or controlled diets and evaluate 1 nutrient at a time, so adjustments must be made to account for differences in bioavailability and nutrient interactions in common foodstuffs as well as animal differences, such as life stage, lifestyle, individual metabolism, and energy needs.

The minimum amount needed also depends on the criteria used to determine adequacy. For example, although balance studies typically are used to determine minimum requirements for protein and amino acids, the amount of protein needed to maintain nitrogen balance is, in fact, not adequate to maintain lean body mass (LBM) or muscle function.[4–6] Studies in both dogs and cats suggest that at least 3 times more protein is needed to maintain protein reserves or LBM compared with that needed to maintain nitrogen balance.[5,7] For adult cats, approximately 5 g protein/kg body weight are needed to maintain LBM compared with approximately 1.5 g protein/kg body weight to maintain nitrogen balance.[5] This is considerably above the recommended intake or minimum requirements cited by the Association of American Feed Control Officials (AAFCO)[8] or the National Research Council (NRC).[9]

Cats require adequate protein and a small amount of essential fatty acids to meet physiologic needs. These are absolute requirements, and no other nutrients can substitute for these. Together, these may constitute up to 50% of dietary calories. Beyond these requirements, cats also need a source of energy, including a source of glucose. Here, there is great flexibility because the energy can come from any of the 3 macronutrients, and glucose can be derived from either protein or carbohydrates. This metabolic flexibility allows cats to thrive on a wide range of nutrient profiles from a wide range of ingredients.

Additional protein and amino acids beyond the minimum provide substrates for endogenous production of glucose as well as the nonessential amino acids. Cats require relatively small amounts of essential fatty acids, including arachidonic acid. Additional fat is used as a source of energy. Cats require a physiologic supply of the carbohydrate glucose, which is the primary energy source for most cells in the body. Adult, nonreproducing cats, however, do not require a dietary source of carbohydrates as long as adequate gluconeogenic substrates are available.

The specific amounts of dietary protein, fats, and carbohydrate needed are dependent on the amounts of the other macronutrients. For example, prey-based diets do not provide adequate glucose from carbohydrates to meet the physiologic needs of cats. The abundant protein in such diets, however, provides the gluconeogenic substrate needed under most circumstances. Although fat and fatty acids provide a rich source of energy calories, containing more than twice as many calories per gram compared with either protein or carbohydrate, they are not an adequate source of glucose. Only a small portion of fats, the glycerol backbone of triglycerides, can be used to produce glucose. Finally, although dietary carbohydrates are not essential, when provided, they can supply a primary source of the glucose needed by cells.

Nutritional Guidelines and Pet Food Labels

Pet food regulations within the United States are managed on a state by state basis. Foods that are produced and sold locally within a given state need only meet the regulatory guidelines, if any, of that state. Most foods sold in multiple states, or internationally, comply with the guidelines published by AAFCO. AAFCO is an organization that includes the state feed control officials from each state as well as Canada and Costa Rica.[8] Although AAFCO does not enforce regulations, they provide model regulations that can be adopted and enforced at the state level. Not all states uniformly do this, so regulations and enforcement can differ among states.

The labels of all foods complying with AAFCO guidelines must provide a guaranteed nutrient analysis, a list of all ingredients in the diet listed in descending order by weight, a nutritional adequacy statement, and the name and contact information for the manufacturer of the food, in addition to other information. The nutritional adequacy statement lists the minimum amount of protein and fat and maximum amount of moisture and crude fiber, on an as-fed basis. Because of the differences in moisture content among foods, especially between dry kibble and canned foods, these nutrients must be converted to dry matter basis prior to comparison. This is relatively simple (% protein/[100 − % moisture]), although it provides only an estimate of the actual content. A more reliable method is to contact the manufacturer and ask for the average nutrient content of interest on a dry matter and an energy basis.

Perhaps the most important information provided on the label is the nutritional adequacy statement. This should state if the food was formulated to provide complete nutrition, based on AAFCO profiles or if the food underwent animal feeding trials to confirm nutritional adequacy. Several foods, especially some wet cat foods, may not carry either of these claims but, rather, may indicate that they are intended only for intermittent or supplemental feeding. Such foods should not be fed as the sole diet nor as a major component of the total diet. Some veterinary therapeutic diets may carry an intermittent feeding claim. In this case, the prescribing veterinarian must understand the limitations with the diet and determine if long-term feeding is appropriate.

The nutrient recommendations provided by AAFCO, as well as by the NRC, generally are based on studies performed with growing animals or with adult animals at maintenance fed purified diets.[8,9] The NRC minimum requirements are defined as the lowest intake of bioavailable nutrients that support a defined physiologic state, such a growth or adult maintenance. Recommended allowances include some estimates to adjust for differences in bioavailability. AAFCO makes further allowances to make practical recommendations for use of common feed ingredients. Due to these differences, the recommendations from the NRC and AAFCO often differ. These recommendations should be taken as a minimum amount to feed rather than an absolute amount. For essentially all nutrients, there is a significant safety margin between minimum needs and any amount likely to cause harm. Although both NRC and AAFCO have separate guidelines for growth and adult maintenance, neither has guidelines to address the unique needs of geriatric animals.[8,9]

Impact of Life Stage on Nutrient Requirements

Adult animals at maintenance have the lowest energy and nutrient requirements compared with animals in other life stages. Late gestation and lactation are recognized as the most demanding life stages from a nutritional perspective, followed by growth. For this reason, foods formulated to address adult maintenance only never should be fed to pregnant or lactating cats or to young, growing kittens. The reverse is not true—there can be situations when it is appropriate to feed kitten food to adult cats, as long as the calorie density of the food is appropriate for the cat. To consider all adult cats as a homogenous group is inappropriate. Individual cats can vary dramatically in their energy requirements, and middle-aged cats differ significantly, as a group, from geriatric cats. Inactive or obese-prone cats should be fed diets with lower calorie density and increased nutrient/calorie ratios, whereas active, thin cats may need higher-calorie diets.

Middle-aged cats (age 6–10 years) are more likely to be obese and their energy requirements lower compared with young adult cats.[10] Cats over 12 years of age tend to lose weight and LBM, have greater energy requirements compared with middle-aged cats, and may have increased protein requirements.[10] Many geriatric cats have a reduced ability to digest fats and protein and show compromised absorption of some vitamins and essential trace nutrients.[11] Given these changes, geriatric cats may benefit from a diet that is more digestible, nutrient enriched, and higher in protein and calories compared with typical adult maintenance dietsor those intended for middle-aged cats. Kitten foods can be a good option for senior cats, unless such a diet would be medically contraindicated; alternatively, senior diets especially designed for cats over age 12 may be considered.

SECTION 2: NUTRITIONAL MYTHS AND MISPERCEPTIONS REGARDING CATS

The fact that cats are carnivores may underlie many of the common misperceptions regarding the dietary needs of cats. Among the more common misperceptions are (1) cats cannot digest or utilize vegetable source proteins; (2) cats cannot digest or utilize dietary carbohydrates; (3) excess carbohydrates in cat foods is a common cause of obesity; and (4) cats must eat wet foods because dry foods cause chronic dehydration.

The perception that cats cannot digest or utilize vegetable source proteins is completely false. It is true that vegetable source proteins, such as soy and corn, wheat, and rice glutens, do not provide all of the essential amino acids that cats require so should not be used as a sole source of protein in a diet. They can be both highly digestible, however, and a good source of protein and many amino acids. Properly cooked and used with complementary amino acid sources, they can contribute available nutrients to a complete, balanced diet.

Cats do have unique features regarding carbohydrate metabolism, including a lack of sweet taste receptors, lack of glucokinase, and relatively lower levels of digestive enzymes. Despite these features, cats are very capable of digesting and metabolizing carbohydrates. Multiple studies have shown the apparent digestibility of carbohydrates in dry commercial and experimental cat foods exceeds 80% to 90%, similar to that shown in dogs.[12–15]

Like other mammals, cats retain the ability to adapt to different macronutrient intakes. Numerous studies have shown that cats metabolize different macronutrients as energy sources, whether from carbohydrates, fat, or protein, based on dietary intake of those nutrients.[16–21] One example is a study wherein cats were fed diets with decreasing amounts of dietary protein (50% down to 7.5% of ME) in exchange for increasing amounts of dietary carbohydrate (11%–54% of ME). Cats metabolized more protein when fed higher-protein diets, whereas they metabolized more carbohydrate when fed the high-carbohydrate diets, sparing dietary protein. As long as minimal protein needs were met, cats were able to adapt their metabolism based on the sources of energy consumed.[18] Gluconeogenesis from protein increases incrementally as dietary protein increases and dietary carbohydrate decreases.[21] Other studies also showed that cats increase fat oxidation when fat is increased in the diet and increase carbohydrate oxidation when that nutrient is increased in the diet[16,20,22]

Excess calories from carbohydrate sometimes are blamed for inducing obesity. In fact, excess calories from any of the macronutrients induce obesity. As a dietary component, carbohydrates have an advantage over dietary fats in that they are much lower in ME. Each gram of carbohydrate provides approximately 3.5 kcal (14.6 kJ) whereas each gram of fat provides approximately 8.5 kcal (35.6 kJ). Thus, replacing dietary fat with more carbohydrates actually reduces the calorie density of foods, which may help reduce the risk for obesity. In cats, consumption of high-fat foods is a significant risk factor for obesity. Multiple studies showed that cats gained more weight and more body fat when allowed to eat or overeat high-fat diets compared with low-fat, high-carbohydrate diets.[23–26] Overconsumption of any diet, however, can contribute to obesity, so total energy intake, rather than dietary carbohydrate, must be limited to manage obesity.

A majority of cats in the United States eat dry commercial cat food either exclusively or as their primary diet.[27,28] The concern that this may cause dehydration is unfounded for the vast majority of cats. Water balance is maintained through a combination of altered intake and excretion via the gastrointestinal and urinary tracts. When fed dry diets, most cats drink more water, whereas those fed wet diets may consume little or no additional water.[29,30] For cats exhibiting chronic, mild dehydration, such as cats with constipation, with conditions that may cause dehydration, or with conditions that may benefit from increased water throughput, such as urinary tract diseases, wet foods or flavored water supplements may provide a valuable source of additional water. Commercial canned foods contain between approximately 65% and 85% water. This exceeds a cat's ability to limit its water intake and forces the cat to excrete the excess water, resulting in increased volume or frequency of urination. To increase fecal water for management of constipation, less-digestible foods with water added or wet foods containing dietary fiber may increase fecal water.[29]

SECTION 3: NUTRITION FOR CATS WITH COMMON DIET-RESPONSIVE CONDITIONS
Age-Related Sarcopenia

Although aging is not a disease, it brings multiple changes to cats, some of which have nutritional implications. Obesity, which can be a problem at any life stage and which, itself, can contribute to disease, is less of a problem in geriatric cats. Instead, weight loss and sarcopenia become more frequent and potentially devastating problems in geriatric cats.

Weight loss occurs in a majority of cats after approximately 12 years of age. Approximately 15% of cats are underweight by 12 years of age, whereas cats over 15 years of age have a 15-fold greater likelihood of being underweight compared with young adult cats.[31,32] Longitudinal studies suggest that this is due to weight loss occurring in apparently healthy senior cats, rather than from attrition of overweight cats.[11,33] In fact, underweight cats at any age are more likely to have a shorter life span.[34] Data also show that weight loss appears to precede the diagnosis of disease in cats, accelerates once the disease has advanced sufficiently to be diagnosed, and is associated with greater mortality.[11,35,36]

Independent of loss of weight, individuals tend to lose LBM with age. Sarcopenia is the age-associated loss of LBM unrelated to disease. It occurs slowly, over years, becoming evident only later in life (**Fig. 1**).[37] In most cases, the loss of LBM is offset by an increase in fat mass, resulting in little or no change in body weight[11,38] The loss of LBM occurs in all species studied, including humans, dogs, and cats.[11,33,37–42] Lean mass was decreased by approximately 33% in healthy cats aged 15 years to 17 years compared with cats aged 5 years to 11 years.[11] Importantly, loss of LBM is associated with increased morbidity and mortality.[33,37] For the reasons discussed previously, it is important that aging cats undergo a thorough nutritional assessment that includes body weight changes, body condition scoring, and muscle scoring, as described in Angela Witzel-Rollins and Maryanne Murphy's article, "Assessing Nutritional Requirements and Current Intake," in this issue. An illustrated muscle condition scoring system from the World Small Animal Veterinary Association can be accessed at https://www.wsava.org/WSAVA/media/Documents/Committee%

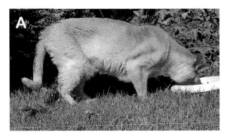 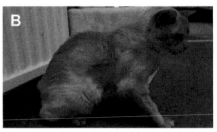

Fig. 1. (*A*) Photo of adult cat in good muscle condition. (*B*) Photo of same cat at 13 years of age with evidence of sarcopenia. Note the generalized loss of muscling despite a normal body condition. (*Courtesy of* M. Chandler, DVM, Lasswade, Scotland.)

20Resources/Global%20Nutrition%20Committee/English/Muscle-Condition-Score-Chart-for-Cats.pdf.

The etiology of sarcopenia is multifactorial and complex (**Box 1**).[38,43–45] Regardless of the mechanisms, the result in sarcopenia is a decrease in LBM, muscle mass, and strength.

Although exercise is the most efficient therapy for managing existing sarcopenia, nutrition also plays a role in development and management of this condition. Specifically, adequate dietary protein, specific amino acids, and vitamin D appear to play a role. Protein supplementation coupled with exercise achieves the best results in sarcopenic people.[46] Other dietary factors that may be important include nutrients impacting metabolism, inflammatory mediators, and acid/base balance.

Insufficient protein intake can contribute to loss of LBM. Multiple studies have confirmed lower protein intakes were associated with greater loss of LBM or muscle function or increased risk for sarcopenia.[4,6,40,47–51] When dietary protein intake is inadequate, mammals gradually deplete proteins from their LBM, in particular skeletal muscle, to support metabolic functions.[4,5]

Because the amount of protein needed to maintain LBM or protein reserves is approximately 3 times that needed to maintain nitrogen balance, diets just meeting minimal standards based on nitrogen balance do not provide sufficient protein to

---

Box 1
Factors contributing to sarcopenia in aging subjects

Inadequate intake of protein or calories

Blunted anabolic response to amino acids and insulin

Altered protein turnover with decreased protein synthesis

Altered protein turnover with increased protein catabolism

Decreased mammalian target of rapamycin (mTOR) pathway function

Chronic increase in inflammatory cytokines

Mitochondrial dysfunction

Increased oxidative stress

Insulin resistance

Decreased neuromuscular junction structure and function

Data from Refs.[38,43–45]

preserve LBM.[5,7] In adult cats, approximately 34% of calories, or approximately 5 g of protein/kg body weight, was needed to maintain LBM compared with approximately 1.5 g protein/kg body weight to achieve nitrogen balance.[5] As discussed previously, aging cats may require even more protein due to age-related inefficiencies in metabolism as well as decreased digestive function.[11,51,52] Aged cats had an average reduction in protein digestion of approximately 6% in 1 study, whereas another study showed that 20% of cats over age 14 had a reduced ability to digest protein.[11,52] The increased need for dietary protein in cats is similar to humans, where there is a growing consensus that older people should consume approximately 50% more protein than the established recommended daily allowance.[6,48,53–55]

In addition to total protein, type of amino acid can play a role in protein turnover. Whey protein appears to be especially useful in this regard. Whey protein is rich in branched-chain amino acids, including leucine. Leucine has important regulatory actions in protein turnover: leucine reduces proteolysis and enhances protein synthesis, among other functions.[45,56] Whey protein also triggers insulin release, which promotes protein synthesis.[56,57] Early research has shown promise, and clinical studies in humans are under way evaluating benefits from leucine and whey protein in sarcopenia.[58] The amino acid lysine also may have an impact on LBM. Lysine deficiency leads to increased protein degradation and decreased protein synthesis in muscle.[59–61] Because lysine is limited (low relative to requirements) in many vegetable source proteins, supplementation may be especially important in diets based on vegetable-source proteins as well as diets low in total protein. One study showed that increasing dietary lysine, independent of total protein, helped reduced loss of LBM in aging cats.[62]

Epidemiologic studies have identified an association between low serum vitamin D concentrations and an increased prevalence of sarcopenia in aging people.[46,50,63] Vitamin D metabolites affect the transcription rate of thousands of genes, including insulin receptors, which promote muscle protein synthesis.[46,64,65] In aged rats, vitamin D deficiency reduced the rate of protein synthesis by 40% compared with vitamin D replete rats.[64] Supplementation with vitamin D resulted in improvements in muscle strength and muscle mass in humans with initially low serum vitamin D.[46,58] Currently, data on vitamin D supplementation to preserve LBM in dogs or cats are lacking.

Anti-inflammatory nutrients, such as long-chain omega-3 fatty acids; antioxidant nutrients, such as vitamins C and E; and trace nutrients, such as magnesium, phosphorus, selenium, and vitamin B_{12}, all are being explored for a potential role in human sarcopenia. In addition, correction of acid/base imbalance is an area of future promise for human and companion animal sarcopenia.

Acidosis is associated with increased protein catabolism, negative nitrogen balance and muscle protein wasting. It appears to promote muscle protein catabolism via the ubiquitin proteasome pathway and to inhibit protein synthesis via promotion of insulin resistance.[66–68] The role of acidosis in LBM wasting is best recognized in patients with chronic kidney disease (CKD), but the same or similar mechanisms may play a role in other conditions, including sarcopenia.[69,70] Correction of acidosis in human subjects with CKD eliminated the muscle protein degradation and improved muscle mass.[69] Even mild metabolic acidosis may contribute to loss of LBM and sarcopenia.[70,71] In a study of men with CKD, in whom arterial pH was adjusted by oral intake of sodium citrate/citric acid and ammonium chloride, decreases in pH within the normal range (7.37–7.44) significantly compromised nitrogen balance.[71]

Although serum bicarbonate may be monitored in pets, evaluation of blood pH or blood gases to quantify acid/base balance rarely is done, especially in healthy aging pets. Future research should evaluate the importance of acid/base balance and blood pH on LBM in aging cats.

Sarcopenia is an active area of research pursuing both nutritional and pharmaceutical treatments. Until more information becomes available, adequate calorie intake should be provided so as to maintain body weight in nonobese geriatric cats. This may require environmental modification to assure access to food, care for any underlying medical conditions or, if needed, use of assisted feeding.[10,72–74] The goal for protein intake should be approximately 5 g/kg to 7 g/kg body weight (approximately 35% to 45% of calories) and should be restricted only if medically essential. Supplementation with the long-chain omega-3 fatty acids, eicosapentaenoic acid (EPA) and docosahexaenoic acid (DHA), should be considered. A recommended dosage is 65 mg EPA + DHA/kg body weight.[72] Veterinarians also may consider supplementing with alkalinizing buffers, such as potassium citrate or sodium bicarbonate, in cats at risk for chronic acidosis.

Diabetes Mellitus

A vast majority of diabetic cats have type 2 diabetes mellitus (DM), with decreased insulin secretion and insulin resistance.[75] Obesity and inactivity, both common in cats, seem to be significant risk factors for type 2 DM.[76] Management involves insulin therapy coupled with appropriate dietary management, which can lead to resolution in 41% to 84% of cats with newly diagnosed DM.[77]

The focus of dietary management in feline DM is to achieve and maintain ideal body condition and to help regulate glycemic control. Cats with type 2 DM may benefit from a high-protein (>45% dry basis), low-carbohydrate (<15% dry basis) (HPLC) diet, although more evidence to support this is needed.[78] The concept behind this dietary approach is to minimize the postprandial glucose influx. Consumption of protein instead of soluble carbohydrates slows absorption and release of glucose into the bloodstream. Consuming multiple small meals reduces the amount of glucose entering the bloodstream at any 1 time. Both of these approaches help reduce the need for insulin.

Evidence to support the value of HPLC diets comes from multiple studies, although all studies had some limitations.[79–82] Many diabetic cats demonstrated decreased insulin requirements or enhanced glycemic control when fed an HPLC diet, and, in many cases, insulin injections could be stopped altogether. Because of the probability that insulin requirements decrease in cats fed HPLC diets, it is critical that these animals be monitored carefully to avoid hypoglycemia.

Obesity causes a significant reduction in insulin sensitivity, making management of DM more difficult. Even moderate increases in body weight can cause significant changes in insulin sensitivity, with a 30% decrease in insulin sensitivity for each kilogram increase in weight in adult cats.[17] It is, therefore, important to try and prevent or correct obesity, which requires a reduction in calorie intake. Unfortunately, HPLC diets tend to be high in fat and calories. Calorie restriction using these diets can result in excessive restriction in total food intake. Instead, a high-protein, low-fat diet, with moderate carbohydrates (15%–25% dry basis) and moderate fiber (5% to 15%, dry basis), may be more appropriate for obese DM cats. Diets with this profile provide some benefit to reduce insulin requirements or enhance DM control while being more appropriate for weight loss.[79,83]

Chronic Kidney Disease

A majority of cats with CKD are 10 years of age or older; cats typically survive many years after a diagnosis of CKD.[84] Although medical therapies, such as angiotensin II receptor blockers, calcium channel blockers, and others, continue to prove beneficial, dietary management remains an important factor in managing cats with CKD.

Although it is well established that renal diets have proved superior to adult mainte-nance diets in managing cats with moderate to severe CKD,[85–87] there remain contro-versies regarding the ideal renal diet. Two of the important goals of such diets are (1) to address the abnormalities in homeostasis produced by renal insufficiency and reduce ongoing renal injury and (2) provide the nutrients needed by these cats over the years they likely will survive with CKD.

The key nutrients often cited for managing CKD include protein, phosphorus, potas-sium, sodium, omega-3 fatty acids, alkalizing buffers, and adequate calorie intake. Maintaining adequate potassium is critical to normal renal function, and low potassium can cause or worsen CKD.[88–90] Although sodium restriction historically has been rec-ommended for CKD patients, evidence in cats suggests not only is this unnecessary but also that excessive restriction can be harmful. When cats with induced CKD were fed sodium-restricted diets, those fed diets with 0.2% sodium (dry basis) developed excessive urine potassium loss and hypokalemia. These cats also showed activation of the renin-angiotensin-aldosterone axis (which can be detrimental in CKD), with no beneficial impact on blood pressure.[91] Additionally, an epidemiologic study indicated that lower-sodium diets were associated with increased risk for developing CKD.[92] Omega-3 fatty acids from fish oil often are recommended for cats with CKD. The only evidence supporting a benefit of this in cats was a retrospective evaluation from cats fed various commercial renal diets: the diet with the highest EPA content was associated with the longest survival.[86]

Alkalinizing buffers are included in renal diets to offset metabolic acidosis. Meta-bolic acidosis affects 53% to 80% of cats with CKD and can cause or contribute to progression of CKD through potassium wasting and other mechanisms.[93–96] Meta-bolic acidosis can cause anorexia, nausea, vomiting, lethargy, and weight loss as well as increased protein catabolism, decreased protein synthesis, and loss of LBM. Correction of acidosis via bicarbonate supplementation in rodents and humans resulted in stabilization of renal function, normalized protein catabolism, or improved markers of nutritional status, including increased LBM.[97] Unfortunately, no data in cats address the potential benefit of independently supplementing bicarbonates.

Phosphorus regulation is disrupted in CKD. Hyperphosphatemia contributes to ongoing damage in the face of existing kidney disease, and dietary phosphorus re-striction may help reduce this ongoing damage.[98–101] In cats, elevations in serum parathyroid hormone and fibroblast growth factor 23, which are involved in phos-phorus homeostasis, as well as elevations in serum phosphate have been identified as risk or prognostic factors for progression of renal disease.[102–106] Serum phosphate was correlated positively with severity of interstitial fibrosis in cats with CKD.[103] Although it is not known if these substances actually contribute to renal injury or simply are markers of ongoing renal injury,[101] restriction in dietary phosphorus does have a positive impact in all species that have been studied. No specific recommendation can be made for an optimum amount of dietary phosphorus due to a lack of data on different phosphorus intakes in CKD, and to the poor association between total phosphorus intake and serum or urine phosphorus. This is, in part, because of the various homeostatic controls over phosphorus and, in part, because of various other dietary factors. Bioavailability of phosphorus sources vary, with highly soluble phos-phate salts being most available and the phosphorus in grains being least available. In addition, dietary calcium, magnesium, and fiber interact with phosphorus, altering uptake from the intestinal tract. Instead of a dietary recommendation, the International Renal Interest Society (IRIS) recommends serum phosphate levels based on the IRIS stage and recommends keeping serum phosphorus in the lower end of the normal range using dietary phosphorus restriction and phosphate binders (http://www.iris-kidney.com/guidelines/recommendations.html).

Studies in multiple species have evaluated the potential role for protein restriction in the management of CKD. It is now recognized that many of these studies were confounded by other dietary variables, such as phosphorus or calorie intake; thus, the conclusions may have been in error. The single best study to determine the role of protein in canine CKD was performed using induced CKD in a factorial study.[107] Based on the intentional study design, the effects of protein restriction were separated from phosphorus restriction. The results clearly showed there were no differences based on protein intake. Studies in other species have confirmed these findings.[98,108]

In cats, only 2 studies have been published that attempted to look at protein independent of other variables. The first study evaluated diets containing either 27.6% or 51.7% protein (dry basis).[109,110] During this 1-year study, a majority of cats fed the high-protein diet developed hypokalemia due to insufficient potassium in that diet. Hypokalemia is an independent risk factor for CKD, thus confounding the study. Although the diet was supplemented with potassium after the first 3 months, markers of renal dysfunction already were notably worse in this group, and some, including proteinuria, actually improved over the remaining months of study after potassium supplementation. At the end of the study, those cats fed the higher-protein diet showed greater renal pathology and had greater serum urea nitrogen concentrations, but the effect of protein versus potassium deficiency could not be confirmed. Other differences between diet groups included calorie intake, with cats fed the lower-protein diet consuming fewer calories. Reduced calorie intake can have a protective effect on kidney function.[111] Because of these confounding factors, it cannot be determined whether the renal pathology observed in this study was due to protein or to other factors. The investigators also reported that cats fed the higher-protein diet had better inulin clearance, had lower serum creatinine, and maintained body weight better than cats fed the lower-protein diet,[109] suggesting possible benefits from the higher-protein diet.

The second cat study controlled both protein intake and calorie intake, and ensured adequate potassium intake.[112] CKD cats fed the high-protein, high-calorie diet maintained body weight whereas those fed low-protein diets lost weight. Similar to the previous study, markers of renal function were better in cats fed the higher-protein diets, although the differences did not achieve statistical significance. Calorie intake, but not protein intake, significantly affected renal lesions. Overall, the results of this study showed no association between protein intake and renal lesions or glomerular filtration rate.[112] Proteinuria, which is a negative prognostic factor in CKD, was not impacted by protein intake in this or another study.[87,112] No clinical studies in cats with naturally occurring CKD have been conducted where dietary protein was the only variable evaluated. Based on the available evidence, protein restriction per se is not warranted in cats with CKD.

Although commercial renal diets generally provide nutrient modifications considered of benefit for patients with CKD, not all historically recommended modifications are beneficial. It is likely that additional research will allow improvements in coming years. At this time, if a commercial renal diet is to be fed, it is recommended to select one of the higher-protein options. As with any dietary change, it is important to reassess the patient periodically to ensure the diet is suitable and intake remains adequate.

Osteoarthritis

Limited scientific data exist regarding dietary care for cats with arthritis. Arthritic cats may have difficulty accessing food or eating due to painful joints; thus, environmental changes to aid food access may be needed. It may be assumed that obesity in cats, as in other mammals, worsens arthritis, so weight management is an important aspect of arthritic care. In addition, the anti-inflammatory long-chain omega-3 fatty acids EPA and DHA have shown promise in arthritic cats.[113,114]

One study showed that, compared with a control diet, a diet containing 188 mg of omega-3 fatty acids/100 kcal ME plus green-lipped mussel extract, glucosamine, and chondroitin sulfate resulted in a significant increase in activity in cats with moderate to severe osteoarthritis.[113] Another study showed that similar amounts of supplementation with the fatty acids alone resulted in improved activity in cats, as perceived by the owners.[114]

Correcting obesity reduces stress on a cat's joints and can reduce inflammatory adipokines, thereby reducing pain. Methods to encourage weight loss include giving less of a cat's normal diet, changing gradually to appropriate amounts of a weight loss diet, and encouraging greater activity, as tolerated. Food calories may be reduced by decreasing fat, increasing protein, increasing fiber, or increasing water content. Fat contains more than twice the ME per gram compared with protein or carbohydrates. Replacing some of the fat with protein or carbohydrate decreases the total calories in the food. Although protein and carbohydrate have approximately the same ME, the actual net energy (energy available for adenosine triphosphate [ATP] production) in protein is lower. The efficiency of capturing the energy in food for ATP production is 90% for fat, 75% for carbohydrate, and 55% for protein.[115] This energy inefficiency is due, in part, to the fact the protein stimulates metabolism and protein turnover, which expends energy. This can be used to advantage in weight loss diets. Cats fed high-protein diets had greater energy expenditure, were able to maintain more LBM, and also were able to lose more weight or maintain weight while consuming more calories, compared with lower-protein diets.[116–118] The addition of fiber to a diet decreases calories, slows gastric emptying, and aids in satiety. Water can dilute calories, allowing a greater volume of food to be fed while reducing calories, but has a limited impact on satiety.

Canned foods have been recommended as a way to control calories for cats. When switched from dry to wet, many cats lose weight over several weeks to months before adjusting to the new diet format. Given the opportunity, however, cats overconsume wet food as readily as dry food, so total food and calorie consumption must be controlled. Use of measuring cups to feed dogs or cats can be unreliable because the amount of food in the cup can vary considerably.[119] Use of smaller measuring devices, such as 1-oz to 2-oz scoops, or weighing food with a kitchen scale can help better control the amount of food provided. Use of smaller bowls also helps owners feed less food.[120,121] Feeding small cans of wet food may help pet owners feed fewer calories, because the amount fed can be judged more accurately.

Use of a feeding ball or food puzzle may be useful as long as a cat's arthritis does not prevent it from interacting with the device and obtaining its food.[122,123] It is important to closely monitor a cat's weight because excessive or unintended weight loss may indicate that a cat no longer can gain access to its food, is experiencing food bowl competition in a multiple-cat household, is bored with the diet, or has developed significant systemic disease. In some cats used to extensive variety, simply limiting the variety, such as may occur with the use of therapeutic diets, also may contribute to reduced intake.

SUMMARY

The iterative process of nutritional management includes the need to reassess patients after changes have occurred. Changes in diet, food intake, or health are some common reasons why alterations may be needed in nutritional management. Diets for cats must not only provide complete nutrition but also meet the needs of individual patients. There is no single diet that is perfect for all cats and veterinarians must consider the needs of the cat as well as the preferences of the owners when making dietary recommendations. This article has touched on many factors that may aid veterinarians in reviewing diets and when making dietary recommendations.

REFERENCES

1. Verbrugghe A, Bakovic M. Peculiarities of one-carbon metabolism in the strict carnivorous cat and the role in feline hepatic lipidosis. Nutrients 2013;5: 2811–35.
2. Plantinga EA, Bosch G, Hendriks WH. Estimation of the dietary nutrient profile of free-roaming feral cats: Possible implications for nutrition of domestic cats. Br J Nutr 2011;106(Suppl. 1):S35–48.
3. Kremen NA, Calvert CC, Larsen JA, et al. Body composition and amino acid concentation of select birds and mammals consumed by cats in northern and central California. J Anim Sci 2013;31:1270–6.
4. Wolfe RR. The underappreciated role of muscle in health and disease. Am J Clin Nutr 2006;84:475–82.
5. Laflamme DP, Hannah SS. Discrepancy between use of lean body mass or nitrogen balance to determine protein requirements for adult cats. J Feline Med Surg 2013;15:691–7.
6. Nowson C, O'Connell S. Protein requirements and recommendations for older people: a review. Nutrients 2015;7:6874–99.
7. Wannemacher RW, McCoy JR. Determination of optimal dietary protein requirements of young and old dogs. J Nutr 1966;88:66–74.
8. Association of American Feed Control Officials. Official Publication. Association of American Feed Control Officials. 2014:149–64.
9. National Research Council Ad Hoc Committee on Dog and Cat Nutrition. Nutrient requirements of dogs and cats. Washington, DC: The National Academies Press; 2006.
10. Laflamme DP, Gunn-Moore D. Nutrition for aging cats. Vet Clin North Am Small Anim Pract 2014;44:761–74.
11. Perez-Camargo G. Cat nutrition: what's new in the old? Comp Cont Educ Small Anim Pract 2004;26(Suppl 2A):5–10.
12. Morris JG, Trudell J, Pencovic T. Carbohydrate digestion by the domestic cat (*Felis catus*). Br J Nutr 1977;37:365–73.
13. Fekete SG, Fodor K, Prohaczik A, et al. Comparison of feed preference and digestion of three different commercial diets for cats and ferrets. J Anim Physiol Anim Nutr 2005;89:199–202.
14. Carciofi AC, Takakura FS, de-Oliveira LD, et al. Effects of six carbohydrate sources on dog diet digestibility and post-prandial glucose and insulin response. J Anim Physiol Anim Nutr 2008;92:326–36.
15. De-Oliveira LD, Carciofi AC, Oliveira MCC, et al. Effects of six carbohydrate sources on diet digestibility and postprandial glucose and insulin responses in cats. J Anim Sci 2008;86:2237–46.
16. Lester T, Czarnecki-Maulden G, Lewis D. Cats increase fatty acid oxidation when isocalorically fed meat-based diets with increasing fat content. Am J Physiol 1999;277:R878–86.

17. Hoenig M, Thomaseth K, Waldron M, et al. Insulin sensitivity, fat distribution, and adipocytokine response to different diets in lean and obese cats before and after weight loss. Am J Physiol Regul Integr Comp Physiol 2007;292:R227–34.

18. Green AS, Ramsey JJ, Villaverde C, et al. Cats are able to adapt protein oxidation to protein intake provided their requirement for dietary protein is met. J Nutr 2008;138:1053–60.

19. Deng P, Ridge TK, Graves TK, et al. Effects of dietary macronutrient composition and feeding frequency on fasting and postprandial hormone responses in domestic cats. J Nutr Sci 2013. https://doi.org/10.1017/jns.2013.32.

20. Gooding MA, Flickinger EA, Atkinson JL, et al. Effects of high-fat and high-carbohydrate diets on fat and carbohydrate oxidation and plasma metabolites in healthy cats. J Anim Physiol Anim Nutr (Berl) 2014;98:596–607.

21. Wester TJ, Weidgraaf K, Hekman M, et al. Upregulation of glucose production by increased dietary protein in the adult cat (Felis catus). FASEB J 2017;31(Suppl 1):792–818.

22. Hoenig M, Jordan ET, Glushka J, et al. Effect of macronutrients, age, and obesity on 6- and 24-h postprandial glucose metabolism in cats. Am J Physiol Regul Integr Comp Physiol 2011;301:R1798–807.

23. Nguyen P, Dumon HJ, Siliart BS, et al. Effects of dietary fat and energy on body weight and composition after gonadectomy in cats. Am J Vet Res 2004;65:1708–13.

24. Backus RC, Cave NJ, Keisler DH. Gonadectomy and high dietary fat but not high dietary carbohydrate induce gains in body weight and fat of domestic cats. Br J Nutr 2007;98:641–50.

25. Farrow HA, Rand JS, Morton JM, et al. Effect of dietary carbohydrate, fat, and protein on postprandial glycemia and energy intake in cats. J Vet Intern Med 2013;27:1121–35.

26. Gooding MA, Atkinson JL, Duncan IJH, et al. Dietary fat and carbohydrate have different effects on body weight, energy expenditure, glucose homeostasis and behavior in adult cats fed to energy requirement. J Nutr Sci 2015;42:e2.

27. Laflamme DP, Abood SK, Fascetti AJ, et al. Pet feeding practices among dog and cat owners in the United States and Australia. J Am Vet Med Assoc 2008;232:687–94.

28. American Pet Products Association, Inc. APPA national pet owners survey 2013-2014. Stamford (CT): American Pet Products Association, Inc.; 2013.

29. Carciofi AC, Bazolli RS, Zanni A, et al. Influence of water content and the digestibility of pet foods on the water balance of cats. Braz J Vet Res Anim Sci 2005;42:429–34.

30. Buckley CMF, Hawthorne A, Colyer A, et al. Effect of dietary water intake on urinary output, specific gravity and relative supersaturation for calcium oxalate and struvite in the cat. Br J Nutr 2011;106:S128–30.

31. Armstrong PJ, Lund EM. Changes in body composition and energy balance with aging. In: Topeka KS, editor. Proceedings of health and nutrition of geriatric cats and dogs. Topeka (KS): Hill's Pet Nutrition, Inc; 1996. p. 11–5.

32. Courcier EA, Mellor DJ, Pendlebury E, et al. An investigation into the epidemiology of feline obesity in Great Britain: results of a cross-sectional study of 47 companion animal practices. Vet Res 2012;171:560.

33. Cupp CJ, Kerr WW. Effect of diet and body composition on life span in aging cats. Proceedings of the Nestle Purina Companion Animal Nutrition Summit: focus on gerontology. Clearwater Beach (FL), March 26–27, 2010. St Louis (MO): Nestlé Purina PetCare; 2010.

34. Teng KT, McGreevy PD, Toriblo JLML, et al. Strong associations of nine-point body condition scoring with survival and lifespan in cats. J Feline Med Surg 2018;20:1110–8.

35. Freeman LM, Lachaud MP, Matthews S, et al. Evaluation of weight loss over time in cats with chronic kidney disease. J Vet Intern Med 2016;30:1661–6.

36. Baez JL, Michel KE, Sorenmo K, et al. A prospective investigation of the prevalence and prognostic significance of weight loss and changes in body condition in feline cancer patients. J Feline Med Surg 2007;9:411–7.

37. Evans WJ. Skeletal muscle loss: cachexia, sarcopenia and inactivity. Am J Clin Nutr 2010;91:1123S–7S.

38. Koopman R, van Loon LJC. Aging, exercise and muscle protein metabolism. J Appl Physiol 2009;106:2040–8.

39. Harper EJ. Changing perspectives on aging and energy requirements: aging, body weight and body composition in humans, dogs and cats. J Nutr 1998; 128:2627–2631S.

40. Kealy RD. Factors influencing lean body mass in aging dogs. Comp Cont Edu Small Anim Pract 1999;21(11K):34–7.

41. Sergi G, Bonometto P, Coin A, et al. Body composition: physiology, pathophysiology and methods of evaluation. In: Mantovani G, editor. Cachexia and wasting: a modern approach. Milano, Italy: Springer-Verlag Italia; 2006. p. 175–83.

42. Adams VJ, Watson P, Carmichael S, et al. Exceptional longevity and potential determinants of successful aging in a cohort of 39 Labrador retrievers: results of a prospective longitudinal study. Acta Vet Scand 2016;58:29.

43. Smith GI, Atherton P, Reeds DN, et al. Dietary omega-3 fatty acid supplementation increases the rate of muscle protein synthesis in older adults: a randomized controlled trial. Am J Clin Nutr 2011;93:402–12.

44. Murton AJ. Muscle protein turnover in the elderly and its potential contribution to the development of sarcopenia. Proc Nutr Soc 2015;74:387–96.

45. Band MM, Sumukadas D, Struthers AD, et al. Leucine and ACE inhibitors as therapies for sarcopenia (LACE trial): study protocol for a randomized controlled trial. Trials 2018;19:6.

46. Robinson SM, Reginster JY, Rizzoli R, et al. Does nutrition play a role in the prevention and management of sarcopenia? Clin Nutr 2018;37:1121–32.

47. Houston DK, Nicklas BJ, Ding J, et al. Dietary protein intake is associated with lean mass change in older, community dwelling adults: the health, aging and body composition (Health ABC) study. Am J Clin Nutr 2008;87:150–5.

48. Mithal A, Bonjour JP, Boonen S, et al. Impact of nutrition on muscle mass, strength, and performance in older adults. Osteoporos Int 2012. https://doi.org/10.1007/s00198-012-2236-y.

49. Sahni S, Mangano KM, Hannan MT, et al. Higher protein intake is associated with higher lean mass and quadriceps muscle strength in adult men and women. J Nutr 2015;145:1569–75.

50. Verlaan S, Aspray TJ, Bauer JM, et al. Nutritional status, body composition, and quality of life in community-dwelling sarcopenic and non-sarcopenic older adults: a case-control study. Clin Nutr 2017;36:267–74.

51. Laflamme DP. Loss of lean body mass in aging cats is affected by age and diet. Eur Society Vet Comp Nutr Annual conference, Ghent, Belgium, September 19–21, 2013 (Abstr).

52. Bermingham EN, Weidgraaf K, Hekman M, et al. Seasonal and age effects on energy requirements in domestic short-hair cats (Felis catus) in a temperate environment. J Anim Physiol Anim Nutr 2012;97:522–30.

53. Gaffney-Stomberg E, Insogna KL, Rodriguez NR, et al. Increasing dietary protein requirements in elderly people for optimal muscle and bone health. J Am Geriatr Soc 2009;57:1073–9.

54. Bauer J, Biolo G, Cederholm T, et al. Evidence-based recommendations for optimal dietary protein intake in older people: a position paper from the PROT-AGE study group. J Am Med Dir Assoc 2013;14(8):542e59.

55. Deutz NE, Bauer JM, Barazzoni R, et al. Protein intake and exercise for optimal muscle function with aging: recommendations from the ESPEN Expert group. Clin Nutr 2014;33(6):929e36.

56. Tishler ME, Desautels M, Goldberg AL. Does leucine, leucyl-tRNA, or some metabolite of leucine regulate protein synthesis and degradation in skeletal and cardiac muscle? J Biol Chem 1982;257:1613–21.

57. Yang Y, Breen L, Burd NA, et al. Resistance exercise enhances myofibrillar protein synthesis with graded intakes of whey protein in older men. Br J Nutr 2012; 108:1780–8.

58. Rondanelli M, Klersy C, Terracol G, et al. Whey protein, amino acids, and vitamin D supplementation with physical activity increases fat-free mass and strength, functionality, and quality of life and decreases inflammation in sarcopenic elderly. Am J Clin Nutr 2016;103:830–40.

59. Wakshlag JJ, Barr SC, Ordway GA, et al. Effect of dietary protein on lean body wasting in dogs: correlation between loss of lean body mass and markers of proteasome-dependent proteolysis. J Anim Physiol Anim Nutr 2003;87:408–20.

60. Sato T, Ito Y, Nagasawa T. Regulation of skeletal muscle protein degradation and synthesis by oral administration of lysine in rats. J Nutr Sci Vitaminol 2013;59:412–9.

61. Wang T, Feugang JM, Crenshaw MA, et al. A systems biology approach using transcriptomic data reveals genes and pathways in porcine skeletal muscle affected by dietary lysine. Int J Mol Sci 2017;18:885.

62. Frantz NZ, Yamka RM, Friesen KG. The effect of diet and lysine:calorie ratio on body composition and kidney health in geriatric cats. Intern J Appl Res Vet Med 2007;5:25–36.

63. Visser M, Deeg DJH, Lips P. Low vitamin D and high parathyroid hormone levels as determinants of loss of muscle strength and muscle mass (sarcopenia): the longitudinal aging study Amsterdam. J Clin Endocrinol Metab 2003;88:5766–72.

64. Chanet A, Salles J, Guillet C, et al. Vitamin D supplementation restores the blunted muscle protein synthesis response in deficient old rats through an impact on ectopic fat deposition. J Nutr Biochem 2017;46:30–8.

65. Salles J, Chanet A, Giraudet C, et al. 1,25(OH)$_2$ vitamin D enhances the stimulating effect of leucine and insulin on protein synthesis rate through Akt/PKB and MTOR mediated pathways in murine C2C12 skeletal myotubes. Mol Nutr Food Res 2013;57(12):2137–46.

66. Mitch WE, Medina R, Grieber S, et al. Metabolic acidosis stimulates muscle protein degradation by activating the adenosine triphosphate-dependent pathway involving ubiquitin and proteasomes. J Clin Invest 1994;93:2127–33.

67. Caso G, Garlick PJ. Control of muscle protein kinetics by acid-base balance. Curr Opin Clin Nutr Metab Care 2005;8:73–6.

68. Garibotto G, Sofia A, Russo R, et al. Insulin sensitivity of muscle protein metabolism is altered in patients with chronic kidney disease and metabolic acidosis. Kidney Int 2015;88:1419–26.

69. Wang X, Mitch WE. Muscle wasting from kidney failure – a model for catabolic conditions. Int J Biochem Cell Biol 2013;45:2230–8.

70. Faure AM, Fischer K, Dawson-Hughes B, et al. Gender-specific association between dietary acid load and total lean body mass and its dependency on protein intake in seniors. Osteoporos Int 2017;28:3451–62.

71. Mehrotra R, Bross R, Wang H, et al. Effect of high-normal compared with low-normal arterial pH on protein balances in automated peritoneal dialysis patients. Am J Clin Nutr 2009;90:1532–40.

72. Freeman LM. Cachexia and sarcopenia: emerging syndromes of importance in dogs and cats. J Vet Intern Med 2012;26:3–17.

73. Ellis SLH, Rodan I, Heath S, et al. AAFP and ISFM Feline Environmental Needs Guidelines. J Feline Med Surg 2013;15:219–30.

74. Johnston L, Freeman L. Recognizing, describing, and managing reduced food intake in dogs and cats. J Am Vet Med Assoc 2017;251:1260–6.

75. Rand JS, Marshall RD. Diabetes mellitus in cats. Vet Clin North Am Small Anim Pract 2005;35:211–24.

76. Slingerland LI, Fazilova VV, Plantinga EA, et al. Indoor confinement and physical inactivity rather than the proportion of dry food are risk factors in the development of feline type 2 diabetes mellitus. Vet J 2009;179(2):247–53.

77. Zini E, Hafner M, Osto M, et al. Predictors of clinical remission in cats with diabetes mellitus. J Vet Intern Med 2010;24:1314–21.

78. Hall TD, Mahony O, Rozanski EA, et al. Effects of diet on glucose control in cats with diabetes mellitus treated with twice daily insulin glargine. J Feline Med Surg 2009;11(2):125–30.

79. Bennett N, Greco DS, Peterson ME, et al. Comparison of a low carbohydrate-low fiber diet and a moderate carbohydrate-high fiber diet in the management of feline diabetes mellitus. J Feline Med Surg 2006;8:73–84.

80. Frank G, Anderson WH, Pazak HE, et al. Use of a high protein diet in the management of feline diabetes mellitus. Vet Ther 2001;2:238–46.

81. Mazzaferro EM, Greco DS, Turner SJ, et al. Treatment of feline diabetes mellitus using an alpha-glucosidase inhibitor and a low-carbohydrate diet. J Feline Med Surg 2003;5:183–9.

82. Marshall R, Rand J, Morton J. Treatment of newly diagnosed diabetic cats with glargine insulin improves glycemic control and results in higher probability of remission that protamine zinc and lente insulins. J Feline Med Surg 2009;11:683–91.

83. Kirk CA. Feline diabetes mellitus: low carbohydrates versus high fiber? Vet Clin North Am Small Anim Pract 2006;36:1297–306.

84. Boyd LM, Langston C, Thompson K, et al. Survival in cats with naturally occurring chronic kidney disease (2000 – 2002). J Vet Intern Med 2008;22:1111–7.

85. Elliott J, Rawlings JM, Markwell PJ, et al. Survival of cats with naturally occurring chronic renal failure, effect of dietary management. J Small Anim Pract 2000;41:235–42.

86. Plantinga EA, Everts H, Kastelein AMC, et al. Retrospective study of the survival of cats with acquired chronic renal insufficiency offered different commercial diets. Vet Rec 2005;157:185–7.

87. Ross SJ, Osborne CA, Kirk CA, et al. Clinical evaluation of dietary modification for treatment of spontaneous chronic kidney disease in cats. J Am Vet Med Assoc 2006;229:949–57.

88. Dow SW, Fettmann MJ, LeCouteur RA, et al. Potassium depletion in cats: renal and dietary influences. J Am Vet Med Assoc 1987;191:1569–75.

89. DiBartola SP, Buffington CA, Chew DJ, et al. Development of chronic renal disease in cats fed a commercial diet. J Am Vet Med Assoc 1993;202:744–851.

90. Theisen SK, DiBartola SP, Radin MJ, et al. Muscle potassium content and potassium gluconate supplementation in normokalemic cats with naturally occurring chronic renal failure. J Vet Intern Med 1997;11:212–7.

91. Buranakarl C, Mathur S, Brown SA. Effects of dietary sodium chloride intake on renal function and blood pressure in cats with normal and reduced renal function. Am J Vet Res 2004;65:620–7.

92. Hughes KL, Slater MR, Geller S, et al. Diet and lifestyle variables as risk factors for chronic renal failure in pet cats. Prev Vet Med 2002;55:1–15.

93. Dow SW, Fettman MJ, Smith KR, et al. Effects of dietary acidification and potassium depletion on acid base balance, mineral metabolism and renal function in adult cats. J Nutr 1990;120:569–78.

94. Polzin DJ, Osborne CA, Ross S, et al. Dietary management of feline chronic renal failure: where are we now? In what direction are we headed? J Feline Med Surg 2000;2:75–82.

95. Elliott J, Syme HM, Reubens E, et al. Assessment of acid-base status of cats with naturally occurring chronic renal failure. J Small Anim Pract 2003;44:65–70.

96. Kraut JA, Madias NE. Metabolic acidosis of CKD: An update. Am J Kidney Dis 2016;67:307–17.

97. Dobre M, Rahman M, Hostetter TH. Current status of bicarbonate in CKD. J Am Soc Nephrol 2015;26:515–23.

98. Lumlertgul D, Burke TJ, Gillum DM, et al. Phosphate depletion arrests progression of chronic renal failure independent of protein intake. Kidney Int 1986;29:658–66.

99. Alfrey AC. Effect of dietary phosphate restriction on renal function and deterioration. Am J Clin Nutr 1988;47:153–6.

100. Uribarri J. Dietary phosphorus and kidney disease. Ann N Y Acad Sci 2013;1301:11–9.

101. Chang AR, Anderson C. Dietary phosphorus intake and the kidney. Annu Rev Nutr 2017;37:321–46.

102. King JN, Tasker S, Gunn-Moore DA, et al. BENRiC (Benazepril in Renal insufficiency in Cats) Study Group. Prognostic factors in cats with chronic kidney disease. J Vet Intern Med 2007;21:906–16.

103. Chakrabarti S, Syme HM, Brown CA, et al. Histomorphometry of feline chronic kidney disease and correlation with markers of renal dysfunction. Vet Path 2012;50:147–55.

104. Finch NC, Syme HM, Elliott J. Parathyroid hormone concentration in geriatric cats with various degrees of renal function. J Am Vet Med Assoc 2012;241:1326–35.

105. Finch NC, Geddes RF, Syme HM, et al. Fibroblast growth factor 23 (FGF23) concentrations in cats with early nonazotemic chronic kidney disease (CKD) and in healthy geriatric cats. J Vet Intern Med 2013;27:227–33.

106. Geddes RF, Elliott J, Syme HM. Relationship between plasma fibroblast growth factor-23 concentration and survival time in cats with chronic kidney disease. J Vet Intern Med 2015. https://doi.org/10.1111/jvim.13625.

107. Finco DR, Brown SA, Crowell WA, et al. Effects of phosphorus/calcium-restricted and phosphorus/calcium-replete 32% protein diets in dogs with chronic renal failure. Am J Vet Res 1992;53:157–63.

108. Koizumi T, Murakami K, Nakayama H, et al. Role of dietary phosphorus in the progression of renal failure. Biochem Biophys Res Commun 2002;295:917–21.

109. Adams LG, Polzin DJ, Osborne CA, et al. Effects of dietary protein and calorie restriction in clinically normal cats and cats with surgically induced chronic renal failure. Am J Vet Res 1993;54:1653–62.

110. Adams LG, Polzin DJ, Osborne CA, et al. Influence of dietary protein/calorie intake on renal morphology and function in cats with 5/6 nephrectomy. Lab Invest 1994;70:347–57.

111. Tapp DC, Kobayashi S, Fernandes G, et al. Protein restriction or calorie restriction? A critical assessment of the influence of selective calorie restriction in the progression of experimental renal disease. Semin Nephrol 1989;9:343–53.

112. Finco DR, Brown SA, Brown CA, et al. Protein and calorie effects on progression of induced chronic renal failure in cats. Am J Vet Res 1998;59:575–82.

113. Lascelles BDX, DePuy V, Thomson A, et al. Evaluation of a therapeutic diet for feline degenerative joint disease. J Vet Intern Med 2010;24:487–95.

114. Corbee RJ, Barnier MMC, van de Lest CHA, et al. The effect of dietary long-chain omega-3 fatty acid supplementation on owner's perception of behavior and locomotion in cats with naturally occurring osteoarthritis. J Anim Physiol Anim Nutr 2013;97:846–53.

115. Flatt JP. Macronutrient composition and food selection. Obes Res 2001;9:256S–62S.

116. Laflamme DP, Hannah SS. Increased dietary protein promotes fat loss and reduces loss of lean body mass during weight loss in cats. Int J Appl Res Vet Med 2005;3:62–8.

117. Wei A, Fascetti AJ, Liu KJ, et al. Influence of a high-protein diet on energy balance in obese cats allowed ad libitum access to food. J Anim Physiol Anim Nutr 2011;95:359–67.

118. Des Courtis X, Wei A, Kass PH, et al. Influence of dietary protein level on body composition and energy expenditure in calorically restricted overweight cats. J Anim Physiol Anim Nutr 2015;99:474–82.

119. German AJ, Holden SL, Mason SL, et al. Imprecision when using measuring cups to weight out extruded dry kibbled food. J Anim Physiol Anim Nutr 2010. https://doi.org/10.1111/j.1439-0396.2010.01063.x.

120. Luedtke ES, Schmidt C, Laflamme D. The effect of food bowl size on the amount of food fed to cats. Proc 11th Annual AAVN Clinical Nutrition & Research Symposium, Denver, CO, June 15, 2011. p. 8.

121. Murphy M, Lusby AL, Bartges JW, et al. Size of food bowl and scoop affects amount of food owners feed their dogs. J Anim Physiol Anim Nutr 2011. https://doi.org/10.1111/j.1439-0396.2011.01144.x.

122. Dantas LM, Delgado MM, Johnson I, et al. Food puzzles for cats: feeding for physical and emotional wellbeing. J feline Med Surg 2016;18:723–32.

123. Sadek T, Hamper B, Horwitz D, et al. Feline feeding programs: Addressing behavioural needs to improve feline health and wellbeing. J feline Med Surg 2018;20:1049–55.

Assessing Nutritional Requirements and Current Intake

Angela Witzel-Rollins, DVM, PhD*, Maryanne Murphy, DVM, PhD

KEYWORDS

• Feline • Nutrition • Diet • Nutritional assessment

KEY POINTS

- Assessing nutritional requirements requires knowledge of the individual patient's age, physiologic status, activity, physical examination findings, and existence of any nutrient-responsive diseases, along with current diet and environmental status.
- Caloric needs are estimated by calculating the resting energy requirement required to maintain normal metabolic functions and multiplying by a life-stage factor based on the status of the individual patient.
- Because fat mass contributes little to energy requirements, ideal weight is used for feeding calculations. When ideal weight is unknown for an overweight patient, it is estimated by assessing current body fat via body condition score or body fat index.
- The entire veterinary team needs to be involved with nutritional assessment and subsequent recommendations to provide the most comprehensive service to patients and their owners, while maintaining practice efficiency.

INTRODUCTION

Nutrition is foundational to good health and disease prevention. As a result, veterinarians have a responsibility to assess and provide recommendations regarding the nutritional status of their patients. A nutritional assessment requires evaluation of the patient, diet history, and environment.[1,2] In busy clinical practices, obtaining thorough diet histories and discussing owner concerns about nutrition can seem daunting and time-consuming. However, implementing a team approach to nutrition by involving the entire clinic staff can streamline the process while providing clients the information they want and need.

Small Animal Clinical Sciences, The University of Tennessee College of Veterinary Medicine, 2407 River Drive, Knoxville, TN 37996, USA
* Corresponding author.
E-mail address: arollins@utk.edu

Vet Clin Small Anim 50 (2020) 925–937
https://doi.org/10.1016/j.cvsm.2020.06.003
0195-5616/20/© 2020 Elsevier Inc. All rights reserved.
vetsmall.theclinics.com

PATIENT ASSESSMENT
Age

Growth
Growing kittens require a calorically dense food with high concentrations of vitamins and minerals, such as calcium, phosphorus, and vitamin D.[3] A diet meeting the Association of American Feed Control Officials (AAFCO) recommendations for growth is best for kittens. The age at which cats should transition from kitten to adult feline food is debatable, but 9 to 12 months is an appropriate age range for most.

Adult and geriatric
The American Association of Feline Practitioners Senior Care Guidelines defines mature/middle-aged cats as those 7 to 10 years, senior cats as 11 to 14 years, and geriatric cats as older than 15 years.[4] Cats from 5 to 10 years old are at highest risk for obesity. After approximately 11 years of age, obesity rates decline dramatically.[5] Although the daily energy needs of many animal species decrease later in life, elderly cats may require more energy to maintain their body weight. There are a couple of explanations for this difference. The activity patterns of pet cats remain relatively similar throughout their lives.[6] Because they spend much of their time resting, sleeping, and grooming, a 4-year-old cat may not move significantly more than a 14-year-old cat. Although activity is somewhat consistent throughout adult life, fat and protein digestion often become impaired as cats reach geriatric ages. Approximately 20% of cats older than 12 years have decreased protein digestibility and 30% have reduced fat absorption.[7] This mitigated digestion may also result in vitamin and mineral deficiencies.[7] To compensate for impaired nutrient absorption, elderly cats tend to eat more food relative to their body weight than younger cats.[6] Many senior feline diets are marketed for cats older than 7 years and are often designed to minimize weight gain. Therefore, senior diets may not be appropriate for all geriatric patients. When developing a nutritional plan for senior and geriatric cats, a full health assessment, including body and muscle condition scoring, is required to screen for other systemic disease. Healthy, geriatric cats with weight loss often benefit from highly digestible, calorically dense diets that are higher in fat and protein.

Physiologic Status

Pregnancy and lactation
Information regarding the specific nutritional needs of pregnant and lactating cats is scarce and most nutritional recommendations are based on the requirements of growing kittens. Nonetheless, optimal nutrition is an important consideration for reproducing females both before and after conception. They should not be underweight or overweight and should receive a diet with ample protein and plentiful essential fatty acids. Malnourished cats can have difficulty conceiving, abort pregnancies, or give birth to malformed or underweight kittens.[8] Conversely, obese queens are more likely to experience stillbirths and require cesarean deliveries.[9]

Pregnant queens typically need 25% to 50% more energy compared with maintenance and will gain weight in a steady, linear fashion from conception to parturition. The weight gained by queens initially goes toward building maternal fat reserves, rather than to growth of fetal or reproductive tissue.[10] Lactating cats require more energy than in any other life stage, needing 2 to 6 times their resting energy requirements (RER). Energy-dense growth formulas or formulas designated for pregnancy and lactation should be fed free choice to pregnant and lactating queens.[8]

Gonadectomy

Spaying and castration can lower the energy needs and increase the appetite of cats.[11] Advising owners to weigh food portions instead of using volume measurements allows more flexibility to reduce caloric intake by 10% to 20% if needed postsurgery. Owners also should be counseled on proper body condition at the time of surgical discharge and may need to choose a food with a lower caloric density to prevent weight gain; however, adult cat foods or those designed for weight loss may not meet nutritional requirements for growth and should not be used before skeletal maturity (9–12 months).

Activity

Although research is lacking, it is reasonable to assume that most outdoor cats have higher overall activity levels compared with indoor cats. Activity also decreases with age in indoor cats.[12] Activity patterns should be assessed for individual patients and food intake increased or decreased accordingly.

Physical Examination

Body condition scoring

Body condition scoring (BCS) is a method for estimating body fat mass using palpation and visual assessment and should be incorporated into every physical examination. One can use either a 5-point or 9-point scale in which 1 is cachexic and 5 or 9 is obese[13,14] (see https://wsava.org/wp-content/uploads/2020/02/Body-Condition-Score-Cat.pdf). Each point on the BCS scales correlates with a percentage of body fat (**Table 1**). Ideally, cats range from 15% to 25% body fat.[15] Many obese cats may exceed the body fat percentages listed in the current BCS systems (>45% body fat). Therefore, additional assessment of body fat index (BFI) may be warranted for overweight and obese cats (**Fig. 1**).[16] The BFI assessment facilitates estimation of body fat percentages in even the most obese cases, aiding client communication (eg, "your cat is 50% body fat and should ideally be closer to 20% fat") and estimations of ideal body weight (see later in this article).

Muscle condition scoring

A muscle condition score (MCS) should be ascribed separately from BCS. For example, an obese cat may have reduced musculature and have a high BCS with a low MCS (**Fig. 2**). Palpation of musculature over the skull, spine, scapula, and wings of the ilia is used to assign a 0 to 3-point score with muscle wasting described as severe (0), moderate (1), mild (2), or normal musculature (3)[17,18] (see https://wsava.org/wp-content/uploads/2020/01/Muscle-Condition-Score-Chart-for-Cats.pdf). Patients with reduced muscle condition should receive further nutritional and medical evaluation to determine the etiology of muscle loss.

Nutrient-Responsive Diseases

Cats with diseases that could benefit from dietary intervention should have an in-depth nutritional evaluation formed (see Dottie. P. Laflamme's article, "Understanding the Nutritional Needs of Healthy Cats and those with Diet-Sensitive Conditions," elsewhere in this issue).

DIET ASSESSMENT
Diet History

Obtaining a thorough and accurate diet history is an important component of the nutritional assessment. Owners should be specifically asked about the following when obtaining a diet history:

Table 1
Descriptions of feline body condition scoring systems and their respective body fat percentages

5-Point Scale	9-Point Scale	% Body Fat	Body Condition Scoring
1	1	≤5	Emaciated: ribs and bony prominences are visible from a distance. No palpable body fat. Loss of muscle mass.
2	2	6–9	Very thin: ribs and bony prominences visible. Minimal loss of muscle mass, but no palpable fat.
	3	10–14	Thin: ribs easily palpable, tops of lumbar vertebrae are visible. Obvious waist and may have an abdominal tuck.
3	4	15–19	Lean: ribs easily palpable, waist visible from above. Abdominal fat may be present or absent. If present, it is comprised of loose skin and no fat within inguinal fat pad.
	5	20–24	Ideal: ribs palpable without excess fat covering. Cats have a visible waist from above and minimal palpable fat within the inguinal fat pad.
4	6	25–29	Slightly overweight: Waist is discernible from above, but not obvious. Fat is palpable within the inguinal fat pad.
	7	30–34	Overweight: Silhouette is straight when viewed from above with no defined waist. Moderately enlarged inguinal fat pad and slight rounding of the abdomen.
5	8	35–39	Obese: Rounding of abdomen when viewed dorsally and laterally. Fat deposit may be obvious in shoulder or abdominal area. Difficult to palpate bony prominences along spine and ribs.
	9	40–45+	Morbidly obese: Large abdominal fat pad and rounded abdomen. Body appears broadened from above. Difficult to impossible to palpate boney prominences.

Note that current body condition scoring systems end at approximately 45% body fat. Morbidly obese cats benefit from additional assessment using the Body Fat Index system (see **Fig. 1**).

- Diet type (eg, wet, dry)
- Name and brand of food
- Flavor/variety of food
- Amount fed per meal
- Number of meals per day
- Treats: type, brand, size, amount fed per day
- Supplements given
- Feeding environment; for example, type of bowl used, location, other household pets that influence eating

Once a diet history is obtained, it is particularly important to quantify current kilocalorie intake in underweight or overweight cats. The kilocalorie content of cat food is available on most company Web sites and is required to meet AAFCO packaging guidelines.

Diet Type

Assessing the quality of diets based on the guaranteed analysis, ingredient lists, or packaging claims is challenging. One method for assessing the quality of a cat food brand is to look for a statement describing if the diet adheres to standards set forth by AAFCO. Foods either can undergo an AAFCO feeding trial or be formulated to

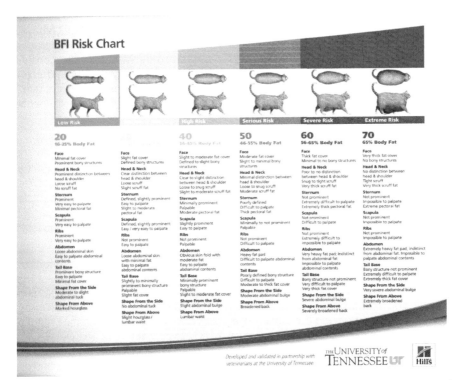

Fig. 1. BFI system for estimating body fat percentage in overweight and obese neutered cats. Cats may have descriptions that fall into 1 or more categories. For example, if a cat has *Scapula*, *Ribs*, and *Tail base* descriptions that fall in the 40 category and *Shape from Above* and *Abdomen* descriptions in the 50 category, one could estimate percent body fat as approximately 45%. The body fat percentage can then be used to estimate ideal body weight with the equation (Current body weight × Current % lean) ÷ 0.8. See text for more information. (Reprinted with permission of the copyright owner, Hill's Pet Nutrition, Inc.)

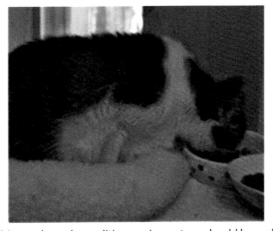

Fig. 2. Body condition and muscle condition scoring systems should be evaluated separately, as some cats can be obese (increased adipose tissue) with significant loss of muscle. (*Courtesy of* M. E. Peterson, DVM, DIP. DACVIM, New York, NY.)

meet AAFCO nutrient requirements. Feeding trials test tolerance and nutrient bioavailability of diets, which is considered superior to formulation alone. In addition to reading the AAFCO statements before recommending a food brand, one should also consider company reputation and prioritize those that have good quality control and safety measures. Determining a company's ability to safely and consistently produce a healthy cat food is not an easy task. The following are some tips to help identify best quality manufacturers:[19]

- Contact the company directly to determine the credentials of the persons formulating their diet.
  - Individuals with advanced degrees or board certification in animal nutrition should perform cat food formulations.
- Ask what steps a company takes to ensure their diets meet post-production safety and nutrient requirements.
- Companies should provide full nutrient profiles of their products when requested.

Some cat owners prefer to avoid commercial cat food and feed their cat homemade diets. Homemade diets that are improperly formulated increase the risk of nutritional imbalances such as taurine deficiency, hypocalcemia, and hypovitaminosis A. If cat owners insist on feeding home-prepared diets, veterinarians should recommend consultation with a board-certified veterinary nutritionist. A list of American College of Veterinary Nutrition and European College of Veterinary and Comparative Nutrition diplomates providing consultations can be found at www.acvn.org and www.esvcn. eu/college, respectively. Feeding diets containing raw meat ingredients is another popular trend that should stimulate veterinarians to have a more detailed nutrition discussion with cat owners (see https://wsava.org/wp-content/uploads/2020/01/WSAVA-Global-Nutrition-Committee-Statement-on-Risks-of-Raw-Meat.pdf).

Nutrient Values

Estimating nutrient values based on a pet food label is challenging. Key nutrients such as calcium and phosphorus are not part of the required labeling in pet food so one may need to look on a company Web site or call the manufacturer to get this value. The percentage of nutrients listed on a bag or can are on an "as-fed" basis, meaning it reflects the percentage of those nutrients with the moisture included. Because of the increased moisture, nutrient percentages listed in canned foods will usually be lower than those listed on dry kibble. To make accurate comparisons, the percentages on the label must be converted to the grams of the nutrient on a calorie basis. This requires some simple math.

1. Find the nutrient of interest on the pet food label (eg, protein)
2. Find the calorie density of the food on the pet food label
   a. Listed as kilocalories per kilogram (kg) of diet
      i. Typical dry cat food will range between approximately 3500 to 4500 kilocalories per kg
      ii. Typical canned cat food will range between approximately 900 to 1100 kilocalories per kg
   b. Divide the kilocalories per kg of diet by 10,000
      i. For example, a food that is 3500 kilocalories per kg/10,000 = 0.3500
3. Take the % of the nutrient of interest on the label and divide by the calorie density/10,000
   a. If the label says a diet is 20% protein, you would now divide 20/0.3500 = 57
   b. This equals 57 g of protein per 1000 calories of food

4. For nutrients listed as mg/kg, ppm, or IU/kg, the kilocalories per kg of diet is divided by 1000
   a. If the label says a diet is 870 IU/kg vitamin E, you would divide 870/3.500 = 249
   b. This equals 249 IU of vitamin E per 1000 calories of food

After converting nutrients from "as-fed" to grams per 1000 kilocalories, remember that the numbers listed on guaranteed analysis are minimums and maximums. Therefore, the amount of protein you calculated is merely an estimation and the true value is likely 10% to 20% higher or lower, depending on the nutrient evaluated.[20] The following is a sample comparison:

Canned Diet A		Dry Diet B	
Guaranteed Analysis		Guaranteed Analysis	
Crude protein (min)	11.5%	Crude protein (min)	34.5%
Crude fat (min)	8.14%	Crude fat (min)	11.6
Moisture (max)	75%	Moisture (max)	10%
Caloric density	1126 kcal/kg	Caloric density	3789 kcal/kg

Calculation for conversion to grams of nutrient per 1000 kcal of diet:
Diet A: 11.5/0.1126 = 102 g of protein per 1000 kcal; 8.14/0.1126 = 72 g of fat per 1000 kcal.
Diet B: 34.5/0.3789 = 91 g of protein per 1000 kcal; 11.6/0.3789 = 30 g of fat per 1000 kcal.

ENVIRONMENTAL ASSESSMENT

The household environment can influence a cat's ability and willingness to eat. For example, interactions with other pets may create competition for food. Some environmental factors such as indoor housing and ad libitum feeding patterns appear more frequently in obese versus lean cats.[21–23] Cats evolved eating many small prey meals per day.[24] Ideally domestic cats would eat in this same manner, with owners offering many small meals instead of 1 to 2 large meals per day. Free choice feeding is acceptable if a cat can maintain ideal body condition. However, overweight and obese cats often benefit from portion-controlled meal feeding. Providing meals through puzzle and food-dispensing toys may be used as an alternative to traditional bowls as a method of environmental enrichment[25] (see Mikel Delgado and Leticia M.S. Dantas' article, "Feeding Cats for Optimal Mental and Behavioral Well-Being," elsewhere in this issue).

EXTENDED EVALUATION

Every cat should receive a basic nutritional assessment evaluating the criteria listed previously (patient, diet fed, environment). If abnormalities or concerns are detected, an extended nutritional examination is warranted. Some examples that may trigger a more in-depth evaluation are found later in this article. This list does not encompass every issue that could prompt an extended nutritional evaluation, but presence of these factors may require changes in feeding strategy.

Patient History

- Growing (<1 year) or senior (>11 years)
- Pregnant or lactating
- Recent castration or ovariohysterectomy

- Gastrointestinal signs such as vomiting, diarrhea, or anorexia
- Change in body weight (increase or decrease)
- Nutritionally responsive diseases
  - For example, chronic kidney disease, obesity, urolithiasis, chronic enteropathy
- Feeding unconventional diets (eg, homemade, raw)
- Use of dietary or herbal supplements

Physical Examination

- Overweight or underweight based on BCS ± BFI (see **Table 1**; **Table 2**)
- Muscle wasting
- Dental disease
- Poor skin or coat quality

Laboratory Evaluation

- Presence of nutritionally responsive disease
- Abnormalities on chemistry/electrolyte panel, complete blood count, and/or urinalysis including, but not limited to
  - Elevated creatinine with inappropriately dilute urine concentration
  - Hypoalbuminemia
  - Hypoglycemia or hyperglycemia with glucosuria
  - Anemia
  - Proteinuria
  - Elevated T4

ESTIMATING CALORIC NEEDS

How many kilocalories per day does a cat need to eat? This is a simple question with a complicated answer. The *daily energy requirement* (DER) of an individual cat is composed of several factors:

- RER is the energy needed to maintain normal metabolic functions (eg, blood flow, cellular metabolism, respiration) and is closely correlated with lean body mass. The RER typically accounts for 60% to 80% of the total DER. Compared with lean mass, fat mass contributes little to the RER. Therefore estimations of

Table 2
Life-stage factors to estimate daily energy requirements (DER)

Life-Stage	Factor to Multiply by Resting Energy Requirement
Intact adult	1.4–1.6
Neutered adult	1.2–1.4
Obese prone	1.0
To promote weight loss	0.8–1.0
Geriatric	1.2–1.6
Gestation	1.6–2.0
Lactation	2.0–6.0
Growth <50% adult weight	3.0
Growth 50%–70% adult weight	2.5
Growth >70% adult weight	2.0

Body weight $(kg)^{0.75} \times 70$ and multiplying by the appropriate life-stage factor listed in the table. Please note these are only guidelines and individual cats may need more or less energy to maintain ideal body condition.

RERs should be based on ideal rather than current weight using the following formula: $RER = BW_{kg}^{0.75} \times 70$

- *Thermic effect of food* is the energy burned through digestion and absorption and typically makes up approximately 10% to 15% of DER.
- *Adaptive thermogenesis* is the energy used to stay warm or cool and varies by environmental temperature.

The best way to determine a patient's DER is to know their kilocalorie intake while at an ideal body weight. For example, if you know a cat has been consuming 220 kilocalories per day for the past 6 months and has an ideal body condition score of 5/9, you can confidently say that cat needs to eat 220 kilocalories per day. However, we often manage cats that are actively gaining or losing weight or their owners are unsure of the amount of food they consume daily. In these cases, the DER can be estimated by calculating the cat's RER for their ideal weight and then multiplying that number by an appropriate life-stage factor (see **Table 2**). **Table 3** also contains estimated energy needs of adult cats based on their ideal weight.

Case example: A 7-year-old, male, castrated domestic short hair weighing 7 kg with a BCS of 8/9 and an ideal weight of approximately 5.5 kg arrives at your clinic for a weight loss program. First, his RER is calculated based on *ideal* weight (5.5 kg) $= 70 (5.5_{kg}^{0.75}) = 251$ kcal/d. You decide to feed a life-stage factor to promote weight loss (0.8). 251 kcal $\times$ 0.8 $=$ 201 kcal/d $=$ DER to achieve weight loss.

Estimating Ideal Body Weight

Because DERs are based on ideal weight, it is important to accurately estimate the patient's target weight. There are several methods that can be used:

- Use previously recorded body weight when patient was noted to be a 5/9 or 3/5 BCS.
- Calculate based on estimation of body fat:
  - After assigning a body condition score, estimate the current fat and lean mass (see **Table 1**). For example, if a cat has a BCS of 7/9, the body fat estimate is 35% to 39%.
  - To determine the patient's lean mass, multiply the cat's current weight by the % lean tissue. If this patient is 38% fat, the lean mass is 62% (100% $-$ 38%).
    - 6 kg cat $\times$ 0.62 $=$ 3.72 kg of *lean* mass. This is what the patient would weigh at 0% body fat.
    - If the target is approximately 20% body fat, then take the lean mass and divide by 0.8 (assuming the lean mass is 80% of the ideal weight).

Table 3
Estimated daily kilocalorie requirements for adult cats

Ideal Weight, kg	Ideal Weight, lb	Obese Prone	Neutered	Intact
3	6.6	160	192–225	225–255
4	8.8	200	240–280	280–320
5	11	235	280–330	330–376
6	13.2	271	325–380	380–433
7	15.4	300	360–420	420–480

Calculated using resting energy requirements (body weight (kg)$^{0.75} \times$ 70) and multiplying by a life-stage factor of 1.0 for obese prone, 1.2 to 1.4 for neutered, and 1.4 to 1.6 for intact cats. Energy requirements for active weight loss may be lower than 1.0. Underweight cats should be allowed to eat as much as they will readily consume until ideal weight is achieved. Please note these are only guidelines and individual cats may need more or less energy to maintain ideal body condition.

- 3.72/0.8 = 4.65 kg is estimated ideal weight.
  - This process is summarized by the following equation:
    - (Current body weight × Current % lean) ÷0.8

PUTTING NUTRITIONAL RECOMMENDATIONS INTO PRACTICE

Incorporating nutritional assessments into everyday practice requires a team effort. Veterinarians, technicians, and front desk staff should all work together to collect accurate information and provide clear, consistent recommendations. The following are suggested steps to incorporate nutritional assessments into practice:

Pet Owner First and Last Name): _____

Street Address: _____

City:_____State:_____ZipCode: _____

Best phone number(s) to reach you: _____

E-mail: _____

PET INFORMATION *(please PRINT)*

Name:_____ Breed: _____

Species: ❑ Canine   ❑ Feline   Gender: ❑ Intact Female   ❑ Spayed Female_____
                                      ❑ Intact Male   ❑ Neutered Male

Age:_____ ❑ YEARS or ❑ MONTHS   Date of Birth:_____/_____/_____(Month/Day/Year)

Who feeds this pet? _____

On average, how many hours per day is the pet home alone? _____
_____

Number of family members at home? Adults:_____Children: _____

Other pets in the house? ❑ YES   ❑ NO   Number of additional pets and species: _____

Where is your pet fed? _____

Does your pet have access to other pet food? ❑ YES ❑ NO

     If YES, please describe: _____
_____

Is there competition for food between pets?   ❑ YES   ❑ NO

     If YES, please describe: _____
_____

Is your pet fed from the same bowl as other pets in the house?   ❑ YES   ❑ NO

     If YES, please describe: _____
_____

Does your pet ever gain access to the trash?   ❑ YES   ❑ NO

     If YES, how often does your pet get into the trash? _____

Does your pet have access to the outdoors?

❑ NO   ❑ Fenced backyard   ❑ Unfenced yard   ❑ Leash walks   ❑ Other: _____

Where does your pet spend most of its time?   ❑ Indoors   ❑ Outdoors   ❑ Both Indoors & Outdoors

Is your pet: ❑ Very active   ❑ Moderately active   ❑ Not very active

Please describe the type or work or exercise (if any) your pet does on average per week. _____

Fig. 3. Diet, activity and household history form. (*Courtesy of* A. Witzel-Rollins, DVM, PhD, DACVN, Knoxville TN.)

Please describe any care not provided by the primary owner *(eg, day care, dog walker, boarding)*. _____

Has your pet experienced any undesired weight gain or weight loss? ❑ YES ❑ NO

If YES, please describe: _____

Have you noticed any change in your pet's bowel movements? ❑ YES ❑ NO

    If YES, please describe: _____

    _____

Does your pet currently have a good appetite? ❑ YES ❑ NO

    If NO, please describe: _____

    _____

Has your pet's appetite recently changed? ❑ YES ❑ NO

    If YES, please describe: _____

    _____

Is your pet vomiting? ❑ YES ❑ NO

    If YES, please describe: _____

Current Supplements (name and dose per day):

1. _____
2. _____
3. _____
4. _____

Fig. 3. *(continued)*.

- Mail or e-mail the nutrition history form with appointment reminder (**Fig. 3**).
- Clients complete nutrition history form before the visit or while in waiting room.
- Veterinary technician reviews the nutrition history form with the owner and calculates current kilocalorie intake.
- Place the nutrition history form in the medical record.
- Veterinarian performs a physical examination and makes nutritional recommendations.
  - Written recommendations should be provided if feeding plan is changed.
- Veterinary technician asks if the client has any questions about the feeding plan and provides informational handouts, brochures, kitchen scales, measuring cups, and so forth, if warranted.
- Front desk staff dispenses recommended food if sold within the hospital and answers any remaining questions.
- If new food is dispensed or recommended, front desk staff or veterinary technician calls or e-mails the owner in a few days to see if the changes are accepted.

The veterinary staff can provide clients with a target kilocalorie goal and ask the owner to calculate their cat's food volume based on the labeled kilocalories per cup or gram. Alternatively, a member of the veterinary team can calculate food volumes for the client. Asking owners to weigh food with a kitchen scale based on the kilocalories per kilogram listed on the product label provides more accuracy and flexibility in feeding plans for cats.

SUMMARY

Nutrition affects the health of every cat. It is our responsibility as veterinarians to provide evidence-based nutritional assessments and plans to every patient at every visit. Otherwise, marketing and misinformation will guide cat owners' decisions, often to the detriment of their pet. To increase efficiency and reinforce messages, veterinary hospitals should incorporate nutritional assessments with a team approach. Every cat should receive a screening assessment, whereas those with nutritional risk factors require evaluation that is more detailed.

DISCLOSURE

A. Witzel-Rollins: Member of the PetSmart Healthy Pet Advisory Council, research funding provided by Vet Innovations Inc, Royal Canin, Hill's Pet Nutrition. M. Murphy: Research funding provided by Royal Canin.

REFERENCES

1. Baldwin K, Bartges J, Buffington T, et al. AAHA nutritional assessment guidelines for dogs and cats. J Am Anim Hosp Assoc 2010;46:285–96.
2. WSAVA Nutritional Assessment Guidelines Task Force Members. WSAVA nutritional assessment guidelines. J Feline Med Surg 2011;13:516–25.
3. NRC. Nutrient requirements of dogs and cats. Washington, DC: The National Academies Press; 2006.
4. Pittari J, RodaN I, Beekman G, et al. American Association of Feline Practitioners: senior care guidelines. J Feline Med Surg 2009;11:763–78.
5. Lund E, Armstrong P, Kirk C, et al. Prevalence and risk factors for obesity in adult cats from private US veterinary practices. Intern J Appl Res Vet Med 2005;3: 88–96.
6. Harper EJ. Changing perspectives on aging and energy requirements: aging and digestive function in humans, dogs and cats. J Nutr 1998;128:2632S–5S.
7. Laflamme DP. Nutrition for aging cats and dogs and the importance of body condition. Vet Clin North Am Small Anim Pract 2005;35:713–42.
8. Gross KL, Becvarova I, Debraekeleer J, Hand MS. Feeding reproducing cats. In: Thatcher CD, Remillard RL, et al, editors. Small animal clinical nutrition. 5th edition. Topeka (KS): Mark Morris Institute; 2010. p. 401.
9. Bilkei G. [Effect of the nutrition status on parturition in the cat]. Berl Munch Tierarztl Wochenschr 1990;103:49–51.
10. Loveridge G, Rivers J. Bodyweight changes and energy intakes of cats during pregnancy and lactation. In: Burgers I, Rivers J, editors. Nutrition of the dog and cat. Cambridge (UK): Cambridge University Press; 1989. p. 113.
11. Flynn MF, Hardie EM, Armstrong PJ. Effect of ovariohysterectomy on maintenance energy requirement in cats. J Am Vet Med Assoc 1996;209:1572–81.
12. Naik R, Witzel A, Albright JD, et al. Pilot study evaluating the impact of feeding method on overall activity of neutered indoor pet cats. J Vet Behav Clin Appl Res 2018;25:9–13.
13. Laflamme D. Development and validation of a body condition score system for cats: a clinical tool. Feline Pract 1997;25:13–8.
14. Toll PW, Yamka RM, Schoenherr WD, et al. Obesity. In: Hand MS. In: Thatcher CD, Remillard RL, et al, editors. Small animal clinical nutrition. Topeka (KS): Mark Morris Institute; 2010. p. 501–42.

15. Cline MG, Witzel AL, Moyers TD, et al. Body composition of lean outdoor intact cats vs lean indoor neutered cats using dual-energy x-ray absorptiometry. J Feline Med Surg 2018;21(6):459–64.

16. Witzel AL, Kirk CA, Henry GA, et al. Use of a morphometric method and body fat index system for estimation of body composition in overweight and obese cats. J Am Vet Med Assoc 2014;244:1285–90.

17. WSAVA Nutritional Assessment Guidelines Task Force Members, Freeman L, Becvarova I, Nick C, et al. WSAVA nutritional assessment guidelines. J Small Anim Pract 2011;52:385–96.

18. Michel KE, Anderson W, Cupp C, et al. Correlation of a feline muscle mass score with body composition determined by dual-energy X-ray absorptiometry. Br J Nutr 2011;106(Suppl 1):S57–9.

19. Committee WGN. WSAVA global nutrition committee: recommendations on selecting pet foods. 2013. Available at: https://www.wsava.org/WSAVA/media/Arpita-and-Emma-editorial/Selecting-the-Best-Food-for-your-Pet.pdf. Accessed July 7, 2020.

20. Shmalberg J. Beyond the guaranteed analysis: comparing pet foods. Today's Veterinary Practice 2013;3(1):43–5.

21. Russell K, Sabin R, Holt S, et al. Influence of feeding regimen on body condition in the cat. J Small Anim Pract 2000;41:12–7.

22. Harper EJ, Stack DM, Watson TD, et al. Effects of feeding regimens on body-weight, composition and condition score in cats following ovariohysterectomy. J Small Anim Pract 2001;42:433–8.

23. Kienzle E, Bergler R. Human-animal relationship of owners of normal and overweight cats. J Nutr 2006;136:1947s–50s.

24. Bradshaw JWS. The evolutionary basis for the feeding behavior of domestic dogs (*Canis familiaris*) and cats (*Felis catus*). J Nutr 2006;136:1927S–31S.

25. Dantas LM, Delgado MM, Johnson I, et al. Food puzzles for cats: feeding for physical and emotional wellbeing. J Feline Med Surg 2016;18:723–32.

Feeding Cats for Optimal Mental and Behavioral Well-Being

Mikel Delgado, PhD[a],*, Leticia M.S. Dantas, DVM, MS, PhD[b]

KEYWORDS

- Feeding behavior • Predation • Food puzzles • Foraging • Domestic cats
- Mental health

KEY POINTS

- Cats naturally eat several small meals per day, but cats in homes are typically either free-fed or fed twice daily.
- Foraging enrichment can encourage natural feeding behaviors, and food puzzles are advised as a form of mental stimulation and behavior modification.
- Free-feeding is likely necessary, but other factors also play a role in the development of obesity.
- Several recommendations for managing feeding issues in cats are offered.
- Diet and food intake have an important role not only in general health but also in mental and behavioral well-being.

INTRODUCTION

Cats that are confined indoors are dependent on their owners to determine when, what, and how they eat, which impacts a cat's welfare on multiple levels. Obesity and behavior problems are common in pet cats,[1–3] and these conditions, although multifactorial, may be related to the ways that cats are fed.[1,4,5] The feeding of cats should follow these key principles:

- How cats are fed should reflect the way that cats naturally eat
- Feeding should promote the physical and mental/behavioral health of the cat
- Cats should be given choices to assess their preferences whenever possible

[a] Department of Medicine and Epidemiology, School of Veterinary Medicine, University of California-Davis, 1 Shields Avenue, 2108 Tupper Hall, Davis, CA 95616, USA; [b] Behavioral Medicine Service, Department of Veterinary Biosciences and Diagnostic Imaging, University of Georgia Veterinary Teaching Hospital, University of Georgia, 501 D.W. Brooks Dr., Athens, GA 30602, USA
* Corresponding author.
E-mail address: mmdelgado@ucdavis.edu

Vet Clin Small Anim 50 (2020) 939–953
https://doi.org/10.1016/j.cvsm.2020.05.003   vetsmall.theclinics.com
0195-5616/20/© 2020 Elsevier Inc. All rights reserved.

HOW CATS EAT

Feral cats are generalist predators,[6] likely able to survive in many environments because of their ability to adapt to variable prey. The natural feeding behavior of feral cats is highly dependent on available resources. Unowned island cats who were not additionally provisioned by humans primarily hunted and ate small rodents[6] and birds,[7] although fish, invertebrates, and reptiles/amphibians were also consumed.[8]

Human provision does not eliminate predatory behavior. One study in a national park found that the native rodent and bird populations were significantly lower in areas in which cats colonies were fed compared with areas in which cats were not observed.[9] Another study found that feral cats hunted and consumed approximately 4 times the amount of prey as housecats. The percentage of feeding from prey for housecats varied from 15% to 90% of their daily intake.[10] The feline diet changes with season and prey availability,[11] and some cats specialize on a particular type of prey, whereas others are generalists.[12] It is unknown whether a cat's preference for varied prey predicts their preference for a varied diet, in terms of meat source, textures, or tastes.

Previous studies have found that more than 40% of cat owners report feeding their cats dry food exclusively, with approximately 30% feeding a diet of at least half canned food.[13] Many cats (40%–60%) are free-fed or fed twice daily,[13,14] with free-feeding more common for obese cats.[14,15]

The caloric intake of the average neutered adult cat varies widely but has been estimated at approximately 55 kcal/kg per day.[16] Because the most common natural prey of both domestic cats and their closest ancestors is mice (30 kcal/mouse), it is likely that this lineage of cats evolved eating several small meals per day. When allowed to choose their own feeding patterns, cats tend to eat between roughly 8 and 16 meals a day.[16,17] It is unknown how feeding relatively infrequent meals impacts the health or behavior of cats, although 1 study of 20 laboratory-housed male cats found increased aggression, and less consumption of food and water when meal-fed compared with when fed ad libitum (unrestricted access to food – time and quantity).[5]

FORAGING AND CONTRAFREELOADING

Because all animals must forage for food, whether by hunting, scavenging, or searching, enrichment that encourages foraging behavior can provide an outlet for natural behaviors. Many captive animals appear to prefer working for food over receiving freely available food, a phenomenon known as contrafreeloading.[18,19]

Because one study found that cats preferred to eat freely available food before lever pressing (working) to receive food,[20] they have been described as "the only species so far tested that showed no contrafreeloading."[18] Due to some methodological issues (small sample size, food restriction, the task required by cats to acquire food) the results of this study should be interpreted with caution, and more studies are clearly needed. Cats naturally work for food, and only approximately a third of cats' hunting attempts lead to a kill.[21] Cats will continue to kill prey (ie, contrafreeload) before consuming previously killed prey.[21,22] Although hunger is not necessary for cats to hunt or play, hunger increases hunting and play,[23,24] and would for example, likely increase a cat's desire to use a foraging toy (food puzzle).

FOOD PUZZLES

Food puzzles have been recommended for cats and dogs as a mode of environmental enrichment,[25–27] as well as one tool in the treatment of pet obesity.[28,29] In theory, food puzzles should increase activity and encourage problem solving.[30] Previous studies of confined companion animals have demonstrated positive effects of foraging toys on behavior, including calmer behavior in shelter dogs[31] and reduced feather-picking in parrots.[32]

Case studies suggest positive effects of food puzzles on the behavior, and well-being of cats,[25] although a recent study found that their use may not increase overall activity.[33] Using a randomized crossover design, 19 housecats were fed from either a bowl or a set of food puzzles while wearing an accelerometer. No differences were found in daily or weekly activity levels between the 2 feeding conditions.

Food puzzles are not commonly used by cat owners. One survey found that fewer than 5% of owners provided food puzzles or hid food around the home to stimulate their cat's foraging behavior.[3] A more recent survey found that 30% of participants used food puzzles, but only occasionally, and another 18% had previously tried, but no longer used food puzzles.[34] It is challenging to quantify how much enrichment owners provide for their cats, and there are few empirically based guidelines for what types and how much enrichment improves the welfare of cats. However, food puzzles should not harm pet cats and may offer benefits for their welfare; current feline care guidelines encourage their routine use.[35]

USING FOOD PUZZLES

- Food puzzles can be used with wet or dry food.
- Mobile puzzles are objects with holes that can be filled with dry food and rolled around to release food.
- Stationary puzzles have a base and wells or cups from which food may be fished out.
- Puzzles can be purchased or homemade.
- The difficulty of the food puzzle should match the abilities of the cat, and at first, the food puzzle should require little effort on the cat's part to release food.
- Food puzzles can be filled with treats at first or introduced to the cat before meals to increase motivation.
- A recent publication offered detailed information on how to introduce food puzzles to cats, suggestions for troubleshooting, and a handout for veterinary clients,[25] and more information is available at: http://foodpuzzlesforcats.com (**Figs. 1–3**).

Other Options to Encourage Foraging Activity

- Divide a cat's food into small, naturally sized portions to place in different locations in the home to stimulate search behavior.
- Toss pieces of dry food across the floor for a cat to chase and retrieve.
- Place food on elevated surfaces, such as cat furniture or tables. The physical condition of a cat (age, joint mobility) should be considered.

FEEDING PRACTICES

Offering small, frequent meals would be most similar to cats' observed preferences.[17,36,37] Owners can allow cats to graze or offer multiple feeding choices (food puzzles, as well as meals). In either case, owners should track the overall daily intake of their cat by weighing food with a scale[38] and following recommendations from their veterinarian. Reassessing the cat's weight, body, and muscle condition will determine how the program is working for the individual (see "Assessing nutritional requirements and current intake" by Witzel-Rollins and Murphy, elsewhere in this issue).

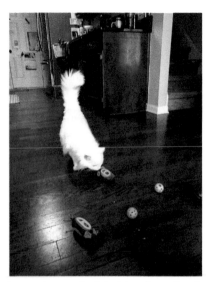

Fig. 1. Mobile food puzzles can be manipulated to release food.

Owners may need education about proper cleanliness of feeding areas, which may impact cat feeding behavior. Many cat owners do not completely or routinely empty and wash bowls, and instead "top off" dry cat food. Saliva and crumbs can quickly accumulate, and a dirty bowl increases bacteria and may be unpleasant to cats; pet food bowls have been ranked among the most bacteria-laded kitchen surfaces.[39,40] Food and water dishes should be washed daily,[41] and food replaced as needed. When wet food is left out for long periods of time, it can become dry, which may reduce its appeal for cats.

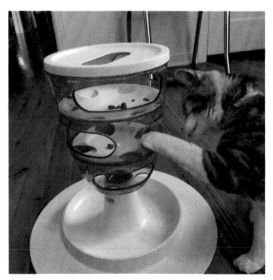

Fig. 2. Example of a stationary food puzzle.

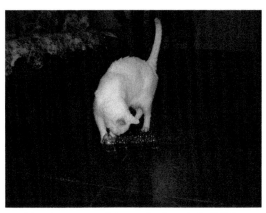

Fig. 3. Gege, 13-year-old male neutered domestic short hair (DSH) cat, using a homemade food toy.

There has been recent attention to a potential issue for cats, labeled "whisker stress,[42]" the assumed discomfort experienced when a cat's whiskers touch the side of a narrow bowl while eating. To date there is no empirical evidence on whether whisker stress occurs[43]; however, owners may choose to offer food in a few different styles of dishes to see if their cat shows a preference.

Another open question is whether cats prefer water separated from their food, a frequent recommendation,[44,45] based on the assumption that dead prey would contaminate a water source. As with "whisker stress," there is no empirical evidence demonstrating a preference for separate food and water areas. Many cats are fed dry food, and dry food increases water consumption,[16,46] so cats may prefer a water source close to their food. Studies are needed, but owners can provide their cats with choices of water and food locations to determine individual preferences.

PROBLEMS RELATED TO FEEDING
Obesity

Although free-feeding is associated with obesity, opportunities to graze may also allow cats to eat in a manner closest to what is natural to them. The relationship between free-feeding and weight gain may be due to the continual availability of calorically dense food, but there are other related factors, such as neuter status, which may reduce a cat's maintenance energy requirements and ability to regulate intake.[47,48] Living in a multi-pet household is associated with a higher body condition score,[4,49,50] which could be due to stress, increased competition for food, or to a larger amount of food being available.

Not all free-fed cats become overweight, thus freely available food is not the only cause of obesity. There has been little exploration of the effects of negative emotions on the feeding behavior of companion animals, although stressors and changes in routine have been associated with anorexia in cats.[51,52] Emotional overeating has been well-established in humans and laboratory animals, and may be caused by frustration, stress, boredom or other factors besides hunger.[53] Recent research suggests a relationship between impulse control and overeating in cats,[54] similar to findings in humans.[55] Unfortunately, obesity and overweight may further reduce an animal's quality of life by restricting their activity and through related physical conditions, such as diabetes mellitus or joint disease.

Obesity may be prevented with an appropriately enriched environment that provides exercise, mental stimulation, and a sense of control and safety. Cats that are at a healthy weight may be able to free feed without excessive weight gain, particularly if owners monitor food intake and their cat's weight (**Fig. 4**). However, cats switched from meal feeding to ad libitum feeding may initially increase their food intake, which can lead to at least short-term weight gain[56,57].

Pickiness

Cats are known to be particular about flavor profiles, textures, shapes, and temperature of food.[58,59] A reduced appetite can be caused by a diversity of pathologic or disease processes and should not be considered "normal behavior" associated with food preferences until health issues have been addressed or ruled out. Cats can be neophobic toward new foods, particularly when they do not find the food palatable,[37] and may instead develop a fixation on one type of food.[59] These cats may sniff at the new food before tasting it or refuse to try it altogether.[37]

One study found behavioral differences between cats eating a preferred versus a less palatable food.[60] When eating less desirable food, cats were more likely to flick their tail, groom their body, flick their ears backwards, and lick their nose without tasting the food. Cats eating a preferred food were more likely to lip-lick.[60]

Owners can prevent pickiness by offering new foods as choices, alongside previously accepted foods.[61] Cats appear to appreciate some variety in foods offered, and may initially show a preference for a novel food, but the effect is usually transient.[62] Accepted foods should be regularly rotated into a feeding regimen to maintain consumption, otherwise, neophobia may be observed during future presentations.[63] Cat owners should also keep in mind that some cats prefer their food at room temperature or warmer.[59]

Begging/Meowing for Food

Cats increase activity and exhibit anticipatory behaviors as feeding time approaches.[64,65] As these behaviors (eg, pacing, meowing, purring) become associated with the delivery of food, they may be reinforced. Some cats may exhibit demanding behavior (eg, meowing, knocking things off shelves) at other times to get food or attention. Cats on restricted intake show more "affectionate" behaviors (such as sitting in a lap) in addition to attention-seeking behaviors (such as begging, following owners, and meowing),[66] likely in an attempt to solicit food from the owner. Some cats may even become aggressive when waiting for food or try to steal human food from counters and tables.[67] Owners are sensitive to the intensity of cats' solicitation behaviors[68]

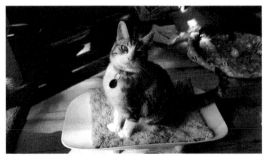

Fig. 4. Cats can be trained to sit on a scale for routine weight monitoring.

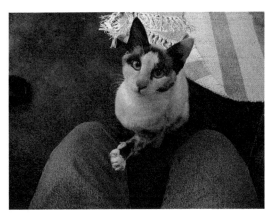

Fig. 5. Cats may engage in attention-seeking behaviors to solicit food from owners.

and may misinterpret these social interactions as hunger, and give the cat more food, which can lead to weight problems[62] (**Fig. 5**).

Providing cats with food on a routine or schedule rather than feeding cats exclusively when they "ask" will reduce begging behavior, although owners will likely observe increased anticipatory behaviors close to scheduled feeding times.[64,65] Cats who have been reinforced for meowing at other times may experience an extinction burst (increased behavior in response to removal of reinforcement) when owners stop feeding the cat on demand.[69] An extinction burst may be avoided by including differential reinforcement of alternative behaviors.[69] One cat with aggressive behaviors around food was successfully treated with a combination of routine, enrichment, training for quiet and calm behaviors, and ignoring demanding behavior that previously led to being fed.[67]

Automated Feeders

If a cat is overly dependent or demanding on their human for food, a timed automated feeder can be implemented. This reduces the connection between the human and the arrival of food and also allows an owner to program multiple feedings per day, at a schedule that works better for their cat (eg, great frequency of small meals) and for them (eg, being able to feed the cat in the middle of the night without the owner having to wake up) (**Fig. 6**).

Multi-pet Households: Multiple Stations For Multiple Cats

Cats are solitary hunters; they hunt small prey[70] that they do not share, aside from mothers with kittens.[36] The ability of natural-occurring groups of cats to exist at high density is directly related to the availability and dispersal of resources, including prey. Cats fed inside homes should also be treated as solitary feeders, and resources should be ample and spaced out sufficiently to prevent competition or stress when eating. Aggression between cats can be influenced by conflict over availability of resources, including food[71,72] (see also "Health: Environment and Feline Health: At Home and in the Clinic in Part I," elsewhere in this issue).

In one survey, approximately half (56.4%) of multi-cat households provided multiple food bowls,[73] although it was not noted whether feeding areas were in proximity to one another, rather than in separate locations. In the same study, almost half of multi-cat households only provided 1 food dish for multiple cats. When cats are

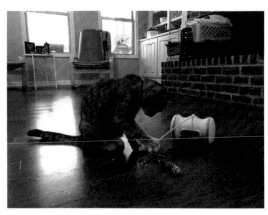

Fig. 6. Nina, 1-year-old female spayed DSH cat, using an automatic feeder.

required to share a feeding bowl or station, a cat may be forced to eat while feeling stress or anxiety, rather than forgo a meal. In some cases, cats may fight at a shared food station both before and during feeding due to crowding,[74] whereas other cats may choose to avoid conflict by waiting to eat until another cat is finished (**Fig. 7**).

Another study found a relationship between aggressive encounters away from the food bowl, feeding order, and agonistic behavior around a feeding station in an owned cat colony.[75] This and a study of an outdoor colony of feral cats in Italy suggested that social interactions around the food bowl are complex.[71,76] Some cats appeared to tolerate eating close to specific individuals, and other cats chose to leave the feeding area and return after other cats had already fed and vacated. In both studies, food was only available from a single, central location.

Although some cats may not mind sharing a food dish, the best way to accommodate multiple cats is to give each cat the choice to eat alone. Some cats will carry food away from the food dish to eat it; this is a normal feline behavior, and cats who hunt often carry their prey away from the kill.[36] Carrying food away from the source can also indicate that the cat has a preferred feeding area. Owners should position bowls

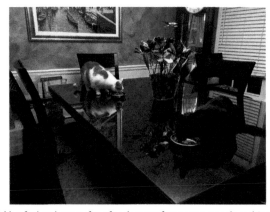

Fig. 7. Cats should be fed at least a few feed apart from one another. (*Courtesy of* S. Globerman, DVM, Marietta, GA.)

to allow cats a vantage point while eating, so they can observe if humans or animals approach while they eat.

MANAGING DIETARY ISSUES IN MULTI-PET HOUSEHOLDS

- Multi-pet households may have animals with different diets or eating preferences, or adversarial relationships.
- Many therapeutic diets provide complete nutrition, so if all cats find it palatable, they can often be transitioned to the same diet.
- The SureFeed is a motorized bowl that can only be accessed by the cat(s) with the correct microchip(s). A microchip-activated flap installed in a door or wall can also limit access to specific cats.
- Other devices are being added to the market (eg, PortionPro Rx, CatsPad) that allow owners to manage feeding while avoiding confining cats, limiting access to food, or punishment/correction.
- These tools can allow cats to eat according to their personal preferences (grazing vs eating larger meals) (**Fig. 8**).

Meal feeding can be part of a cat's daily routine. Knowing when to expect food and having a routine are known to reduce sickness behaviors in cats.[51] Meal feeding may increase the cat-owner bond and allows the owner to use food as reinforcement for behaviors, such as asking a cat to sit quietly in a desired location (eg, a mat). Feeding a large meal before bedtime and after an exercise session can reduce nighttime activity, a common complaint of cat owners.[36] A complementary recommendation to prevent or modify night activity is for the cat owner to introduce food puzzles and leave them available overnight so the cat can self-feed, while using other feeding methods during the day.

USING FOOD IN BEHAVIOR THERAPY INTERVENTIONS: APPLICATIONS IN CLINICAL BEHAVIORAL MEDICINE AND FELINE MENTAL HEALTH CARE

As previously explained in this article, diet and food intake have a role not only in general health but also in mental and emotional well-being. Specific nutrients cause changes in brain structure, chemistry, and physiology, leading to behavioral changes.[77] Besides the usefulness of food as a tool in veterinary behavior therapy,

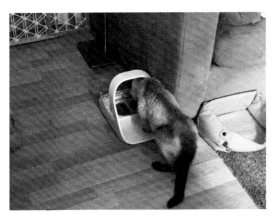

Fig. 8. Senior cat using a microchip-activated feeder. (*Courtesy of* I. Johnson, CCBC, Marietta, GA.)

this understanding allowed for the production of prescription diets that are part of mental health treatments for animals, including cats.[78] Besides providing precursors to important mood-regulating neurotransmitters (such as tryptophan for serotonin synthesis), food ingestion regulates receptors and causes release of neurotransmitters associated with pleasure and calmness.

Overall, food is a fundamental aid in 3 main types of interventions commonly used in veterinary psychiatry and psychological care: the application of environmental enrichment and meeting basic behavioral needs, counterconditioning therapy, and differential reinforcement of alternative behaviors. These interventions are of benefit not only to owned cats but also to cats living in shelters and laboratories.[79,80] The efficacy of these tools is generally related to food value,[81] with more palatable reinforcers leading to increased response.[82]

The literature citing benefits of environmental enrichment for brain health is extensive and beyond the scope of this article. Benefits can be externally measured and are part of assessment, treatment evaluation, and prognosis of feline patients (such as increases in behavioral diversity, presentation of normal species-specific behaviors, utilization and exploration of the environment, ability to cope with stressors, reductions in the frequency and intensity of abnormal and pathologic behaviors, and decreased clinical signs of anxiety).[27,52] However, benefits at the neuroanatomical and neurochemical levels are also well-known (from changes in cortical thickness, size of synaptic contacts, number of dendritic spines and dendritic branching, to increased brain weight).[83]

In 2013, the American Association of Feline Practitioners and the International Society of Feline Medicine published their Feline Environmental Needs Guidelines that recommended, among other techniques, the use of food puzzles for feline well-being.[84] This recommendation has been supported by several other publications and studies. Consequently, in behavioral medicine and veterinary psychiatry, environmental enrichment in the form of food toys, puzzles, and games are an important aid for all feline patients regardless of their diagnoses. However, it can be particularly helpful for specific conditions such as separation anxiety disorder (eg, by giving the cat options of rewarding and stimulating activities not related to interacting with and the presence of the owner), generalized anxiety disorder (eg, by decreasing clinical signs of hypervigilance and arousal), and for cases of inter-cat conflict (eg, by taking the cats' focus away from each other and toward a rewarding and relaxing activity, which might also promote counterconditioning between cats).[25,85]

Counterconditioning therapy is commonly used as part of the treatment and management of fear, phobias, and other anxiety disorders. It is based on classic conditioning (ie, learning through association), which is involved in the development of fear responses.[86] Classic counterconditioning does not require a specific response from the animal, but instead depends on changing an animal's emotional or motivational state in the presence of a conditioned stimuli. Because food affects neurophysiology and neuroendocrinology and therefore the cat's emotional state, the association of high value food and/or food toys and puzzle with specific situations and conditioned stimuli (eg, another animal, sounds) can decrease stress, fear, and anxiety (**Fig. 9**).

Counterconditioning is ideally paired with systematic desensitization (ie, progressive exposure) and it is tailored for every individual cat with gradual steps based on the cat's body language, facial expression and emotional responses. A few examples of this type of therapy are to decrease fear of veterinary visits, the carrier and car rides, people, appliances, and other animals.[87] Counterconditioning is key when integrating or re-integrating cats in a multi-cat household.[25,88]

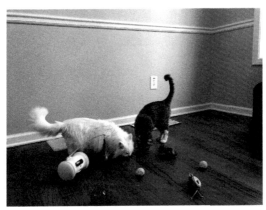

Fig. 9. Food puzzles are instrumental in behavior therapy, promoting counter conditioning between cats, encouraging positive social behavior and decreasing conflict.

Differential reinforcement of alternative behaviors (DRA) is based on both classic conditioning and operant conditioning. This type of therapy replaces dysfunctional behaviors with actions that are more appropriate for a situation. The general guidelines involve removing the reinforcers for unwanted behaviors when possible/applicable, teaching acceptable alternative behaviors in the same context, and using positive reinforcement to maintain desired behaviors long term. Again, food (especially when high value) is a powerful reward for most cats, as the changes achieved are not only external (behavioral) but also happen at a neurochemical level. When applied properly and consistently, these interventions can lead to long-lasting behavioral and emotional change. This form of therapy is fundamental for the treatment and management of cats whose stress response escalates into aggression. For example, DRA is used to teach avoidance to replace or substitute threatening signals and aggression between cats.[88] Differential reinforcement is also effective for the treatment of obsessive-compulsive disorders, by modifying stereotypical behaviors while reinforcing other, functional responses.[85] Details on the use of food rewards, food puzzles, and toys for veterinary mental health and behavioral care is covered extensively in the most current literature.

DISCLOSURE

Dr. Delgado was supported by funding from Maddie's Fund and the National Center for Advancing Translational Sciences, National Institutes of Health, through grant number UL1 TR001860 and linked award TL1 TR001861 to MD. The content is solely the responsibility of the authors and does not necessarily represent the official views of the NIH. The funding sources had no role in study design or in the collection, analysis, or interpretation of data.

REFERENCES

1. Lund EM, Armstrong PJ, Kirk CA, et al. Prevalence and risk factors for obesity in adult cats from private US veterinary practices. Intern J Appl Res Vet Med 2005; 3:88–96.
2. Colliard L, Paragon BM, Lemuet B, et al. Prevalence and risk factors of obesity in an urban population of healthy cats. J Feline Med Surg 2009;11:135–40.

3. Strickler BL, Shull EA. An owner survey of toys, activities, and behavior problems in indoor cats. J Vet Behav 2014;9:207–14.
4. Russell K, Sabin R, Holt S, et al. Influence of feeding regimen on body condition in the cat. J Small Anim Pract 2000;41:12–8.
5. Finco D, Adams D, Crowell W, et al. Food and water intake and urine composition in cats: influence of continuous versus periodic feeding. Am J Vet Res 1986;47: 1638–42.
6. Bonnaud E, Bourgeois K, Vidal E, et al. Feeding ecology of a feral cat population on a small Mediterranean island. J Mammal 2007;88:1074–81.
7. Kirkpatrick RD, Rauzon MJ. Foods of feral cats Felis catus on Jarvis and Howland Islands, central Pacific Ocean. Biotropica 1986;18:72–5.
8. Bonnaud E, Medina F, Vidal E, et al. The diet of feral cats on islands: a review and a call for more studies. Biol Invasions 2011;13:581–603.
9. Hawkins CC, Grant WE, Longnecker MT. Effect of house cats, being fed in parks, on California birds and rodents. Paper presented at: Proceedings of the 4th International Urban Wildlife Symposium. Tucson, AZ, May 1-5, 1999.
10. Liberg O. Food habits and prey impact by feral and house-based domestic cats in a rural area in southern Sweden. J Mammal 1984;65:424–32.
11. Jones E, Coman BJ. Ecology of the feral cat, Felis catus (L.), in south-eastern Australia. Wildl Res 1981;8:537–47.
12. Dickman CR, Newsome TM. Individual hunting behaviour and prey specialisation in the house cat Felis catus: implications for conservation and management. Appl Anim Behav Sci 2015;173:76–87.
13. Laflamme DP, Abood SK, Fascetti AJ, et al. Pet feeding practices of dog and cat owners in the United States and Australia. J Am Vet Med Assoc 2008;232:687–94.
14. Kienzle E, Bergler R. Human-animal relationship of owners of normal and overweight cats. J Nutr 2006;136:1947S–50S.
15. Harper E, Stack D, Watson T, et al. Effects of feeding regimens on bodyweight, composition and condition score in cats following ovariohysterectomy. J Small Anim Pract 2001;42:433–8.
16. Kane E, Rogers Q, Morris J. Feeding behavior of the cat fed laboratory and commercial diets. Nutr Res 1981;1:499–507.
17. Mugford RA. External influences on the feeding of carnivores. In: Kare M, Maller O, editors. The chemical senses and nutrition. New York: Academic Press; 1977. p. 25–50.
18. Inglis IR, Forkman B, Lazarus J. Free food or earned food? A review and fuzzy model of contrafreeloading. Anim Behav 1997;53:1171–91.
19. Osborne SR. The free food (contrafreeloading) phenomenon: a review and analysis. Anim Learn Behav 1977;5:221–35.
20. Koffer K, Coulson G. Feline indolence: cats prefer free to response-produced food. Psychon Sci 1971;24:41–2.
21. Leyhausen P. Cat behaviour. New York: Garland; 1979.
22. Adamec RE. The interaction of hunger and preying in the domestic cat (Felis catus): an adaptive hierarchy? Behav Biol 1976;18:263–72.
23. Hall SL, Bradshaw JWS. The influence of hunger on object play by adult domestic cats. Appl Anim Behav Sci 1998;58:143–50.
24. Biben M. Predation and predatory play behaviour of domestic cats. Anim Behav 1979;27:81–94.
25. Dantas LM, Delgado MM, Johnson I, et al. Food puzzles for cats: feeding for physical and emotional wellbeing. J Feline Med Surg 2016;18:723–32.
26. Whelan F. Environmental enrichment for pets. Vet Nursing J 2010;25:27–8.

27. Ellis SL. Environmental enrichment: practical strategies for improving feline welfare. J Feline Med Surg 2009;11:901–12.

28. Laflamme DP. Understanding and managing obesity in dogs and cats. Vet Clin North Am Small Anim Pract 2006;36:1283–95.

29. Clarke D, Wrigglesworth D, Holmes K, et al. Using environmental and feeding enrichment to facilitate feline weight loss. J Anim Physiol Anim Nutr 2005;89:427.

30. Meehan CL, Mench JA. The challenge of challenge: can problem solving opportunities enhance animal welfare? Appl Anim Behav Sci 2007;102:246–61.

31. Herron ME, Kirby-Madden TM, Lord LK. Effects of environmental enrichment on the behavior of shelter dogs. J Am Vet Med Assoc 2014;244:687–92.

32. Lumeij JT, Hommers CJ. Foraging 'enrichment'as treatment for pterotillomania. Appl Anim Behav Sci 2008;111:85–94.

33. Naik R, Witzel A, Albright JD, et al. Pilot study evaluating the effect of feeding method on overall activity of neutered indoor pet cats. J Vet Behav 2018;25:9–13.

34. Delgado M, Bain MJ, Buffington CT. A survey of feeding practices and use of food puzzles in owners of domestic cats. J Feline Med Surg 2020;22(2):193–8.

35. Sadek T, Hamper B, Horwitz D, et al. Feline feeding programs: addressing behavioural needs to improve feline health and wellbeing. J Feline Med Surg 2018;20:1049–55.

36. Beaver BV. Feline behavior: a guide for veterinarians. St Louis (MO): Saunders; 2003. p. 212–46.

37. Bradshaw J, Casey R, Brown S. Feeding behaviour. In: Bradshaw JWS, Casey RA, Brown SL, editors. The behaviour of the domestic cat. Wallingford, UK: CAB International; 2012. p. 113–27.

38. German A, Holden S, Mason S, et al. Imprecision when using measuring cups to weigh out extruded dry kibbled food. J Anim Physiol Anim Nutr 2011;95:368–73.

39. National Science Foundation. NSF International Household Germ Study. Ann Arbor (MI): National Science Foundation; 2011.

40. National Science Foundation. Cleaning the germiest home items. Ann Arbor (MI): National Science Foundation; 2019.

41. Case LP. Canine and feline nutrition: a resource for companion animal professionals. Maryland Heights (MO): Mosby; 2010.

42. Kingson JA. Feline food issues? 'Whisker Fatigue' may be to blame. New York Times 2017.

43. Sweeney C. Did the *New York Times* publish fake news about cats? Boston: Boston Magazine; 2017.

44. Rochlitz I. A review of the housing requirements of domestic cats (*Felis silvestris catus*) kept in the home. Appl Anim Behav Sci 2005;93:97–109.

45. Ellis S, RE. Five-a-Day Felix. A report into improving the health and welfare of the UK's domestic cats. 2017. Available at: icatcare.org. Accessed March 6, 2020.

46. Anderson R. Water balance in the dog and cat. J Small Anim Pract 1982;23: 588–98.

47. Flynn M, Hardie E, Armstrong P. Effect of ovariohysterectomy on maintenance energy requirement in cats. J Am Vet Med Assoc 1996;209:1572–81.

48. Nguyen PG, Dumon HJ, Siliart BS, et al. Effects of dietary fat and energy on body weight and composition after gonadectomy in cats. Am J Vet Res 2004;65: 1708–13.

49. Robertson I. The influence of diet and other factors on owner-perceived obesity in privately owned cats from metropolitan Perth, Western Australia. Prev Vet Med 1999;40:75–85.

50. Allan F, Pfeiffer D, Jones B, et al. A cross-sectional study of risk factors for obesity in cats in New Zealand. Prev Vet Med 2000;46:183–96.
51. Stella J, Croney C, Buffington T. Effects of stressors on the behavior and physiology of domestic cats. Appl Anim Behav Sci 2013;143:157–63.
52. Amat M, Camps T, Manteca X. Stress in owned cats: behavioural changes and welfare implications. J Feline Med Surg 2016;18:577–86.
53. McMillan FD. Stress-induced and emotional eating in animals: A review of the experimental evidence and implications for companion animal obesity. J Vet Behav 2013;8:376–85.
54. Moesta A, Bosch G, Beerda B. Choice impulsivity and not action impulsivity may be associated with overeating in cats. Paper presented at: Proceedings of the 12th International Veterinary Behavior Meeting. Washington DC, July 30 - August 1, 2019.
55. Giel KE, Teufel M, Junne F, et al. Food-related impulsivity in obesity and binge eating disorder—a systematic update of the evidence. Nutrients 2017;9:1170.
56. Durenkamp N. The effects of ad libitum feeding of low-or high-palatable feed on the physical activity, bodyweight and feeding patterns of domestic cats [Master Thesis]. Wageningen, Netherlands: Department of Animal Sciences, Wageningen University; 2015.
57. Goggin J, Schryver H, Hintz H. The effects of ad libitum feeding and caloric dilution on the domestic cat's ability to maintain energy balance. Feline Pract 1993; 21:7–11.
58. Zaghini G, Biagi G. Nutritional peculiarities and diet palatability in the cat. Vet Res Commun 2005;29:39–44.
59. German A, Heath S. Feline obesity: a medical disease with behavioral influences. In: Feline behavioral health and welfare. St. Louis (MO): Elsevier Health Sciences; 2015. p. 148–61.
60. Savolainen S, Telkanranta H, Junnila J, et al. A novel set of behavioural indicators for measuring perception of food by cats. Vet J 2016;216:53–8.
61. Zoran DL, Buffington CT. Effects of nutrition choices and lifestyle changes on the well-being of cats, a carnivore that has moved indoors. J Am Vet Med Assoc 2011;239:596–606.
62. Bradshaw JW. The behaviour of the domestic cat. Wallingford, UK: CABI; 2012.
63. Bradshaw JW, Goodwin D, Legrand-Defretin V, et al. Food selection by the domestic cat, an obligate carnivore. Comp Biochem Physiol A Physiol 1996;114: 205–9.
64. Deng P, Iwazaki E, Suchy SA, et al. Effects of feeding frequency and dietary water content on voluntary physical activity in healthy adult cats. J Anim Sci 2014;92: 1271–7.
65. Bradshaw JW, Cook SE. Patterns of pet cat behaviour at feeding occasions. Appl Anim Behav Sci 1996;47:61–74.
66. Levine ED, Erb HN, Schoenherr B, et al. Owner's perception of changes in behaviors associated with dieting in fat cats. J Vet Behav Clin Appl Res 2016;11:37–41.
67. Mongillo P, Adamelli S, Bernardini M, et al. Successful treatment of abnormal feeding behavior in a cat. J Vet Behav Clin Appl Res 2012;7:390–3.
68. McComb K, Taylor AM, Wilson C, et al. The cry embedded within the purr. Curr Biol 2009;19:R507–8.
69. Lerman DC, Iwata BA. Prevalence of the extinction burst and its attenuation during treatment. J Appl Behav Anal 1995;28:93–4.
70. Bradshaw JW. The evolutionary basis for the feeding behavior of domestic dogs (Canis familiaris) and cats (Felis catus). J Nutr 2006;136:1927S–31S.

71. Crowell-Davis SL, Curtis TM, Knowles RJ. Social organization in the cat: a modern understanding. J Feline Med Surg 2004;6:19–28.
72. Dantas-Divers LM, Crowell-Davis SL, Alford K, et al. Agonistic behavior and environmental enrichment of cats communally housed in a shelter. J Am Vet Med Assoc 2011;239:796–802.
73. Alho AM, Pontes J, Pomba C. Guardians' knowledge and husbandry practices of feline environmental enrichment. J Appl Anim Welf Sci 2016;19:115–25.
74. Laundré J. The daytime behaviour of domestic cats in a free-roaming population. Anim Behav 1977;25:990–8.
75. Knowles RJ, Curtis TM, Crowell-Davis SL. Correlation of dominance as determined by agonistic interactions with feeding order in cats. Am J Vet Res 2004; 65:1548–56.
76. Bonanni R, Cafazzo S, Fantini C, et al. Feeding-order in an urban feral domestic cat colony: relationship to dominance rank, sex and age. Anim Behav 2007;74: 1369–79.
77. Wurtman R. Effects of nutrients on neurotransmitter release. In: Marriott BM, editor. Food components to enhance performance. Washington, DC: National Academy Press; 1994. p. 239–62.
78. Overall K. Pharmacological approaches to changing behavior and neurochemistry: roles for diet, supplements, nutraceuticals, and medication. In: Overall K, editor. Manual of clinical behavioral medicine for dogs and cats. St Louis (MO): Mosby; 2013. p. 458–512.
79. Gourkow N, Fraser D. The effect of housing and handling practices on the welfare, behaviour and selection of domestic cats (Felis sylvestris catus) by adopters in an animal shelter. Anim Welf 2006;15:371–7.
80. McCune S, Smith C, Taylor V, et al. Enriching the environment of the laboratory cat. In: Smith CP, Taylor V, Nicol C, editors. Environmental enrichment information resources for laboratory animals. Washington, DC: United States Department of Agriculture; 1995. p. 27–42.
81. Domjan M. The principles of learning and behavior. Nelson Education; 2014.
82. Shah K, Bradshaw C, Szabadi E. Relative and absolute reinforcement frequency as determinants of choice in concurrent variable interval schedules. Q J Exp Psychol 1991;43:25–38.
83. Rosenzweig MR, Bennett EL. Psychobiology of plasticity: effects of training and experience on brain and behavior. Behav Brain Res 1996;78:57–65.
84. Ellis SL, Rodan I, Carney HC, et al. AAFP and ISFM feline environmental needs guidelines. J Feline Med Surg 2013;15:219–30.
85. Overall K. Undesirable, problematic, and abnormal feline behavior and behavioral pathologies. In: Overall K, editor. Clinical behavioral medicine of dogs and cats. St Louis (MO): Mosby; 2013. p. 360–456.
86. Mazur JE. Learning and behavior. Upper Saddle River (NJ): Prentice Hall; 2002.
87. Pratsch L, Mohr N, Palme R, et al. Carrier training cats reduces stress on transport to a veterinary practice. Appl Anim Behav Sci 2018;206:64–74.
88. Dantas L. Living with multiple cats - creating harmony in the multicat household (in press). In: Herron M, Horwitz D, Siracusa C, et al, editors. Decoding your cat. Boston: Houghton Mifflin Harcourt; 2020. p. 93–114.

Stem Cell Therapy and Cats
What Do We Know at This Time

Tracy L. Webb, DVM, PhD

KEYWORDS

• Feline • Mesenchymal stem cells • Regenerative medicine

KEY POINTS

- For liability purposes, veterinary clinicians must be aware of all regulations regarding the use of stem cells and other regenerative therapies in their practice area.
- Stem cell therapy is complex, and veterinarians should be aware of stem cell terminology and biology to accurately assess potential therapies for their patients.
- Many variables can affect stem cell function, which provides a source of promise but must be considered when comparing different study outcomes and applications.
- Only a few studies have been published to date evaluating mesenchymal stem cells as a therapeutic option for cats.
- Mesenchymal stem cells show promise for use in chronic inflammatory diseases in cats, although additional studies are needed.

INTRODUCTION

Although stem cells were originally mentioned in the literature back in the 1800s and have been used clinically for decades in bone marrow transplant therapies, investigation into other disease applications has greatly expanded in recent years. The significant need for new therapies to treat diseases for which there are no current therapies, significant side effects with some current therapies, and nonresponders has spurred the interest and hope in stem cells and other regenerative therapies in both human and veterinary medicine.

Unfortunately, this hope has led to many unproven and unsafe practices using regenerative therapies, the dangerous results of which caused Google to institute an advertisement ban for unproven and unapproved stem cell therapies in 2019. In fact, there currently are no veterinary US Food and Drug Administration (FDA)-approved regenerative therapies. The FDA's Center for Veterinary Medicine released a guidance in June of 2015 stating that cell-based therapies are considered new animal drugs.[1] In July of 2017, the American Veterinary Medical Association released a policy entitled "Therapeutic Use of Stem Cells and Regenerative Medicine" listing specific guidelines for the use of stem cells and other regenerative

Clinical Sciences, Colorado State University, 1678 Campus Delivery, Fort Collins, CO 80523, USA
E-mail address: Tracy.webb@colostate.edu

Vet Clin Small Anim 50 (2020) 955–971
https://doi.org/10.1016/j.cvsm.2020.06.002
0195-5616/20/© 2020 Elsevier Inc. All rights reserved.
vetsmall.theclinics.com

therapies starting with the requirement to follow the FDA Guidance for Industry #218.[2] Veterinarians who engage in the use of stem cells or other regenerative therapies in the United States must know and follow these and any additional applicable guidelines and policies; veterinarians in other countries must know and follow applicable policies where they practice. It is important to note that regulatory agencies like the US FDA protect the public and medical fields by working to ensure that drugs are safe and effective, and drug products that are unapproved lack the benefits of this oversight. Additionally, drugs that are not approved by the US FDA are not covered by the American Medicinal Drug Use Clarification Act and therefore cannot be used off-label (as they have no approved label) or for compassionate use.[3]

Although regenerative medicine is an exciting field with much interest in the potential it holds, it is also very complex and outside the realm of most current veterinary education. Lack of knowledge about the intricacies of the products and regulations combined with a strong desire to help patients can lead to misunderstanding among owners and clinicians. The American Veterinary Medical Association policy on the Therapeutic Use of Stem Cells and Regenerative Medicine states that "[v]eterinarians have few guidelines and limited resources for differentiating valid and effective therapies from those that have insufficient data support. Therefore, it is incumbent upon veterinarians engaged in regenerative therapies to be well versed in the emerging science of the field to successfully select the specific therapeutic protocols, processes, equipment, and vendors most likely to result in clinical benefit for their patients."[2] Accordingly, the goal of this article is to provide clinicians with a basic review of stem cells and a summary of the currently available data on their clinical use in cats.

STEM CELL PRIMER
What Is Regenerative Medicine?

Regenerative medicine is a very broad term that is perhaps misleading for much of the work that is done in the field. Regenerative medicine includes both the idea of regenerating tissue, that is, repairing or making new tissue in the true sense of the word, and also other means of renewing tissue through immune modulation. Although stem cells are probably the most well-known of the regenerative therapies and are the focus of this article, many other therapies are included in regenerative medicine. These therapies are sometimes combined, making study details particularly important in this field.

What Are Stem Cells?

Found in all multicellular organisms, stem cells are cells that are able to differentiate into specialized cells and self-renew, that is, make more of themselves. Stem cells come in several types, which are differentiated by source, how they are derived, and their potency (**Fig. 1**).

The 3 main types of stem cells are embryonic stem cells (ESC), induced pluripotent stem cells, and adult stem cells. ESC are derived from the inner cell mass of preimplantation stage embryos and have been the subject of significant controversy. They are pluripotent, which means they can differentiate into all adult cell types, but cannot make a new embryo. Induced pluripotent stem cells are also pluripotent, but they are derived from adult tissues such as skin fibroblasts using viral vectors or other methods of gene transfer and are therefore less controversial than ESC. Finally, adult or tissue-derived stem cells are derived from many different tissue types from placenta to adipose tissue to teeth.

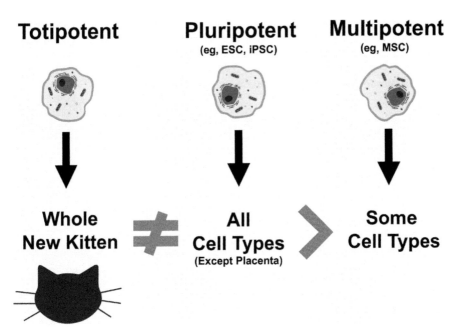

Fig. 1. Examples of stem cell potency. Cell potency is a measure of the differentiation capacity of a cell. Totipotent cells are very early stage cells (eg, zygote) and the most potent as they are capable of making both the embryo and placenta. Pluripotent cells (eg, ESC), are derived from the inner cell mass of the blastocyst and therefore can generally make all cells of the embryo. Cell potency continues to decrease through multipotent cells (eg, MSC), which can make several cell types, through oligopotent, unipotent, and finally to a nullipotent cell, which is a terminally differentiated cell. In recent years, techniques have been developed to transform cells with decreased potency into pluripotent cells (eg, induced pluripotent cells [iPSC]).

Adult stem cells are multipotent and have more limited self-renewal capacity than ESC and induced pluripotent stem cells. They can be found in almost all adult tissues, remaining in specialized niches to contribute to tissue repair during the animal's life. Adult stem cells include hematopoietic stem cells (HSC) and mesenchymal stem cells (MSC). HSC are derived mainly from bone marrow, produce all cells in the blood, and are the cells used in bone marrow transplantation. Until recently, HSC were thought to be the only functional stem cells in adult animals.[4]

MSC have been studied since the 1970s, but interest in their use has accelerated in recent years owing to discovery of their immunomodulatory and trophic abilities.[4] Although MSC can differentiate into cell types of mesenchymal lineage, they are also able to affect the activity of many cells in the immune system. Owing to their potent immunosuppressive abilities, they are immune evasive and can be used allogenically or even xenogenically, that is, in another species than the donor.[4] Additionally, MSC have been found to have paracrine effects and the ability to home to areas of inflammation and injury, where they have trophic capabilities, supporting tissue repair through inhibition of fibrosis and apoptosis and stimulation of tissue-specific stem cell mitosis and revascularization.[4] Of note, MSC are sometimes called mesenchymal stromal cells, multipotent stromal cells, or even medicinal signaling cells in an attempt to better describe their biology and function.

Feline MSC were first mentioned in the literature in 2002.[5] Although research has been done in the pluripotent cells types, most of the clinical work in cats has been in MSC, which are the focus of the rest of this article.

How Are Mesenchymal Stem Cells Harvested or Acquired?

As mentioned, MSC can be found in almost any tissue of the body. The tissue from which MSC are derived, however, may influence MSC properties. Many details involved in MSC collection and use can impact their eventual number and function (**Box 1**).[6] Donor characteristics and disease status are of particular importance both to prevent disease transmission and because they can significantly affect cell growth and/or function as has been found with age and feline foamy virus infection in cats.[7,8] Owing to the high number of variables influencing MSC properties, transparency in reporting specific study details is necessary for accurate comparisons between studies. Once understood, these variables can be used to optimize MSC treatment efficacy and safety.

MSC can be harvested in many ways. They can be derived from peripheral blood samples, bone marrow aspirates, lipoaspiration, surgical resection or biopsy, or simple tissue collection in the case of placenta or cord blood. Some tissues, such as bone marrow and adipose tissue, are easy to obtain, nonessential in small quantities, accessible, and contain large numbers of MSC and therefore are used most commonly. The samples then must undergo some form of processing to collect or

---

Box 1
Examples of factors influencing MSC function

Species

Donor characteristics

Donor disease status

Tissue type

Tissue location

Tissue collection methods

Tissue processing methods

Media composition

Culture methods

Cell characteristics

Cell storage methods

Suspending agents

Cell transportation details

Injection protocol

Injection route

Timing of injection(s)

Cell dose

Recipient characteristics

Recipient disease type and status

release the MSC (**Fig. 2**). In many cases, this process involves washing of the tissues and then blunt tissue dissection and chemical lysis or digestion followed by centrifugation to separate the MSC from the other tissue components. In the case of adipose tissue, the resultant cell pellet is called the stromal vascular fraction (SVF). The SVF contains a small number of MSC and several other components, including preadipocytes, endothelial cells, pericytes, immune cells, smooth muscle cells, and fibroblasts.[9] SVF is sometimes used directly as an autologous regenerative therapy and may be called stem cell therapy, although it is technically different than culture-expanded MSC.

For MSC selection and expansion, the blood or SVF is plated into plastic flasks in specific media and maintained in incubators. MSC are plastic adherent, so other cells are washed away in the culture process through repeated media changes. Cell expansion takes several days to weeks, and the characteristics of the cells are monitored closely for appropriate morphology, growth, and signs of contamination. Cells are passaged, or chemically removed from the flasks, and placed into a larger surface area to allow continued expansion of MSC numbers. MSC that become too confluent or are from a higher passage number can lose their function, become senescent, and stop dividing.

The culture conditions and media components used can significantly impact the resultant MSC type, number, and function. Varying the culture conditions or media components can be used to purposefully program cells for specific functions. Cells from different species can have different morphology, growth characteristics, and require different cell culture techniques for optimal growth.

Once MSC have been expanded, they are tested to ensure they are the desired cell type and safe for clinical use. MSC are defined by their plastic adherence and spindle-shaped morphology (**Fig. 3**). Although there are no specific cell markers to determine that a cell is an MSC, the cells are stained to look for presence and absence of several surface markers called clusters of differentiation that are consistent with an MSC. Additionally, the cells are exposed to several factors to induce differentiation of the cells into bone, cartilage, and fat. As MSC cultures are heterogeneous, not all cells will express the surface markers or undergo trilineage differentiation.

Before injection, the MSC should be tested for viability and presence of bacterial contamination. In the case of allogeneic use, the tissue donor should be tested for the presence of infectious disease. Although not yet standardized in the field, functional testing should be considered. MSC function can be determined by measuring their immunosuppressive capabilities and by measuring the secretome or bioactive factors secreted by the cells.

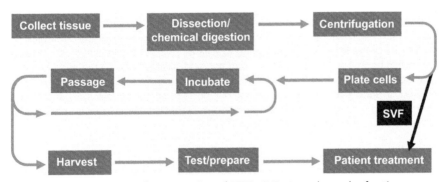

Fig. 2. General process map for generation of MSCs. SVF, stromal vascular fraction.

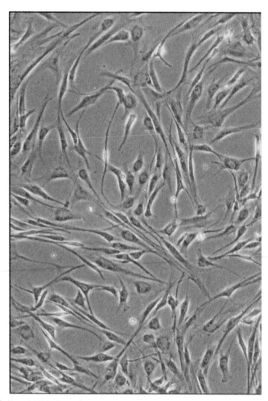

Fig. 3. Photo of feline MSCs in culture.

HOW ARE MESENCHYMAL STEM CELLS USED?

Once the MSC are obtained and tested, they have to be administered to the recipient. MSC have been administered by both systemic and local routes, often depending on the desired outcome of the therapy. For example, immunomodulatory effects may be obtained by systemic delivery in some diseases and local tissue engraftment may not be necessary. Intravenous (IV) delivery, however, is known to lead to pulmonary trapping of the cells, which may or may not ultimately impact therapeutic outcomes.[10] In localized disease or injury or areas in which new tissue growth is desired, the delivery of cells to the specific area may be ideal.

In addition to the route, other methods have been found to impact cell availability and function as well as safety. For example, cryopreservation of cells enables the availability of treatments without having to wait for cell culture. However, cryopreservation has been found to affect MSC function and safety in some studies.[11] The relevance of cryopreservation techniques and MSC therapeutic outcomes continues to be studied. In fact, every detail including, but not limited to, needle size, suspending agent, speed of injection, and incorporation of biomaterials may play a role in safety and efficacy of the delivered MSC (see **Box 1**).

Clinical Applications

Before discussing clinical application of feline stem cells, the current regulatory landscape must be considered. As mentioned in the Introduction, stem cells are categorized as drugs by the US FDA. Because no FDA-approved veterinary stem cell product currently exists, in most circumstances stem cells can only be used in client-owned animals with an investigational exemption under very specific conditions.[1,2] A cell-based therapy for horses was recently approved for use in the European Union, and hopefully other products will be available for clinical use in the not too distant future.

As a therapeutic option, MSC have much to offer feline medicine. Cats have many diseases for which new therapies are needed, and they develop deleterious side effects to many current medications. Additionally, the potential for single or intermittent treatment options would allow improved compliance in cats that resist therapeutic interventions. However, to date, there have been fewer than 10 clinical trials published evaluating MSC use in less than 100 feline patients with naturally occurring disease (**Table 1**). These trials have evaluated MSC in diseases for which there is currently no acceptable or definitive treatment, including chronic kidney disease (CKD), chronic enteropathy, focal chronic gingivostomatitis (FCGS), and feline eosinophilic keratitis (FEK).

Chronic kidney disease

Five publications describing 7 clinical trials using MSC in cats have been for CKD. CKD affects a significant number of cats, and there is no current definitive treatment aside from renal transplantation. The ability of MSC to differentiate into renal tubular epithelium and secrete bioactive substances that have anti-inflammatory, angiogenic, anti-apoptotic, and antifibrotic properties make them promising options for treatment of CKD, and positive results have been obtained in experimental models of disease.[12,13] The significance of naturally occurring disease models and potential species-specific differences are highlighted by the positive changes seen in induced renal disease in rodents treated with MSC compared with the comparative lack of efficacy seen in feline studies thus far.

The first 3 publications on the use of MSC in cats with CKD describe 5 clinical trials that were performed by the same research group, hereafter numbered study 1 through study 5 for clarity. The initial study (study 1), published in 2011, was the first publication looking at MSC treatment in clinical cats.[14] This study investigated a single, ultrasound-guided intrarenal injection of autologous bone marrow- or adipose-derived MSC (Ad-MSC). The authors noted that feline Ad-MSC were much easier to generate from the study cats then bone marrow-derived MSC. Dose escalation was used owing to a lack of available safety information. Six cats were enrolled in the study: 2 healthy controls and 4 CKD-affected cats. Over the 2-month study period, the only adverse event noted was transient microscopic hematuria in 1 healthy cat, but the study protocol was challenging on the cats. Two of the CKD-affected cats showed possible improvement in glomerular filtration rate and serum creatinine, but these changes were small and not statistically significant.

Studies 2 through 4, published together in 2013, built on the information gained from the 2011 study as well as additional information from rodent models showing improvement with multiple stem cell doses.[15,16] These pilot studies evaluated 3 IV injections of MSC suspended in saline and heparin given once every 2 weeks with variable doses and cell preparations. Study 2 included 6 cats that received 2×10^6 allogeneic, cryopreserved Ad-MSC. In this manner, clinically affected animals did not have to undergo a procedure for adipose tissue collection as tissue was collected from healthy, specific pathogen-free cats. Additionally, cryopreservation of the cells allowed easy scheduling for patients. Study 3 included 5 cats that received twice the dose of allogeneic, cryopreserved Ad-MSC. These cats developed self-limiting clinical signs associated

Table 1
List of published clinical trials using feline MSC

Disease	Cell Type	Storage	MSC Dose	Vehicle	Route	Treatment No./ Time Between	Animal No. (MSC Treated)	Control Group	Adverse Events	Outcome Summary	Study Length	Reference
CKD	Autologous BM-MSC or Ad-MSC	Fresh	$1-4 \times 10^6$ (dose escalation)	PBS	Intrarenal	1/n/a	4	n/a	None	Possible mild improvement in creatinine and GFR; demanding protocol	$\geq$2 mo	Quimby et al,[14] 2011
CKD	Allogeneic Ad-MSC	Cryo-preserved	2×10^6	HBSS + heparin	IV	3/14 d	6	n/a	None	Mildly decreased creatinine	2 mo	Quimby et al,[15] 2013
	Allogeneic Ad-MSC	Cryo-preserved	4×10^6	HBSS + heparin	IV	3/14 d	5	n/a	Vomiting (n = 2) and increased respiratory rate and effort (n = 4) with 1st injection and (n = 1) with third injection	No difference in renal parameters	2 mo	

CKD	Allogeneic Ad-MSC	Fresh	4×10^6	DPBS + heparin	IV	3/14 d	5	n/a	None	No difference in renal parameters	2 mo	Quimby et al,[17] 2015
CKD	Allogeneic Ad-MSC	Fresh	2×10^6/kg BW	DPBS + heparin	IV	3/14 d	6	Yes (crossover)	None	No difference in renal parameters	2 mo	
CKD	Allogeneic amniotic membrane-derived MSC	Fresh (re-cultured)	2×10^6	0.9% NaCl	IV	2/21 d	9	n/a	Vomiting (n = 1)	Mildly decreased creatinine	2 mo	Vidane et al,[18] 2017
CKD	Autologous SVF	First fresh, second cryo-preserved	Unknown (TNCC = 1.5–5.7 $\times 10^6$)	PBS	Intra-arterial	2/14 d	5	n/a	Bruising/discomfort harvest site (n = 1), Horners syndrome (n = 1)	Safe but challenging protocol; mildly increased creatinine in 3 cats	3 mo	Thomson et al,[19] 2019
Chronic enteropathy	Allogeneic Ad-MSC	Fresh	2×10^6/kg BW	DPBS + heparin	IV	2/14 d	10	Yes	None	88.9% showed improvement from modest to complete resolution of clinical signs	3 mo	Webb and Webb,[28] 2015

(continued on next page)

Table 1
(continued)

Disease	Cell Type	Storage	MSC Dose	Vehicle	Route	Treatment No./ Time Between	Animal No. (MSC Treated)	Control Group	Adverse Events	Outcome Summary	Study Length	Reference
Chronic gingivo-stomatitis	Autologous Ad-MSC	Fresh (re-cultured)	2×10^7 + pretreatment diphenhydramine	Unknown	IV	2/30 d	7	n/a	Immediate, self-limiting transfusion reaction (n = 2)	71.4% response rate; no recurrence	≥6 mo	Arzi et al,[24] 2016
Chronic gingivo-stomatitis	Allogeneic Ad-MSC	Fresh (re-cultured)	2×10^7	Unknown	IV	2/30 d	7	n/a	None	57% response rate by 20 mo; no recurrence	≥6 mo	Arzi et al,[25] 2017
Eosinophilic keratitis	Allogeneic Ad-MSC	Cryo-preserved	2×10^6	DMEM	Subconjunctival	2/60 d	5	n/a	None	100% response rate by 6 mo; no recurrence	11 mo	Villatoro et al,[31] 2018

Abbreviations: BM-MSC, bone marrow-derived MSC; DMEM, Dulbecco's Modified Eagle Medium; DPBS, Dulbecco's phosphate-buffered saline; GFR, glomerular filtration rate; HBSS, Hank's balanced salt solution; IV, intravenously; PBS, phosphate-buffered saline.

Data from Refs.[14,15,17–19,24,25,28,31]

with the injections, including increased respiratory rate and effort (n = 4) and vomiting (n = 2). Study 4 enrolled 5 cats who were treated with 4×10^6 allogeneic, fresh Ad-MSC. None of the cats treated with fresh cells developed any adverse events. Unfortunately, none of the cats in studies 2, 3, or 4 had any discernible clinically relevant improvement in measures of renal function. Cats in study 2 had a statistically significant decrease in serum creatinine, but the change (<0.5 mg/dL; <44.21 μmol/L) was deemed of questionable clinical significance by the study authors.

In 2016, the same group published a randomized, placebo-controlled, blinded cross-over study in cats with CKD.[17] In this study (study 5), 4 cats received the same 3 injection protocol with a higher dose (2×10^6 MSC/kg body weight) of MSC; 2 cats crossed over from the placebo group and also received MSC. No adverse events were noted, but, as before, no significant changes in renal function were noted by study end. Similar to the previous studies, cats in this study were followed for 2 months.

The following year, Vidane and colleagues[18] published a study evaluating allogeneic combined amniotic membrane-derived MSC in cats with CKD. Nine cats received 2 IV doses of 2×10^6 fresh, recultured MSC in saline 21 days apart. Owners reported that the cats showed improved welfare, food intake, and social interaction, although no specific data were provided, no control group was included to rule out placebo effect, and weight did not change during the 8-week study period. Serum creatinine decreased significantly by study end from 2.43 to 2.1 mg/dL, a change of 0.33 mg/dL (29.18 μmol/L). Again, the clinical relevance of a less than 0.5 mg/dL (44.21 μmol/L) change in creatinine is uncertain.[15] No other renal function parameters changed significantly during the 2-month study. The only adverse event reported was vomiting by 1 cat during the MSC injection.

The final study investigating MSC therapy for feline CKD was published in 2019 by Thomson and colleagues.[19] Five cats with stage III International Renal Interest Society kidney disease were treated with 2 intra-arterial renal infusions of autologous SVF 2 weeks apart. The number of MSC in the SVF is unknown, because only the total nucleated cell count was reported. Based on the literature, the percentage of stromal progenitor cells in human SVF may be a small, and SVF contains many other cell types.[9,20] The first SVF dose was fresh and the second was cryopreserved. Additionally, the cell count for the 2 doses varied. Adverse events included temporary bruising and discomfort at tissue harvest site (n = 1) and development of Horner's syndrome after carotid arterial catheterization (n = 1), which resolved in 3 days. At the 3-month study end, the serum creatinine was noted to increase in 3 cats with a median change of +0.5 mg/dL (44.21 μmol/L). No control group was included to compare outcomes, and the study was not powered to determine efficacy. The authors noted that the technique is feasible, but technically challenging. A phase II study is stated to be underway to determine treatment efficacy.

Thus far, these varied studies have investigated use of MSC in 40 cats with CKD and have shown relatively disappointing results despite promise demonstrated in experimental models.[12,13,16] Certainly, chronic, naturally occurring disease varies significantly from induced models of disease in rodents, possibly contributing to the different outcomes. Although similar in many ways, MSC from different species are known to have differences.[6,21] Additionally, none of the study periods extended past 3 months, and more recent MSC trials using allogeneic cells in cats with other chronic diseases required up to 20 months for efficacy to be noted.[22–25] Larger studies with inclusion of control groups and longer follow-up are needed to determine the efficacy of MSC in feline CKD. Techniques to preactivate MSC, use of MSC-derived extracellular vesicles, alternate delivery techniques, as well as the development and use of new methods to diagnose and monitor disease may help optimize MSC therapy and improve outcomes in feline CKD.

Chronic enteropathy and inflammatory bowel disease

Interestingly, the first indications that stem cell therapy could be useful in inflammatory bowel disease (IBD) were incidental findings. Reports from the early 1990s from human patients with IBD that received hematopoietic stem cell transplants for other indications noted that their IBD went into long-term remission.[26] Although often successful, hematopoietic stem cell transplants are a substantial undertaking requiring conditioning chemotherapy. Once the significant immunosuppressive properties of MSC were identified through application in graft-versus-host disease, their application to other inflammatory, and autoimmune disorders such as IBD was investigated.

IBD causes significant morbidity in affected individuals, and an increasing prevalence of IBD has been noted in humans. In affected people and animals, long-term immunosuppressive medications are required to decrease symptoms, and many individuals are refractory to treatment. In 2005, an initial study investigating the use of autologous Ad-MSC for refractory fistulating Crohn's disease showed a 75% response rate.[27] Since then, additional studies have been performed investigating MSC therapy for IBD. In 2018, darvadstrocel (Alofisel) became the first allogeneic stem cell therapy to receive approval in Europe, which is for treatment of refractory perianal fistulas secondary to Crohn's disease in humans.

After the success seen in rodent and human literature, a proof-of-concept study evaluating MSC in cats with chronic enteropathy was conducted and published in 2015.[28] The study was randomized and placebo controlled, with the owners blinded to treatment. Seven cats received 2 allogeneic IV infusions of 2×10^6 fresh-cultured Ad-MSC/kg body weight suspended in saline and heparin given 14 days apart. Three of the control cats crossed over and also received MSC in a nonblinded fashion. There were no adverse events, and 5 of the 7 initial MSC-treated cats had significant improvement or complete resolution of clinical signs according to the owners with the 2 remaining cats showing modest but persistent improvement. Of the 3 crossover cats, the owners reported that 1 showed marked improvement, 1 reported no change, and 1 was lost to follow-up. The cats were followed for 2 to 3 months with no recurrence of symptoms noted. Interestingly, routine sections of the intestine obtained at necropsy from 1 of the MSC-treated cats with biopsy-confirmed IBD did not have histologic evidence of significant IBD identified. Owing to the positive pilot study results, a follow-up study is in progress in cats with confirmed IBD comparing MSC treatment to standard prednisolone therapy.

Chronic gingivostomatitis

FCGS is a severe, chronic inflammatory disease affecting the gingiva and mucosa of unknown etiology (see Da Bin Lee DVM and Colleagues' article, "An Update on Feline Chronic Gingivostomatitis," in this issue). The cause is likely multifactorial and arises from an inappropriate immune response to oral antigenic stimulation.[29] Treatment generally involves dental extractions and immunosuppressive therapy, although a significant number of cats remain refractory to treatment. Clinical signs include severe oral pain, dysphagia, and secondary effects of these issues and can dramatically affect quality of life.[29]

Thus far, 2 studies have been published by Arzi and colleagues[24] evaluating the potential for MSC to treat refractory FCGS. The first study evaluated the use of autologous Ad-MSC in cats with FCGS. Seven cats were pretreated with diphenhydramine before receiving 2 relatively high doses of (2×10^7) fresh cultured Ad-MSC IV 1 month apart. Two cats developed immediate transfusion reactions characterized by short-term, self-limiting tachypnea, urination, vomiting, and apathy. Although 2 cats did not respond to MSC therapy, 5 of the 7 cats (71.4%) showed complete remission or marked improvement. Clinical response took up to 4 months and was correlated with a lower pretreatment percentage of a subset of CD8 lymphocytes and higher levels of IL-6 after treatment. Although outside the normal clinical diagnostics, these findings provide both a means of identifying cats that will best respond to MSC therapy and evidence of mechanism of action of MSC in FCGS.

In the second study, allogeneic, fresh-cultured Ad-MSC were administered to a similar population of 7 cats.[25] The cats received the same dose of cells IV twice, 1 month apart. No adverse events were noted. 4 of the 7 cats (57%) showed complete remission or marked improvement. The response was delayed compared with the cats who received autologous cells, taking up to 20 months to induce a stable response. Interestingly, changes in CD8 cells and IL-6 were not associated with clinical response to MSC treatment as was seen in the cats treated with autologous cells, and the authors proposed that allogeneic cells may work through an alternate mechanism. The nonresponders were noted to have more significant inflammation than the responders, prompting speculation that treatment earlier in the disease process may be beneficial. Although no control group was included in either study, spontaneous resolution of FCGS has not been reported.[24] As with IBD, the promising results with MSC therapy in these initial cases of refractory FCGS are being investigated further and will hopefully lead to improved disease understanding and additional treatment options for affected cats.

Feline eosinophilic keratitis

FEK is a chronic, progressive inflammatory disease affecting the cornea and/or conjunctiva in cats.[30] FEK is suspected to be caused by an immune-mediated response to an unknown antigenic stimulus. Many, but not all, of the affected cats are polymerase chain reaction positive for feline herpes virus-1.[30] Diagnosis involves the presence of characteristic raised, vascularized corneal mass with gritty plaques on the corneal surface, and cytologic evidence of corneal eosinophils with or without mast cells (**Fig. 4**). Corneal ulceration is found in approximately 25% of the cases.[30] Treatment involves intensive and long-term antibiotics, corticosteroids, and immunosuppressive therapy. Recurrence, side effects, and refractory cases are common. FEK can be

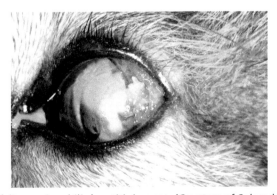

Fig. 4. Photo of feline eosinophilic keratitis in a cat. (*Courtesy of* Colorado State University Comparative Opthalmology, Fort Collins, CO.)

painful and lead to vision loss through associated infection and progressive corneal scar tissue formation.[30]

A study was published recently investigating the use of MSC for FEK.[31] Five cats with refractory, unilateral FEK received 2 injections of 2×10^6 allogeneic, early passage, cryopreserved Ad-MSCs subconjunctivally 2 months apart. Cells were derived from a single, female specific pathogen-free cat. No adverse events were noted, and all cats showed complete remission at 6 months that was stable through the 11-month study period. The treated cats did not receive any immunomodulatory or anti-inflammatory medication for 2 weeks before study enrollment and through study completion. A control group was not included, but spontaneous resolution of FEK has never been reported.[30]

The results of this study show the potential of local application of MSC in refractory, inflammatory disease. Although only a small number of patients were enrolled, all of the treated cats showed sustained resolution of signs with no obvious side effects after receiving the allogeneic, cryopreserved cells. The fact that 2 local injections given 2 months apart resulted in long-term clinical response for a disease that generally requires long-term therapy with immunosuppressive medications, sometimes multiple times a day, is very intriguing. Similar to the FCGS studies, signs took several months to completely resolve in some cases.

Allergic asthma

Although use of MSC in allergic asthma has only been investigated in cats with experimentally induced disease thus far, the results are intriguing and briefly presented. Allergic asthma is an inflammatory disease of the airway affecting many animal species, including cats. Many affected animals require life-long immunosuppressive medications to decrease clinical signs, and severe respiratory distress can still occur, necessitating emergency treatment. Investigation of MSC therapy in mice with allergen-induced airway inflammation has shown significant improvement.[32]

A 2014 study followed 5 cats with experimentally induced asthma for 1 year after receiving 6 IV infusions of cryopreserved, allogeneic Ad-MSC (between 3.64×10^6 and 2.5×10^7) administered every 14 days.[22] Unlike the rodent studies, no differences were noted in airway eosinophilia and airway hyper-responsiveness between MSC-treated and untreated cats. However, measures of airway remodeling, that is, lung attenuation and bronchial wall thickening, were lower in MSC-treated cats compared with untreated controls 6 months after the last MSC treatment. These differences were not sustained at study end (month 12).

A second study by the same group evaluated the efficacy of serially administered allogeneic, cryopreserved Ad-MSC in cats with induced allergic asthma.[23] Four cats were given a total of 5 IV injections of MSC, from 2×10^6 to 1×10^7 cells per injection over a more variable time frame. Eosinophil number returned to normal and airway hyperresponsiveness was decreased in MSC-treated cats but not until study day 133. At 9 months, lung attenuation and bronchial wall thickening scores were significantly decreased with MSC treatment compared with untreated cats.

These studies in allergic airway disease demonstrate several important concepts. First, they show the safety of multiple IV injections of allogeneic MSC. The cats in these studies received up to 6 injections of allogeneic, cryopreserved MSC, at least twice as many as in other published studies. One cat in the 2 studies was noted to develop a scrotal sarcoma 1 month after study completion; however, the relationship to MSC treatment is unknown. Second, the studies again demonstrate potential differences in models of disease in larger animals versus rodents. Finally, the studies further emphasize the importance of long-term follow-up in feline MSC studies to determine safety and efficacy as well as potential optimization strategies such as dosing intervals.

SUMMARY

Regenerative medicine is a complex field of research, with much hope that regenerative therapies such as stem cells may provide new treatment options for many frustrating disease processes. Further study is needed in many areas of stem cell biology including, but not limited to, evaluation of mechanisms of action, donor characteristics, cell culture conditions, and dosing and delivery methods, which may differ between diseases. Advances in biomaterials for cell differentiation and delivery, 3-dimensional cultures and bioreactors, preconditioning strategies, gene therapy, and extracellular vesicle biology hold promise for improved outcomes in stem cell therapies. However, species-specific differences in MSC function and disease characteristics may mean that work done in other species may not be applicable to cell therapy in cats.

MSC therapy shows significant promise in inflammatory feline diseases such as chronic gingivostomatitis, FEK, and chronic enteropathy. Although some immediate reactions have been noted, thus far there have been no proven long-term side effects reported in the literature for MSC therapy in cats. However, there are only a few available studies, most of which are small, proof-of-concept evaluations using variable strategies.

It is worth noting that several studies report positive owner evaluations of their cats after receiving MSC, often regardless of evidence of target disease improvement. Although the placebo effect likely plays a large role in cases where the owner is not blinded to treatment, it is also possible that the MSC are helping with other common, concurrent conditions, such as osteoarthritis.[33] High-quality, controlled, studies with larger patient numbers and long-term follow-up are needed to truly evaluate the safety and efficacy of feline MSC for disease applications. Continued research will hopefully help to determine the true potential of MSC therapy in feline medicine and lead to development of safe and effective products for clinical use in cats.

ACKNOWLEDGMENTS

The author thanks Maddi Funk for her artistic help with figure creation.

DISCLOSURE

The author has nothing to disclose.

REFERENCES

1. U.S. Department of Health and Human Services Food and Drug Administration Center for Veterinary medicine guidance for industry #218: cell-based products for animal use. 2015. Available at: https://www.fda.gov/media/88925/download. Accessed October 1, 2019.
2. American Veterinary Medical Association policy on therapeutic use of stem cells and regenerative medicine. 2017. Available at: https://www.avma.org/KB/Policies/Pages/Therapeutic-Use-of-Stem-Cells-and-Regenerative-Medicine.aspx. Accessed October 1, 2019.
3. Public Law 103-396: Animal Medicinal Drug Use Clarification Act of 1994.
4. Caplan AI. Are all adult stem cells the same? Regen Eng Transl Med 2015;1:4.

5. Martin DR, Cox NR, Hathcock TL, et al. Isolation and characterization of multipotent mesenchymal stem cells from feline bone marrow. Exp Hematol 2002;30:879.

6. Uder C, Bruckner S, Winkler S, et al. Mammalian MSC from selected species: features and applications. Cytometry A 2018;93(1):32.

7. Zalic LB, Webb TL, Webb P, et al. Comparison of proliferative and immunomodulatory potential of adipose-derived mesenchymal stem cells from young and geriatric cats. J Feline Med Surg 2017;19(10):1096.

8. Arzi B, Kol A, Murphy B, et al. Feline foamy virus adversely affects feline mesenchymal stem cell culture and expansion: implications for animal model development. Stem Cells Dev 2015;24(7):814.

9. Han S, Sun HM, Hwang KC, et al. Adipose-derived stromal vascular fraction cells: update on clinical utility and efficacy. Crit Rev Eukaryot Gene Expr 2015; 25(2):145.

10. Eggenhofer E, Benseler V, Kroemer A, et al. Mesenchymal stem cells are short-lived and do not migrate beyond the lungs after intravenous infusion. Front Immunol 2002;3:297.

11. Moll G, Geißler S, Catar R, et al. Cryopreserved or fresh mesenchymal stromal cells: only a matter of taste or key to unleash the full clinical potential of MSC therapy? Adv Exp Med Biol 2016;951:77.

12. Fang Y, Tian X, Bai S, et al. Autologous transplantation of adipose-derived mesenchymal stem cells ameliorates streptozotocin-induced diabetic nephropathy in rats by inhibiting oxidative stress, pro-inflammatory cytokines and the p38 MAPK signaling pathway. Int J Mol Med 2012;30:85.

13. Ezquer F, Giraud-Billoud M, Carpio D, et al. Proregenerative microenvironment triggered by donor mesenchymal stem cells preserves renal function and structure in mice with severe diabetes mellitus. Biomed Res Int 2015;2015:164703.

14. Quimby JM, Webb TL, Gibbons DS, et al. Evaluation of intrarenal mesenchymal stem cell injection for treatment of chronic kidney disease in cats. J Feline Med Surg 2011;13(6):418.

15. Quimby JM, Webb TL, Habernicht L, et al. Safety and efficacy of intravenous infusion of allogeneic cryopreserved mesenchymal stem cells for treatment of chronic kidney disease in cats: results of three sequential pilot studies. Stem Cell Res Ther 2013;4(2):48.

16. Semedo P, Corea-Costa M, Antonio Cenedeze M, et al. Mesenchymal stem cells attenuate renal fibrosis through immune modulation and remodeling properties in a rat remnant kidney model. Stem Cells 2009;27:3063.

17. Quimby JM, Webb TL, Randall E, et al. Assessment of intravenous adipose-derived allogeneic mesenchymal stem cells for the treatment of feline chronic kidney disease: a randomized, placebo-controlled clinical trial in 8 cats. J Feline Med Surg 2015;8(2):165.

18. Vidane AS, Pinheiro AO, Casals JB, et al. Transplantation of amniotic membrane-derived multipotent cells ameliorates and delays the progression of chronic kidney disease in cats. Reprod Domest Anim 2017;52(Suppl 2):316.

19. Thomson AL, Berent AC, Weisse C, et al. Intra-arterial renal infusion of autologous mesenchymal stem cells for treatment of chronic kidney disease in cats: phase 1 clinical trial. J Vet Intern Med 2019;33(3):1353.

20. Bourin P, Bunnell BA, Casteilla L, et al. Stromal cells from the adipose tissue-derived stromal vascular fraction and culture expanded adipose tissue-derived stromal/stem cells: a joint statement of the International Federation for Adipose Therapeutics (IFATS) and Science and the International Society for Cellular Therapy (ISCT). Cytotherapy 2013;15(6):641.

21. Carrade DD, Borjesson DL. Immunomodulation by mesenchymal stem cells in veterinary species. Comp Med 2013;63(3):207.
22. Trzil JE, Masseau I, Webb TL, et al. Long term evaluation of mesenchymal stem cell therapy in a feline model of chronic allergic asthma. Clin Exp Allergy 2014; 44(12):1546.
23. Trzil JE, Masseau I, Webb TL, et al. Intravenous adipose-derived mesenchymal stem cell therapy for the treatment of feline asthma: a pilot study. J Feline Med Surg 2015;18(12):981.
24. Arzi B, Mills-Ko E, Verstraete FJ, et al. Therapeutic efficacy of fresh, autologous mesenchymal stem cells for severe refractory gingivostomatitis in cats. Stem Cells Transl Med 2016;5(1):75.
25. Arzi B, Clark KC, Sundaram A, et al. Therapeutic efficacy of fresh, allogeneic mesenchymal stem cells for severe refractory feline chronic gingivostomatitis. Stem Cells Transl Med 2017;6(8):1710.
26. Duijvestein M, van den Brink GR, Hommes DW. Stem cells as potential novel therapeutic strategy for inflammatory bowel disease. J Crohns Colitis 2008;2(2):99.
27. Garcia-Olmo D, Garcia-Arranz M, Herreros D, et al. A phase I clinical trial of the treatment of Crohn's fistula by adipose mesenchymal stem cell transplantation. Dis Colon Rectum 2005;48:1416.
28. Webb TL, Webb CB. Stem cell therapy in cats with chronic enteropathy: a proof-of-concept study. J Feline Med Surg 2015;17(10):901.
29. Winer JN, Arzi B, Verstraete FJM. Therapeutic management of feline chronic gingivostomatitis: a systematic review of the literature. Front Vet Sci 2016;3:54.
30. Spiess AK, Sapienza JS, Mayordomo A. Treatment of proliferative feline eosinophilic keratitis with topical 1.5% cyclosporine: 35 cases. Vet Opthalmol 2009; 12(2):132.
31. Villatoro AJ, Claros S, Fernandez V, et al. Safety and efficacy of the mesenchymal stem cell in feline eosinophilic keratitis treatment. BMC Vet Res 2018;14(1):116.
32. Takeda K, Webb TL, Ning F, et al. Mesenchymal stem cells recruit CCR2+ monocytes to suppress allergic airway inflammation. J Immunol 2018;200(4):1261.
33. Marino CL, Lascelles BD, Vaden SL, et al. Prevalence and classification of chronic kidney disease in cats randomly selected from four age groups and in cats recruited for degenerative joint disease studies. J Feline Med Surg 2014; 16(6):465.

An Update on Feline Chronic Gingivostomatitis

Da Bin Lee, DVM[a], Frank J.M. Verstraete, DrMedVet, MMedVet[a,b], Boaz Arzi, DVM[b,*]

KEYWORDS

- Feline • Gingivostomatitis • Surgical therapy • Medical therapy • Oral mucosa
- Inflammation

KEY POINTS

- Feline chronic gingivostomatitis seems to be a manifestation of an aberrant immune response to chronic antigenic stimulation.
- Multicat environments play an important role and are associated with this multifactorial disease.
- The current standard of care involves dental extractions of at least all premolar and molar teeth, with or without medical management, rather than medical therapy alone.
- Future regenerative therapies, currently in development, show promise for management of feline chronic gingivostomatitis.

INTRODUCTION

Feline chronic gingivostomatitis (FCGS) is a severe, immune-mediated, oral mucosal inflammatory disease of cats. The typical location of the ulcerative and/or proliferative inflammatory lesions is lateral to the palatoglossal folds, previously referred to as the fauces.[1–3] Clinically, a proliferative and ulcerative phenotype of the disease can be observed (**Fig. 1**). Occasionally, the proliferative form of the disease is so severe as to prevent retraction of the tongue (**Fig. 2**). Although FCGS is a familiar condition encountered in veterinary practice, with a reported prevalence ranging from 0.7% to 12.0%,[4–6] there is much confusion regarding the cause and subsequent treatment of the disease.[6,7] This article reviews the current knowledge on the etiopathogenesis of FCGS and describes the leading treatment modalities.

ETIOPATHOGENESIS

The cause of FCGS remains elusive despite extensive investigations. A multitude of conditions and infectious agents have been implicated without proof of causation,

[a] Dentistry and Oral Surgery Service, William R. Pritchard Veterinary Medical Teaching Hospital, University of California - Davis, 1 Garrod Drive, Davis, CA 95616, USA; [b] Department of Surgical and Radiological Sciences, School of Veterinary Medicine, University of California - Davis, 1 Garrod Drive, Davis, CA 95616, USA
* Corresponding author.
E-mail address: barzi@ucdavis.edu

Vet Clin Small Anim 50 (2020) 973–982
https://doi.org/10.1016/j.cvsm.2020.04.002
0195-5616/20/© 2020 Elsevier Inc. All rights reserved.

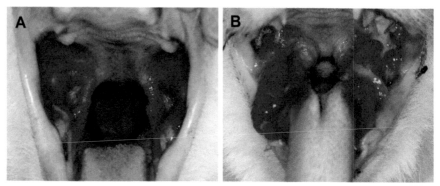

Fig. 1. The hallmark of FCGS is inflammation in the caudal oral cavity in the area lateral to the palatoglossal folds. Ulcerative (*A*) and proliferative (*B*) phenotypes can be observed.

including infectious pathogens such as feline calicivirus (FCV), feline herpesvirus (FHV-1), feline immunodeficiency virus (FIV), feline leukemia virus (FeLV), and various bacteria, as well as noninfectious factors such as dental disease, environmental stress, and hypersensitivity.[8–23] Little or no new information has been forthcoming in this regard.

Systemic and Local Consequences of Feline Chronic Gingivostomatitis

The chronic inflammatory nature of the disease is suggested by the predominant presence of lymphocytes and plasma cells in affected oral tissues, with fewer neutrophils, Mott cells, and mast cells.[24,25] Immunohistochemical staining has revealed the infiltration of cluster of differentiation (CD) 3+ T lymphocytes within the epithelium and subepithelial stroma, and restriction of CD20+ B lymphocytes mainly to the subepithelial stroma (**Fig. 3**).[26,27]

Increased levels of CD8+ (cytotoxic) T cells, compared with CD4+ (helper) T cells, have been detected locally as well as in the systemic circulation, suggesting that the inflammatory response seen in FCGS is a cytotoxic cell-mediated immune response to antigenic stimulation likely from intracellular pathogens such as viruses.[7,26,27]

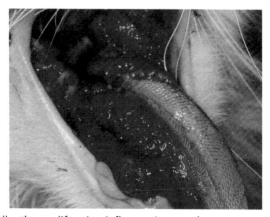

Fig. 2. Occasionally, the proliferative inflammation can be so severe as to prevent the tongue from retracting into its normal and functional position.

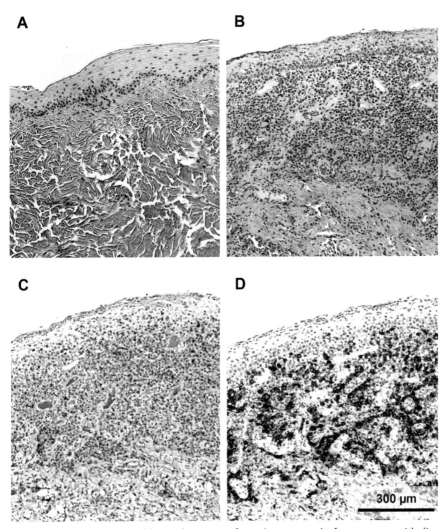

Fig. 3. On histology, the healthy oral mucosa of cats is composed of squamous epithelium with a rare presence of inflammatory cells (*A*). However, in cats affected by FCGS, ulceration of the squamous epithelium is observed with profound inflammatory infiltration comprising mostly granulocytes, lymphocytes, plasma cells, and mast cells (*B*) (hematoxylin-eosin [H&E] staining, original magnification ×10). Immunohistochemistry of FCGS mucosal inflammation indicates that most of the T lymphocytes (CD3 cells) are present in the epithelium (C) and most of the B lymphocytes (CD20 cells) are present in the submucosa (D) (original magnification ×10).

Moreover, in 2 studies, a decreased CD4/CD8 ratio was found in most cats diagnosed with FCGS, with a normal percentage of CD4+ T cells and an increased percentage of CD8+ T cells in circulation.[26,27] In humans, a low CD4/CD8 ratio is typically associated with immune dysfunction, immune senescence, and chronic inflammation, and is seen in immunodeficiency or autoimmune diseases such as human immunodeficiency virus/acquired immunodeficiency syndrome, systemic lupus erythematosus, and neoplasia, supporting the notion that an aberrant immune response is also involved in FCGS.[28] Interestingly, systemic administration of autologous mesenchymal stem cells (MSCs) in cats has been shown to normalize the CD4/CD8 ratio because of normalization of the percentage of CD8+ T cells, reinforcing the finding that CD8+ T cells play a noteworthy role in the pathophysiology of FCGS.[27]

Potential Viral Causes

FCV, FHV-1, FIV, and FeLV have been implicated in FCGS. Demonstration of causal relationships have not been successful, but, of these agents, FCV seems to have the most consistent evidence of being associated with FCGS.[9,12,18–20,29–31] A recent study found the incidence of FCV to be significantly higher in cats with FCGS (60%) compared with control cats (24%) as well as cats with feline resorptive lesions (23%).[32] Regardless, well-known risk factors for these viruses include free-roaming behavior and living in multicat environments such as shelters, shared households, and breeding catteries. This finding is worth exploring given that the etiopathogenesis of FCGS is likely multifactorial.

Environmental Stressors

A recent study investigated the association of multicat environments and outdoor access with the prevalence of FCGS.[33] It was revealed that the prevalence of FCGS was higher in multicat than single-cat households, and that each additional cat in the household increased the odds of FCGS by more than 70%. Association between outdoor access and FCGS was lacking, suggesting that factors relating to multicat environments may be necessary in addition to an infectious cause to trigger the development of FCGS. Examples mentioned in the article include the favoring of high rates of viral evolution and cyclic reinfections in susceptible individuals caused by chronic exposure to viruses shed by chronic carriers in multicat environments, as well as the stress of living in such environments.[33,34]

Feline Chronic Gingivostomatitis and Periodontitis

The association between FCGS and periodontitis has been proved in a retrospective case-control study where full-mouth dental radiographs of 101 cats with FCGS and 101 control cats with other oral diseases were evaluated.[10] This study revealed that not only do cats with FCGS have generalized, advanced periodontitis but they are also significantly more likely to have external inflammatory root resorption. The findings underscore that dental radiography plays an essential role in the diagnosis and evaluation of cats with FCGS, and that the treatment of associated periodontitis, likely contributing to persistent oral inflammation, is integral in the treatment of FCGS.

Bacterial Burden in Feline Chronic Gingivostomatitis

Bacterial organisms are thought to play a role in the pathogenesis of FCGS. The oral microbial diversity is less in cats with FCGS than in healthy cats, with the predominant species being *Pasteurella multocida* subsp. *multocida*.[17] Consistent with previous studies, a recent study found higher abundance of gram-negative and anaerobic bacteria in FCGS and periodontitis.[21] The phylum Bacteroidetes and the genus *Peptostreptococcus* were more abundant in cats with FCGS than in healthy cats and cats with periodontitis. The findings suggest that *Filifactor* and *Peptostreptococcus* may play a role in periodontitis of FCGS. In contrast with the study mentioned previously, this study found higher bacterial diversity in the oral microbiota of cats with FCGS and periodontitis, suggesting a possible role of bacterial biofilms in the pathophysiology both of these oral diseases.

Feline Chronic Gingivostomatitis and Esophagitis

It has recently been found that esophagitis seems to occur concurrently with FCGS.[35] In a controlled study involving 58 cats with FCGS, evidence of esophagitis was found via esophagoscopy in 98% of cats with FCGS, compared with control cats. Interestingly, none of the cats showed clinical signs of gastrointestinal disease. In addition, microscopic evidence of inflammation and metaplasia was found on histopathologic evaluation of grossly normal-appearing tissues. Endoscopic reexamination of 2 cats that were treated for FCGS and no longer showed clinical signs of that disease also showed macroscopic healing of esophagitis. One cat that had a relapse of FCGS showed worsening of esophagitis despite appropriate treatment of esophagitis. Prior medications, salivary and esophageal lumen pH, and chronicity of FCGS signs do not correlate with the degree of esophagitis. The investigators speculated that the virulent oral microbiota of cats with FCGS is transmitted to the esophagus via the saliva, where the production of certain proinflammatory cytokines may contribute to the development of esophagitis. In light of the findings of this study, diagnosis and treatment or empiric treatment of esophagitis may be considered in cats affected by FCGS, especially considering that both diseases share some clinical signs (ie, ptyalism, nausea, and inappetence).[35]

LEADING TREATMENT MODALITIES

In general, there are 2 approaches to the treatment of FCGS: surgical and medical. However, on its own, medical treatment typically does not have favorable long-term outcomes, making the current standard of care surgical intervention by means of dental extractions with or without additional medical management. A wide range of therapies has been suggested. However, only the most common and promising (based on scientific evidence) modalities are discussed in this article.

Pain Management

Regardless of modality, all treatment options require adequate pain management. Appropriate therapy depends on factors including comorbidities (eg, renal or hepatic disease), concurrent medications being administered (eg, corticosteroids), patient compliance, and the owner's perception of oral pain. Typically, long-term pain management includes administration of opioids (eg, buprenorphine) complemented with gabapentin. A recent randomized, prospective, blinded, controlled, crossover study showed that buccal administration of buprenorphine had a significant effect on reducing pain scores with low interindividual variations in plasma concentration in cats with FCGS.[36]

Surgical Treatment

A few studies have shown that partial- (all premolar and molar teeth) or full-mouth extraction provides the best long-term results.[37–39] These studies report substantial improvement or resolution of FCGS in approximately 70% to 80% of cats, with approximately 20% to 30% of cats showing minimal or no improvement.

A retrospective case series involving 95 cats with FCGS treated with full-mouth or partial-mouth extractions with concurrent medical management revealed that 28.4% of cats achieved complete resolution, 39% achieved substantial clinical improvement, 26.3% had little improvement, and 6.3% had no improvement (refractory).[37] Of the patients that achieved substantial improvement or complete resolution, most (68.8%) required medical management with antimicrobial, antiinflammatory, or analgesic medications for a finite period after the 2-week immediate postoperative period. Those that had little or no improvement still required medical management at the final recheck examination. A more recent study of 56 cats treated with dental extractions for FCGS showed that 51.8% achieved clinical cure or very significant improvement within a median time of 38 days.[38]

Moreover, extent of dental extractions seems to have no impact on outcome.[37,38] Therefore, partial-mouth extraction (plus other teeth that independently have indications for extraction, such as severe periodontitis, retained tooth roots, or resorptive lesions) as the first stage of treatment is the highest evidence-based recommendation. It also has the advantages of reduction in anesthetic time, surgeon fatigue, and surgical trauma. If there is no positive response within 1 to 4 months after partial-mouth extraction, full-mouth extractions may be pursued as the second stage of treatment based on the findings of Druet and Hennet.[37]

Medical Management

As already mentioned, most cats with FCGS require medical management in addition to surgical treatment, and some depend on lifelong medications. Because FCGS is an immune-mediated inflammatory disease, the basis of medical therapy has been immunosuppression or immunomodulation.[5]

Corticosteroids

Prednisolone is often used as a short-acting corticosteroid to control inflammation. In a randomized, double-blinded, prospective, controlled study of calicivirus-positive cats with FCGS refractory to dental extractions, it was used as the control (at 1 mg/kg/d tapering over 3 weeks) to recombinant feline interferon omega.[40] In the study, 23% of 11 cats that received treatment with prednisolone achieved substantial improvement, of which 7% achieved clinical remission.[40] Because of the potential deleterious side-effects of long-term corticosteroid administration, it should only be used as needed for symptomatic treatment, on a tapering course.

Recombinant feline interferon omega

Interferons (IFNs) are a group of signaling proteins that have the ability to interfere with viral replication.[40] Recombinant feline interferon omega (rFeIFN-ω) is marketed for use in canine parvovirus, FeLV, and FIV infections. Interferons also have antiviral activity against FHV-1, FCV, and feline coronavirus.[41] Oromucosal absorption of IFN has been shown to stimulate immunomodulation via oropharyngeal lymphoid tissues, whereas gastrointestinal absorption destroys the glycoprotein.[42,43] In a controlled, randomized, double-blinded study of oromucosal administration of rFeIFN-ω for 3 months in 19 cats, substantial improvement was seen in 45%, of which 10% achieved clinical remission. However, the results were not statistically significant between the 2 groups, implying that rFeIFN-ω is at least as effective as short-term prednisolone in the treatment of FCV-positive cats with refractory FCGS.[40] A recent controlled study showed that subcutaneous administration of rFeIFN-ω may be effective for the treatment of FCGS in FCV-positive cats by inhibiting the replication of FCV.[44] Furthermore, a novel rFeIFN (rFeIFN-α15) has been produced via transgenic silkworms that may carry a lower allergy risk, compared with the baculovirus expression system in silkworms by which the current form of rFeIFN-ω is produced.[45]

Cyclosporine

Cyclosporine provides immunosuppressive effects primarily via inhibition of T-cell activation by reducing interleukin-2 expression, a proinflammatory cytokine involved in a positive feedback loop that increases T-cell numbers.[46,47] It may also have inhibitory effects on B-cell reproduction.[48] In a small retrospective case series that examined the efficacy of oral cyclosporine in 8 cats not previously treated with extractions, 4 (50%) of the cats were reported to achieve clinical remission, whereas the rest had partial to fairly good improvement.[49] In a randomized, controlled, double-blinded, prospective clinical trial where oral cyclosporine was administered to 9 cats that had previously been treated with extractions, there was a statistical significance in the number of cats experiencing significant clinical improvement over the 6-week study period between the treatment group (77.8%) and the placebo group (14.3%).[50] Long-term observation was continued in 11 cats, of which 5 (45.5%) were clinically cured after receiving cyclosporine for 3 or more months.[50]

Mesenchymal stem cells

Mesenchymal stem cells (MSCs) are fibroblastlike, multipotent stem cells that have immunomodulatory effects through inhibition of T-cell proliferation, alteration of B-cell function, downregulation of major histocompatibility complex II on antigen-presenting cells, and inhibition of dendritic cell maturation.[27,51–53] The efficacy of both autologous and allogeneic, fresh, adipose-derived MSCs administered intravenously has been studied in cats with refractory FCGS.[26,27]

Treatment with autologous adipose-derived MSCs in 7 cats resulted in a positive response rate of 71.4% reflected by clinical remission in 42.8%, substantial improvement in 28.6% of the cats, and no response in 28.6% of cats over a follow-up period of 6 to 24 months.[27]

A subsequent clinical trial examining the efficacy of allogeneic adipose-derived MSCs in 7 cats resulted in lower clinical efficacy with delayed clinical and histologic resolution compared with autologous therapy.[26] Of the 7 cats, 28.6% achieved clinical remission, 28.6% achieved substantial improvement, and 42.8% were nonresponders.[26]

Clinical trials involving MSCs are currently ongoing and have expanded into a multicenter study to include control cats and to further investigate mechanism of action, biomarkers, efficacy of therapy before surgical treatment, as well as efficacy in cats with comorbidities[52] (for more on MSC in feline medicine, see Webb's article, "Stem Cell Therapy and Cats: What Do We Know at this Time?" in this issue).

SUMMARY

Although the exact etiopathogenesis of FCGS remains unclear, it seems to be a manifestation of an inappropriate immune response to antigenic stimulation, potentially potentiated or exacerbated by viral infection. Furthermore, environmental stressors such as multicat environments seem to be an important contributing factor. The current first line of treatment involves dental extractions of at least the premolar and molar teeth as opposed to medical therapy alone. Following surgical treatment, outcome can be divided into approximate thirds for cats achieving remission, substantial improvement, and little to no improvement. Most cats that undergo surgical treatment need concurrent medical therapy for control of inflammation, some requiring lifelong medical management. New modalities such as MSC therapy show promise. In addition, the importance of analgesic therapy cannot be overemphasized.

DISCLOSURE

The authors have no financial disclosures to acknowledge.

REFERENCES

1. Available at: https://avdc.org/avdc-nomenclature/AVDC. Accessed August 15, 2019.

2. Lommer MJ. Oral inflammation in small animals. Vet Clin North Am Small Anim Pract 2013;43(3):555–71.

3. Arzi B, Murphy B, Baumgarth N, et al. Analysis of immune cells within the healthy oral mucosa of specific pathogen-free cats. Anat Histol Embryol 2011;40(1):1–10.

4. Healey KA, Dawson S, Burrow R, et al. Prevalence of feline chronic gingivostomatitis in first opinion veterinary practice. J Feline Med Surg 2007;9(5):373–81.

5. Winer JN, Arzi B, Verstraete FJM. Therapeutic management of feline chronic gingivostomatitis: a systematic review of the literature. Front Vet Sci 2016;3:54.

6. Girard N, Servet E, Biourge V, et al. Periodontal health status in a colony of 109 cats. J Vet Dent 2009;26(3):147–55.

7. Harley R, Gruffydd-Jones TJ, Day MJ. Immunohistochemical characterization of oral mucosal lesions in cats with chronic gingivostomatitis. J Comp Pathol 2011;144(4):239–50.

8. Lommer MJ, Verstraete FJM. Radiographic patterns of periodontitis in cats: 147 cases (1998-1999). J Am Vet Med Assoc 2001;218(2):230–4.

9. Lommer MJ, Verstraete FJM. Concurrent oral shedding of feline calicivirus and feline herpesvirus 1 in cats with chronic gingivostomatitis. Oral Microbiol Immunol 2003;18(2):131–4.

10. Farcas N, Lommer MJ, Kass PH, et al. Dental radiographic findings in cats with chronic gingivostomatitis (2002-2012). J Am Vet Med Assoc 2014;244(3):339–45.

11. White SD, Rosychuk RA, Janik TA, et al. Plasma cell stomatitis-pharyngitis in cats: 40 cases (1973-1991). J Am Vet Med Assoc 1992;200(9):1377–80.

12. Reubel GH, George JW, Higgins J, et al. Effect of chronic feline immunodeficiency virus infection on experimental feline calicivirus-induced disease. Vet Microbiol 1994;39(3–4):335–51.

13. Pedersen NC. Inflammatory oral cavity diseases of the cat. Vet Clin North Am Small Anim Pract 1992;22(6):1323–45.

14. Diehl K, Rosychuk RA. Feline gingivitis-stomatitis-pharyngitis. Vet Clin North Am Small Anim Pract 1993;23(1):139–53.

15. Dolieslager SM, Bennett D, Johnston N, et al. Novel bacterial phylotypes associated with the healthy feline oral cavity and feline chronic gingivostomatitis. Res Vet Sci 2013;94(3):428–32.

16. Dolieslager SM, Lappin DF, Bennett D, et al. The influence of oral bacteria on tissue levels of Toll-like receptor and cytokine mRNAs in feline chronic gingivostomatitis and oral health. Vet Immunol Immunopathol 2013;151(3–4):263–74.

17. Dolieslager SM, Riggio MP, Lennon A, et al. Identification of bacteria associated with feline chronic gingivostomatitis using culture-dependent and culture-independent methods. Vet Microbiol 2011;148(1):93–8.

18. Dowers KL, Hawley JR, Brewer MM, et al. Association of Bartonella species, feline calicivirus, and feline herpesvirus 1 infection with gingivostomatitis in cats. J Feline Med Surg 2010;12(4):314–21.

19. Quimby JM, Elston T, Hawley J, et al. Evaluation of the association of Bartonella species, feline herpesvirus 1, feline calicivirus, feline leukemia virus and feline immunodeficiency virus with chronic feline gingivostomatitis. J Feline Med Surg 2008;10(1):66–72.

20. Belgard S, Truyen U, Thibault JC, et al. Relevance of feline calicivirus, feline immunodeficiency virus, feline leukemia virus, feline herpesvirus and Bartonella henselae in cats with chronic gingivostomatitis. Berl Munch Tierarztl Wochenschr 2010;123(9–10):369–76.

21. Rodrigues MX, Bicalho RC, Fiani N, et al. The subgingival microbial community of feline periodontitis and gingivostomatitis: characterization and comparison between diseased and healthy cats. Sc Rep 2019;9(1):12340.
22. Waters L, Hopper CD, Gruffydd-Jones TJ, et al. Chronic gingivitis in a colony of cats infected with feline immunodeficiency virus and feline calicivirus. Vet Rec 1993;132(14):340–2.
23. Lee M, Bosward KL, Norris JM. Immunohistological evaluation of feline herpesvirus-1 infection in feline eosinophilic dermatoses or stomatitis. J Feline Med Surg 2010;12(2):72–9.
24. Arzi B, Murphy B, Cox DP, et al. Presence and quantification of mast cells in the gingiva of cats with tooth resorption, periodontitis and chronic stomatitis. Arch Oral Biol 2010;55(2):148–54.
25. Rolim VM, Pavarini SP, Campos FS, et al. Clinical, pathological, immunohistochemical and molecular characterization of feline chronic gingivostomatitis. J Feline Med Surg 2017;19(4):403–9.
26. Arzi B, Clark KC, Sundaram A, et al. Therapeutic efficacy of fresh, allogeneic mesenchymal stem cells for severe refractory feline chronic gingivostomatitis. Stem Cells Transl Med 2017;6(8):1710–22.
27. Arzi B, Mills-Ko E, Verstraete FJM, et al. Therapeutic efficacy of fresh, autologous mesenchymal stem cells for severe refractory gingivostomatitis in cats. Stem Cells Transl Med 2016;5(1):75–86.
28. McBride JA, Striker R. Imbalance in the game of T cells: what can the CD4/CD8 T-cell ratio tell us about HIV and health? PLoS Pathog 2017;13(11):e1006624.
29. Knowles JO, McArdle F, Dawson S, et al. Studies on the role of feline calicivirus in chronic stomatitis in cats. Vet Microbiol 1991;27(3–4):205–19.
30. Addie DD, Radford A, Yam PS, et al. Cessation of feline calicivirus shedding coincident with resolution of chronic gingivostomatitis in a cat. J Small Anim Pract 2003;44(4):172–6.
31. Poulet H, Brunet S, Soulier M, et al. Comparison between acute oral/respiratory and chronic stomatitis/gingivitis isolates of feline calicivirus: pathogenicity, antigenic profile and cross-neutralisation studies. Arch Virol 2000;145(2):243–61.
32. Thomas S, Lappin DF, Spears J, et al. Prevalence of feline calicivirus in cats with odontoclastic resorptive lesions and chronic gingivostomatitis. Res Vet Sci 2017; 111:124–6.
33. Peralta S, Carney PC. Feline chronic gingivostomatitis is more prevalent in shared households and its risk correlates with the number of cohabiting cats. J Feline Med Surg 2019;21(12):1165–71.
34. Buffington CA. External and internal influences on disease risk in cats. J Am Vet Med Assoc 2002;220(7):994–1002.
35. Kouki MI, Papadimitriou SA, Psalla D, et al. Chronic gingivostomatitis with esophagitis in cats. J Vet Intern Med 2017;31(6):1673–9.
36. Stathopoulou TR, Kouki M, Pypendop BH, et al. Evaluation of analgesic effect and absorption of buprenorphine after buccal administration in cats with oral disease. J Feline Med Surg 2018;20(8):704–10.
37. Jennings MW, Lewis JR, Soltero-Rivera MM, et al. Effect of tooth extraction on stomatitis in cats: 95 cases (2000-2013). J Am Vet Med Assoc 2015;246(6):654–60.
38. Druet I, Hennet P. Relationship between feline calicivirus load, oral lesions, and outcome in feline chronic gingivostomatitis (caudal stomatitis): retrospective study in 104 cats. Front Vet Sci 2017;4:209.
39. Hennet P. Chronic gingivo-stomatitis in cats: long-term follow-up of 30 cases treated by dental extractions. J Vet Dent 1997;14:15–21.

40. Hennet PR, Camy GA, McGahie DM, et al. Comparative efficacy of a recombinant feline interferon omega in refractory cases of calicivirus-positive cats with caudal stomatitis: a randomised, multi-centre, controlled, double-blind study in 39 cats. J Feline Med Surg 2011;13(8):577–87.

41. Ueda Y, Sakurai T, Kasama K, et al. Pharmacokinetic properties of recombinant feline interferon and its stimulatory effect on 2',5'-oligoadenylate synthetase activity in the cat. J Vet Med Sci 1993;55(1):1–6.

42. Cummins JM, Krakowka GS, Thompson CG. Systemic effects of interferons after oral administration in animals and humans. Am J Vet Res 2005;66(1):164–76.

43. Schellekens H, Geelen G, Meritet JF, et al. Oromucosal interferon therapy: relationship between antiviral activity and viral load. J Interferon Cytokine Res 2001;21(8):575–81.

44. Matsumoto H, Teshima T, Iizuka Y, et al. Evaluation of the efficacy of the subcutaneous low recombinant feline interferon-omega administration protocol for feline chronic gingivitis-stomatitis in feline calicivirus-positive cats. Res Vet Sci 2018;121:53–8.

45. Minagawa S, Nakaso Y, Tomita M, et al. Novel recombinant feline interferon carrying N-glycans with reduced allergy risk produced by a transgenic silkworm system. BMC Vet Res 2018;14(1):260.

46. Robson D. Review of the properties and mechanisms of action of cyclosporine with an emphasis on dermatological therapy in dogs, cats and people. Vet Rec 2003;152(25):768–72.

47. Matsuda S, Koyasu S. Mechanisms of action of cyclosporine. Immunopharmacology 2000;47(2–3):119–25.

48. Winslow MM, Gallo EM, Neilson JR, et al. The calcineurin phosphatase complex modulates immunogenic B cell responses. Immunity 2006;24(2):141–52.

49. Vercelli A, Raviri G, Cornegliani L. The use of oral cyclosporin to treat feline dermatoses: a retrospective analysis of 23 cases. Vet Dermatol 2006;17(3):201–6.

50. Lommer MJ. Efficacy of cyclosporine for chronic, refractory stomatitis in cats: A randomized, placebo-controlled, double-blinded clinical study. J Vet Dent 2013;30(1):8–17.

51. Clark KC, Fierro FA, Ko EM, et al. Human and feline adipose-derived mesenchymal stem cells have comparable phenotype, immunomodulatory functions, and transcriptome. Stem Cell Res Ther 2017;8(1):69.

52. Quimby JM, Borjesson DL. Mesenchymal stem cell therapy in cats: Current knowledge and future potential. J Feline Med Surg 2018;20(3):208–16.

53. Taechangam N, Iyer SS, Walker NJ, et al. Mechanisms utilized by feline adipose-derived mesenchymal stem cells to inhibit T lymphocyte proliferation. Stem Cell Res Ther 2019;10(1):188.

Precision/Genomic Medicine for Domestic Cats

Reuben M. Buckley, PhD, Leslie A. Lyons, PhD*

KEYWORDS

- Precision medicine • Genomic medicine • Direct-to-consumer genetic testing

KEY POINTS

- In veterinary health care, precision/genomic medicine should be considered at the level of species, population/breed, and the individual.
- Precision/genomic medicine will develop as a standard-of-care in veterinary medicine.
- Direct-to-consumer genetic testing implements precision/genomic medicine.

PRECISION/GENOMIC MEDICINE

Precision/genomic medicine (P/GM) is the practice of disease treatment and prevention that considers individual variability with regard to genetics, environment, and lifestyle.[1] Historically, health care has evolved around the needs of the population with a one-size-fits-all approach. For example, 2 patients displaying the same symptoms would typically be diagnosed with the same disease and therefore receive the same drug for treatment. Ideally, the drug prescribed would have shown strong efficacy across a broad population, rather than an alternative drug that may have had higher levels of efficacy in some but with only small effects in most. A P/GM approach would instead focus on each patient's individual characteristics for both diagnosis and treatment. In the preceding example, genetic markers may have indicated that one of the patients would have responded well to the alternative drug, potentially leading to a speeder recovery with fewer side effects for that patient.

The practice of P/GM requires a detailed profile of each patient's molecular characteristics and an understanding of how those characteristics affect disease processes and the treatment options in question. In this context, genomics is potentially the most valuable tool available for PM.[2] Each individual's genome is a unique combination of DNA variants, in which the DNA variants themselves were inherited from the individual's parents, are often found in others within the population through shared ancestry, and can contribute in various amounts to physiological processes. Moreover, genomics,

Department of Veterinary Medicine and Surgery, College of Veterinary Medicine, University of Missouri - Columbia, E109 Vet Med Building, 825 East Campus Loop, Columbia, MO 65211, USA
* Corresponding author.
E-mail addresses: Lyonsla@Missouri.edu; felinegenome@missouri.edu

Vet Clin Small Anim 50 (2020) 983–990
https://doi.org/10.1016/j.cvsm.2020.05.005
0195-5616/20/© 2020 Elsevier Inc. All rights reserved.
vetsmall.theclinics.com

or genomic medicine, provides the framework necessary for PM. Because individual DNA variants are distributed across populations, these variants can be correlated with specific medically relevant traits, such as a DNA marker that indicates a positive response to a specific drug or susceptibility to a disease. Also, because each individual has a unique combination of these DNA variants, knowledge generated from such correlations can be translated into a precise individualized molecular profile that can guide diagnosis and treatment. The P/GM approach applies to cats as well.[3–5]

The entire repertoire of approximately 21,000 genes of a domestic cat influences its overall biology,[6] physiology, health, and appearance; however, for many genetic diseases, only a limited number of genes and variants influence the disease, trait, or health problem.[7] By considering the DNA variation present in an individual's disease/trait-causing genes, genetically defined therapies, targeted at specific genes, can then be identified and applied.[3,5] The therapies are targeted on a perturbed biological pathway, with the intention of correcting the disturbance, or activating an alternative pathway, which will rectify the adverse health condition. In cancers, the genetic profile of the tumor's DNA can be used to help select more appropriate cancer treatments, attacking the tumors more directly and efficiently. PM implies individualized treatment that should be more efficient and more effective, which should improve quality and quantity of life for the specific patient. Already becoming an active approach for canine cancers, cats too will benefit from P/GM.[8–10]

Although P/GM is a new term, it is not necessarily a new concept and has been gradually infiltrating veterinary medicine for years.[10] Although the goal of P/GM has been to focus on individual characteristics, throughout history, steps have been taken to refine our understanding at increasingly higher levels of resolution. Discussed in the following sections, are several different levels of interpreting patient characteristics that have been used to inform a P/GM approach within feline veterinary medicine.

Species-Level Precision Medicine

Although a new "buzz word," P/GM is not really a new concept and is a routine aspect of veterinary medicine. Unlike human medicine, veterinary medicine has the added complication of treatment for widely different species. Trial and error in the use of acetaminophen demonstrated this valuable drug for many species, is toxic in cats.[11,12] Glucuronidation is catalyzed by the UDP-glucuronosyltransferases (UGTs), a superfamily of conjugative liver enzymes that transfer glucuronic acid to a nontoxic, more water-soluble, and readily excreted glucuronide metabolite. UDP-glucuronosyltransferase 1A6 (*UGT1A6*), the major species-conserved phenol detoxification enzyme, is a pseudogene in domestic cats, thus nonfunctional, and cats also are reported to have a less diverse pattern of UGT1A isoform expression compared with other species.[13] Such differences most likely reflect the highly carnivorous diet of Felid species and resultant minimal exposure to phytoalexins, which are usually found in plant tissue.[14,15] Slow glucuronidation of acetaminophen and other drugs, such as acetylsalicylic acid (aspirin),[16] account for the slow clearance and extreme sensitivity of cats to the toxicity of these drugs. Therefore, species-specific factors, such as dietary requirements and genetics, contribute to a cat's inability to metabolize certain drugs that are effective in most other species.

Population-Level Precision/Genomic Medicine

Regularly, medical interventions are leveraged at the level of groups within a population defined by shared characteristics, such as, age, ethnicity, race, and sex. Such groupings are useful, as certain diseases are known to be more prominent in specific groups, allowing for enhanced detection or monitoring in susceptible groups. The same principles are also used in veterinary medicine, where domestic animals have the added benefit of breeds or breed structure, which were created by strictly enforcing and documenting mating patterns among individuals that carry traits desired by breeders. Importantly, individuals within the same breed share extremely high degrees of common ancestry and are often easily recognized by the presence of distinctive features, such as coat texture or stature. One example of P/GM leveraged at the population level in cats is the genetics and detection of various blood types. Importantly, blood type incompatibilities leading to transfusion reactions and neonatal isoerythrolysis have been recognized in cats for decades and are of particular concern for specific breeds and populations.[17,18] Genetic variants in the cat control the function and efficiency of the enzyme *cytidine monophospho-N-acetylneuraminic acid hydroxylase (CMAH)*, which converts neurominic acid to acetyl acid, thereby changing a cat's blood group from Type B to Type A.[19] Serologic, cross-matching and now genetic testing predicts the red blood cell antigens and hence identifies potential incompatibilities. Thus, every time a transfusion donor was decided or a breeding was conducted using blood type information, the veterinarian or breeder was performing a rudimentary form of P/GM for the cat.

Individual-Level Precision Medicine

Individual genetic tests
To apply P/GM at the individual level, genetic analyses of well-recognized candidate genes can be individually scanned in hopes of finding causal DNA variants for a disease, condition, or novel phenotype. Knowing the gene involved with the presentation may direct the treatment plan for the patient. These specific candidate gene analyses are well proven and are generally conducted in 2 steps, which are reviewed in "Direct-to-Consumer Genetic Testing for Domestic Cats" by Lyons and Buckley, elsewhere in this issue.

Whole genome and whole exome sequencing
Although genetic testing and candidate gene screening are aspects of P/GM, whole genome (WGS) and or whole exome sequencing (WES) are the newest techniques to advance the concept. Highly accurate and robust genome assemblies are the backbone of WGS/WES, as high-quality reference genome assemblies facilitate accurate comparisons between patient and healthy control genomes. The new long-read assembly, Felis_catus_9.0, the genome sequence of an Abyssinian named Cinnamon, is one of the strongest assemblies for any species,[4] besides humans and mice. A second requirement for effective P/GM is the establishment of a database that has a robust collection of DNA variants that are normally found in cat genomes. The 99 Lives Cat Genome Sequencing Initiative has collated both published and yet unpublished cat genomic data to establish an extensive dataset of known DNA variants in cats (http://felinegenetics.missouri.edu/99lives). The 99 Lives project has evaluated approximately 300 domestic cat genomes to produce a cat DNA variant dataset with more than 70 million variants. In addition, research support groups, such as the National Center for Biotechnology Information (www.ncbi.nlm.nih.gov), Ensembl (www.ensembl.org), and the University of California–Santa Cruz (https://genome.ucsc.edu/) use other information, such as RNA sequencing data, to periodically improve the annotation of the cat genome by improving the positioning and descriptions of genes and their exon-intron boundaries. Hence, armed with a strong reference genome, good annotation, and an expanding variant database, significant advancements in applications of P/GM in cats is technically feasible. Several cat diseases

have already been discovered by using WGS and the required supportive resources.[5,20–23]

Today, any cat with a suspected genetic disease can have its DNA submitted for WGS/WES. Institutions such as the University of Missouri College of Veterinary Medicine perform this task regularly for both cats and dogs. Once sequencing is complete and data become available, bioinformatics tools can be used to compare the patient's DNA with the reference genome and variant datasets to detect and prioritize potentially harmful mutations specific to the patient. Here, annotation information is used to determine in which gene the variant resides and the possible impact that variant has on the protein produced by that gene. In summary, the tools are available, the cost is reasonable, and WGS/WES and bioinformatic processing can each be accomplished within a week. Therefore, genetics can support bedside to benchtop and back to bedside diagnosis or treatment within a reasonable timeframe and support the health care of cats in a precise and individually focused manner.

GENOME ORGANIZATION

Among higher eukaryotes, very little of the genome codes for proteins,[24] indicating the vast majority of DNA variants, have an unknown biological impact. To use genomic technologies efficiently in PM, a basic understanding of genome organization is required. The domestic cat haploid genome, which is typical of most mammalian genomes, consists of approximately 2.6 billion base pairs (2.6 gigabases or Gb) spread across 18 autosomes and 1 pair of X and Y sex chromosomes.[4] The genes themselves are distributed across these chromosomes. Organization also takes place on the level of individual genes, which are composed of exons, introns, and 5′ and 3′ untranslated regions (UTRs) (**Fig. 1**). Exons contain the genetic information that is translated into proteins, the molecules that perform most tasks within a cell. Together, all exons combined account for less than 50 Mb of DNA or less than 2% of DNA in the entire genome.[25] Exons within the same gene are separated by introns. Introns vary widely in size and are usually much larger than exons. Together, all introns combined account for approximately 40% of the entire genome. After transcription, introns are spliced out of the messenger RNA transcript, leaving the remaining transcribed exons to essentially be stitched together before undergoing translation. The remaining DNA found outside of genes is referred to as "intergenic" and comprises less than 60% of the entire genome. Often found within intergenic regions and introns, usually within the immediate vicinity of genes, are DNA elements known as regulatory regions, these elements help determine how much product of any given gene is produced. Although regulatory regions can be an important factor in some traits, such as a retroelement insertion into one of the introns of *KIT* that causes white spotting in coats,[26] they are difficult to define and remain poorly annotated in the cat.

The final component to consider for mammalian genome organization is the mitochondrial DNA. Discussions of the cat genome generally omit the mitochondrial DNA (mtDNA), as it consists only of a small number of genes involved in controlling cellular energy. In total, the mitochondrial genome is approximately 17 kb in length and is only inherited through the maternal lineage.[27] No mtDNA disease causing variants have been identified in cats but many are associated with diseases in humans, indicating the mtDNA should also be considered in health studies.

CHOOSING BETWEEN WHOLE GENOME AND WHOLE EXOME SEQUENCING

Two sequencing approaches assist the identification of new DNA variants: WGS that captures DNA variants across the vast majority of the genome, and WES that captures

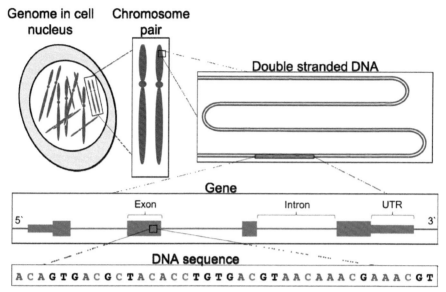

Fig. 1. The hierarchical organization of mammalian genomes. DNA in mammalian genomes is organized at several different levels of resolution. At the highest level of organization is the entire genome, which mostly resides within the cell's nucleus and is packaged into individual chromosome pairs. Cats have 19 chromosome pairs; 1 copy of each pair is inherited maternally and the other copy is inherited paternally. Chromosomal DNA itself is double stranded. A vast majority of the DNA is intergenic (*blue*) and the function of this DNA is relatively unknown. Genes (*orange*) account for less than 10% of the genomic DNA. Distributed throughout the DNA sequence are specific sequences that indicate the presence of genes and gene features such as exons (large *orange boxes*), introns (sequence between exons), and the 3' and 5' UTRs (smaller *orange boxes*). During transcription (the production of messenger RNA from DNA), intron sequences are removed from the transcripts, leaving only the exons behind, which are in turn translated into proteins. Knowledge of these sequence features is important for deciding which technologies to use for a genetic test. WES will capture only the exons, the small portion of the genome that is translated into proteins, whereas whole genome sequencing will capture almost the entire DNA sequence of the genome.

DNA variants only within exons and their immediate flanking regions. The most important questions to ask when considering each approach are (1) how likely will the causative variant be sequenced and identified, (2) which individuals are available for sequencing, (3) what is the cost of each approach, and (4) how useful will the results be for future research and analysis? For sequencing and identifying candidate causative variants, although WGS will most likely sequence the variant, identifying a single candidate from all other variants is challenging and depends on the quality of genome annotation. Because regulatory regions in the cat remain poorly annotated, most meaningful variants will be in exons, and therefore also captured by WES. However, WES is usually not able to detect copy number changes or large structural variants, such as the deletion in *UGDH* that causes feline dwarfism or the *KIT* variants that cause white spotting.[4,26] Independent of the expanded range of sequences WGS captures, a variety of analyses demonstrate a number of metrics showing WGS generally outperforms WES,[28,29] including diagnostic successes, which is approximately 36% for WES and approximately 41% for WGS.[30] In terms of cost, WES can be performed for less than $250 per cat and WGS can be performed for approximately $1000 per cat. Also, because WES captures only approximately 2% of the genome, WES file sizes are much smaller than WGS file sizes, requiring significantly less computational resources and time to process and analyze. The final question regards the future usefulness of the data. Because many P/GM approaches require a data set of known variation, this means after an individual's genome is sequenced, their genome data can be added to a variant dataset and used to influence future cases. Here WGS provides far more utility than WES, in addition to capturing all of the exons, WGS captures the intergenic and intronic regions that require significantly more investigation to understand their influences on health.

Ultimately, when deciding on a sequencing strategy, individuals must also consider their available budget, available computational resources, and be aware there is a strong possibility they may not find a candidate variant.

FUTURE OF PRECISION/GENOMIC MEDICINE

P/GM is also known as P4 Medicine, implying health care that is predictive, personalized, preventive, and participatory.[31–36] Lower technological costs, improved bioinformatics, and improved genomic resources, such as genome assemblies, annotations, and variant databases, all afford veterinary health care to encompass P/GM. Besides simply knowing the gene causing a health problem and then treating the symptoms, the ultimate hope for P/GM is to apply drugs that specifically target the pathway of the gene, leading to remediation of the defect and "cure" of the disease. Besides more personalized treatments, the DNA variants of the individual are also important during clinical trials and drug development. Many drugs have failed clinical trials because of poor effects or adverse reactions in patients. As the role of DNA variation becomes clearer, some clinical trials may have failed because of the specific genetics of the patient; that was not the right drug for that individual but may be a very effective drug for others. Thus, many drugs may have been shelved before the understanding of the specific reactions of patients due to their background DNA profiles. By linking standardized, electronic health care records across clinics and to genomic datasets, cohorts of patients can be well defined and ascertained to investigate common and more complex health problems that also involve the environment and lifestyle. P/GM is feasible in companion animals; however, efficiency and robust datasets, including genetic and clinical phenotypes, need to grow and improve to move P/GM to a standard-of-care.

REFERENCES

1. Collins FS, Varmus H. A new initiative on precision medicine. N Engl J Med 2015; 372:793–5.
2. Aronson SJ, Rehm HL. Building the foundation for genomics in precision medicine. Nature 2015;526:336–42.
3. Ontiveros ES, Ueda Y, Harris SP, et al. Precision medicine validation: identifying the MYBPC3 A31P variant with whole-genome sequencing in two Maine Coon cats with hypertrophic cardiomyopathy. J Feline Med Surg 2019;21:1086–93.
4. Buckley RM, Davis BW, Brashear WA, et al. A new domestic cat genome assembly based on long sequence reads empowers feline genomic medicine and identifies a novel gene for dwarfism. PLoS Genetics 2020.
5. Mauler DA, Gandolfi B, Reinero CR, et al. Precision medicine in cats: novel Niemann-Pick type C1 diagnosed by whole-genome sequencing. J Vet Intern Med 2017;31:539–44.

6. Pontius JU, Mullikin JC, Smith DR, et al. Initial sequence and comparative analysis of the cat genome. Genome Res 2007;17:1675–89.

7. Nicholas FW. Online Mendelian Inheritance in Animals (OMIA): a comparative knowledgebase of genetic disorders and other familial traits in non-laboratory animals. Nucleic Acids Res 2003;31:275–7.

8. Lorch G, Sivaprakasam K, Zismann V, et al. Identification of recurrent activating HER2 mutations in primary canine pulmonary adenocarcinoma. Clin Cancer Res 2019;25:5866–77.

9. Katogiritis A, Khanna C. Towards the delivery of precision veterinary cancer medicine. Vet Clin North Am Small Anim Pract 2019;49:809–18.

10. Lloyd KC, Khanna C, Hendricks W, et al. Precision medicine: an opportunity for a paradigm shift in veterinary medicine. J Am Vet Med Assoc 2016;248:45–8.

11. Finco DC, Duncan JR, Schall WD, et al. Acetaminophen toxicosis in the cat. J Am Vet Med Assoc 1975;166:469–72.

12. Leyland A. Probable paracetamol toxicity in a cat. Vet Rec 1974;94:104–5.

13. Court MH, Greenblatt DJ. Molecular genetic basis for deficient acetaminophen glucuronidation by cats: UGT1A6 is a pseudogene, and evidence for reduced diversity of expressed hepatic UGT1A isoforms. Pharmacogenetics 2000;10:355–69.

14. Court MH, Greenblatt DJ. Molecular basis for deficient acetaminophen glucuronidation in cats. An interspecies comparison of enzyme kinetics in liver microsomes. Biochem Pharmacol 1997;53:1041–7.

15. Court MH, Greenblatt DJ. Biochemical basis for deficient paracetamol glucuronidation in cats: an interspecies comparison of enzyme constraint in liver microsomes. J Pharm Pharmacol 1997;49:446–9.

16. Davis LE, Westfall BA. Species differences in biotransformation and excretion of salicylate. Am J Vet Res 1972;33:1253–62.

17. Giger U, Bucheler J, Patterson DF. Frequency and inheritance of A and B blood types in feline breeds of the United States. J Hered 1991;82:15–20.

18. Malik R, Griffin DL, White JD, et al. The prevalence of feline A/B blood types in the Sydney region. Aust Vet J 2005;83:38–44.

19. Bighignoli B, Niini T, Grahn RA, et al. Cytidine monophospho-N-acetylneuraminic acid hydroxylase (CMAH) mutations associated with the domestic cat AB blood group. BMC Genet 2007;8:27.

20. Gandolfi B, Grahn RA, Creighton EK, et al. COLQ variant associated with Devon Rex and Sphynx feline hereditary myopathy. Anim Genet 2015;46:711–5.

21. Jaffey JA, Reading NS, Giger U, et al. Clinical, metabolic, and genetic characterization of hereditary methemoglobinemia caused by cytochrome b5 reductase deficiency in cats. J Vet Intern Med 2019;33(6):2725–31.

22. Lyons LA, Creighton EK, Alhaddad H, et al. Whole genome sequencing in cats, identifies new models for blindness in AIPL1 and somite segmentation in HES7. BMC Genomics 2016;17:265.

23. Oh A, Pearce JW, Gandolfi B, et al. Early-onset progressive retinal atrophy associated with an IQCB1 variant in African black-footed cats (*Felis nigripes*). Sci Rep 2017;7:43918.

24. Sakharkar MK, Chow VT, Kangueane P. Distributions of exons and introns in the human genome. In Silico Biol 2004;4:387–93.

25. Lander ES, Linton LM, Birren B, et al. Initial sequencing and analysis of the human genome. Nature 2001;409:860–921.

26. David VA, Menotti-Raymond M, Wallace AC, et al. Endogenous retrovirus insertion in the KIT oncogene determines white and white spotting in domestic cats. G3 (Bethesda) 2014;4:1881–91.

27. Lopez JV, Cevario S, O'Brien SJ. Complete nucleotide sequences of the domestic cat (*Felis catus*) mitochondrial genome and a transposed mtDNA tandem repeat (Numt) in the nuclear genome. Genomics 1996;33:229–46.

28. Belkadi A, Bolze A, Itan Y, et al. Whole-genome sequencing is more powerful than whole-exome sequencing for detecting exome variants. Proc Natl Acad Sci U S A 2015;112:5473–8.

29. Meienberg J, Bruggmann R, Oexle K, et al. Clinical sequencing: is WGS the better WES? Hum Genet 2016;135:359–62.

30. Clark MM, Stark Z, Farnaes L, et al. Meta-analysis of the diagnostic and clinical utility of genome and exome sequencing and chromosomal microarray in children with suspected genetic diseases. NPJ Genom Med 2018;3:16.

31. Auffray C, Charron D, Hood L. Predictive, preventive, personalized and participatory medicine: back to the future. Genome Med 2010;2:57.

32. Cesario A, Auffray C, Russo P, et al. P4 medicine needs P4 education. Curr Pharm Des 2014;20:6071–2.

33. Hood L. Systems biology and p4 medicine: past, present, and future. Rambam Maimonides Med J 2013;4:e0012.

34. Hood L, Flores M. A personal view on systems medicine and the emergence of proactive P4 medicine: predictive, preventive, personalized and participatory. Nat Biotechnol 2012;29:613–24.

35. Hood L, Friend SH. Predictive, personalized, preventive, participatory (P4) cancer medicine. Nat Rev Clin Oncol 2011;8:184–7.

36. Tian Q, Price ND, Hood L. Systems cancer medicine: towards realization of predictive, preventive, personalized and participatory (P4) medicine. J Intern Med 2012;271:111–21.

Direct-to-Consumer Genetic Testing for Domestic Cats

Leslie A. Lyons, PhD*, Reuben M. Buckley, PhD

KEYWORDS

- Direct to consumer • Genomic testing • DTC • Genetic testing • Precision medicine

KEY POINTS

- Over 25 DNA variants (including blood type variants) are found in cat breeds and 55 in random bred cats that should be monitored for health care and to support breeding strategies.
- Whole genome DNA sequencing can be conducted in cats as a form of a genetic test to help identify new causes of suspected inherited diseases.
- Genetic test results from large panel assays should be validated by a single disease test when considering health care decisions.

DIRECT-TO-CONSUMER GENETIC TESTING
Individual Genetic Tests

If a feline patient is suspected of having an inherited disease or trait, veterinarians can seek genetic testing to support a diagnosis, that hopefully will direct and refine treatment. Genetic testing for diagnosing a disease is a form of precision/genomic medicine (P/GM), as the results will be specific to only this patient and the treatment can be tailored to the disease and the patient. To apply personalized P/GM to a specific cat, genetic analyses of well-recognized candidate genes of a given health concern or trait can be individually scanned in hopes of finding a causal DNA variant for the disease, condition, or novel phenotype. Knowing the gene and or mutation involved with the clinical presentation may direct the treatment plan for the patient. These specific candidate gene analyses are well-proven and are generally conducted in 2 steps.

Step 1: to be financially efficient and support diagnosis, all known variants that have been suggested or demonstrated to cause a similar disease in previous cases are usually tested in the patient. The genetic tests available for cats are presented in **Tables 1** and **2**. **Table 1** presents all the genetic diseases with identified mutations known to be health problems in cat breeds. **Table 2** presents diseases that have been identified in random bred cats or are not common for any specific breed. The veterinarian and the

Department of Veterinary Medicine & Surgery, College of Veterinary Medicine, University of Missouri - Columbia, E109 Vet Med Building, 825 East Campus Loop, Columbia, MO 65211, USA
* Corresponding author.
E-mail addresses: Lyonsla@Missouri.edu; felinegenome@missouri.edu

Vet Clin Small Anim 50 (2020) 991–1000
https://doi.org/10.1016/j.cvsm.2020.05.004
0195-5616/20/© 2020 Elsevier Inc. All rights reserved.

owner need to select a genetic testing provider that offers the desired test. Because buccal swabs can be used for most genetic testing, veterinarians and cat owners can submit samples and receive rapid results from laboratories throughout the world. In North America, genetic laboratories such as the University of California–Davis Veterinary Genetics Laboratory, Mars Optimal Selection, Genetic Veterinary Services, Inc. (CatScan), and others offer a vast number of cat disease tests and have strong customer service.

The earliest direct DNA variant tests were offered to cats of the Korat breed for 2 different forms of gangliosidosis (see **Table 1**). Although knowing the DNA variants and genes at the time did not support effective treatments, breeders could take preventive measures and select appropriate matings that would not produce sick cats. These early DNA tests generally required a blood sample collected by a veterinarian, who submitted the samples to a research laboratory, such as the Scott-Ritchey Research Center at Auburn University (www.vetmed.auburn.edu/research/scott-ritchey-research-center/). Thus, veterinarians were directly involved with health and mating decisions, supporting a veterinarian-researcher-client-patient network of information flow. Once DNA could be isolated from buccal swabs, the breeders themselves would directly submit samples. At this point, testing for cats became more direct-to-consumer (DTC) because many of the tests of interest were just for aesthetic traits, like coat colors and fur types.

In cats, many diseases have more than one known variant in a given gene. For example, a cat presenting with a suspected methemoglobinopathy can be assayed for the 2 DNA variants known for this disease in the gene, CYB5R3 (see **Table 2**).[1] If the cat is positive for the DNA variant, the disease is now very likely confirmed and treatment with methylene blue could be recommended. However, in other circumstances, diseases with similar clinical presentations could be caused by variants in different genes, thus thorough clinical diagnoses are always imperative. If a cat has a presentation suggestive of a type of porphyria, 2 genes can be assayed (UROS and HMBS), including more than 8 variants (see **Table 1**). Four different genes and variants are known to cause progressive retinal atrophy in cats (see **Table 1**), whereas at least 17 variants for different types of lysosomal storage diseases are known (see **Table 2**). For some diseases, only 1 variant is known and the screening process is simple, but for other diseases, the screening processes become costly and are more complex. Therefore, efficient assays (multiplexing) that can accurately test several DNA variants at one time, have become an important tool for genetic testing in cats, equating to P/GM.

Candidate Gene Scanning

Step 2: the second type of DNA evaluation for a patient with a well-recognized genetic disease or trait is known as the "candidate gene" approach. If a known disease-causing DNA variant was previously excluded via genetic testing as the cause for a health concern, then only that specific variant in that specific gene had been eliminated. This same gene may still be involved in the new case, but the patient may have a novel DNA variant, which is not yet described in the literature. If strong clinical phenotyping is available, a particular candidate gene can be implicated and genetically scanned for a specific disease. For example, if a cat has bilateral cystic kidneys, and the known DNA variant causing polycystic kidney disease in the cat is absent in the patient, then the known gene (polycystin-1 [PKD1]) can be scanned by direct sequencing to determine if a novel DNA variant can be found to associate with the disease in the new patient.[2]

Table 1
The genes and DNA variants of inherited diseases common to domestic cat breeds

Disease/ Trait (Alleles) OMIA Entry	MOI[a]	Phenotype (Breed Affected)[b]	Gene	Mutation[c]
AB Blood Type (A⁺, AB, b) 000119–9685	AR	Determines Type B (Various breeds)	*CMAH*	c.139G > A, c.142G > A, c.179G > T, c.268T > A, c.364C > T, c.933delA, c.1193G > T, c.1322delT, c.1603G > A
Autoimmune lymphoproliferative Disease (ALPS) 002064–9685	AR	Non-neoplastic lymphoproliferative disease (British Shorthair)	*FASL*	c.413_414insA
Craniofacial Defect 001551–9685	AR	Craniofacial Defect (Burmese)	*ALX1*	c.496delCTCT-CAGGACTG
Dwarfism 000299–9685	AD	Shortening of long bones	*UGDH*	3.3 Kb deletion
Fold (Fd, fd⁺) 000319–9685	AD	Ventral ear fold, osteochondrodysplasia	*TRPV4*	c.1024G > T
Gangliosidosis 1 000402–9685	AR	Lipid storage disorder (GM1) (Korat, Siamese, S.E. Asia)	*GLB1*	c.1448G > C
Gangliosidosis 2 01462–0985	AR	Lipid storage disorder (GM2) (Burmese)	*HEXB*	c.1356_1362delGTTCTCA
Gangliosidosis 201462–0985	AR	Lipid storage disorder (GM2) (Korat)	*HEXB*	c.39delC
Glycogen Storage Dis. IV 000420–9685	AR	Glycogen storage disorder (GSD) (Norwegian Forest Cat)	*GBE1*	IVS11 + 1552_IVS12–1339 del6.2kb ins334 bp
Hypertrophic Cardiomyopathy 000515–9685	AD	Cardiac disease (hypertrophic cardiomyopathy) (Maine Coon)	*MYBPC*	c.91G > C
Hypertrophic Cardiomyopathy 000515–9685	AD	Cardiac Disease (hypertrophic cardiomyophathy) (Ragdoll)	*MYBPC*	c.2460C > T
Hypokalemia 001759–9685	AR	Potassium deficiency (HK) (Burmese)	*WNK4*	c.2899C > T
Manx (M, m⁺) 000975–9685	AD	Absence/short tail	*TBX1*	c.998delT, c.1169delC, c.1199delC, c.998_1014dup17delGCC

(continued on next page)

Table 1
(continued)

Disease/ Trait (Alleles) OMIA Entry	MOI[a]	Phenotype (Breed Affected)[b]	Gene	Mutation[c]
Progressive Retinal Atrophy 001244–9685	AR	Late-onset blindness (rdAC) (Abyssinian)	CEP290	IVS50 + 9T > G
Progressive Retinal Atrophy 000881–9685	AD	Early-onset blindness (rdy) (Abyssinian)	CRX	c.546delC
Progressive Retinal Atrophy 001613–9685	AR	Mid-onset blindness (Bengal)	KIF3B	c.1000G > A
Progressive Retinal Atrophy 001222–9685	AR	Early onset blindness (Persian)	AIPL1	c.577C > T
Polycystic Kidney Disease 000807–9685	AD	Kidney cysts (PKD) (Persian)	PKD1	c.10063C > A
Pyruvate Kinase Def. 000844–9685	AR	Hemopathy (PK Deficiency) (Abyssinian)	PKLR	c.693 + 304G > A
Spasticity 001621–9685	AR	Congenital myasthenic syndrome (CMS) (Devon Rex)	COLQ	c.1190G > A
Spinal Muscular Atrophy 000939–9685	AR	Muscular atrophy (SMA) (Maine Coon)	LIX1-LNPEP	Partial gene deletions

[a] Mode of inheritance of the non–wild-type variant.
[b] The breed affected represents the breed in which the DNA variant was identified. Other breeds may be affected if they have common ancestry, especially other breeds in a breed family. Not all transcripts for a given gene may have been discovered or well documented in the cat, DNA variants presented as interpreted from original publication. A "+" implies the wild-type allele when known. In reference to the variant allele, AD implies autosomal dominant, AR implies autosomal recessive, co-D implies co-dominant. OMIA: Online Mendelian Inheritance in Animals (http://omia.angis.org.au/home/) entries provides links to citations and clinical descriptions of the phenotypes and the diseases.
[c] Variants as presented in publications. Confirm variant positions if designing assays.

However, genes vary widely in size, with each gene, on average, having approximately 8.8 exons and 7.8 introns, covering approximately 10,000 to 15,000 base pairs (bp) of coding DNA within an overall region of 47,000 bp.[3] For small genes, such as *melanocortin receptor 1 (MC1R)*, which consists of one exon and is only approximately 600 bp in length, the candidate gene approach is fairly simple. For other genes, such as *PKD1*, which are larger with more than 40 exons, scanning is far more time-consuming and tedious to explore. The advancement of short-read sequencing

Table 2
The genes and DNA variants of uncommon inherited domestic cat diseases[a]

Disease	OMIA Entry	Gene	Mutation[b]
11b-hydroxylase Def. (congenital adrenal hyperplasia)	001661–9685	CYP11B1	Exon 7G > A
Dihydropyrimidinase deficiency	001776–9685	DPYS	c.1303G > A
Chediak-Higashi syndrome	000185–9685	LYST	20 Kb duplication
Copper metabolism	001071–9685	ATP7B	c.1585G > A, c.3890C > G
Cystinuria, type 1A	000256–9685	SLC3A1	c.1342C > T
Cystinuria, type B	002023–9685	SLC7A9	c.706G > A, c.881T > A, c.1175C > T
Ehlers-Danlos syndrome	002165–9685	COL5A1	c.3420delG
Factor XII deficiency	000364–9685	FXII	c.1321delC; c.1631G > C; c.1549C > T
Fibrodysplasia ossificans progressiva	000388–9685	ACVR1	c.617G > A
Gangliosidosis 1	000402–9685	GLB1	c.1448G > C
Gangliosidosis 2	001462–9685	HEXB	c.1467_1491inv
Gangliosidosis 2	001462–9685	HEXB	c.667C > T
Gangliosidosis 2	001427–9685	GM2A	c.390_393GGTC
Glaucoma 3, primary congenital	002017–9685	LTBP2	c.1998insGGAG
Hemophilia B	000438–9685	F9	c.247G > A, c.1014C > T
Hypertrophic Cardiomyopathy	002212–9685	MYH7	c.5647G > A
Hyperoxaluria	000821–9685	GRHPR	G > A I4 acceptor site
Hypogonadotropic hypogonadism	002219–9685	TAC3	c.220G > A
Hypothyroidism	000536–9685	TPO	c.1333G > A
Hypotrichosis, congenital with short life expectancy	001949–9685	FOXN1	c.1030_1033delCTGT
Inflammatory linear verrucous epidermal nevi	002185–9685	NSDHL	c.397A > G
Leukocyte adhesion deficiency	000595–9685	ITGB2	c.46_58 + 11del
Lipoprotein lipase deficiency	001210–9685	LPL	c.1234G > A
Methemoglobinopathy	002131–9685	CYB5R3	c.625G > A; c.232-1G > C
Mucolipidosis II	001248–9685	GNPTAB	c.2644C > T
Mannosidosis, alpha	000625–9685	LAMAN	c.1749_1752delCCAG
Mucopolysaccharidosis I	000664–9685	IDUA	c.1107_1109delCGA; c.1108_1110GAC
Mucopolysaccharidosis VI	000666–9685	ARSB	c.1427T > C; c.1558G > A
Mucopolysaccharidosis VII	000667–9685	GUSB	c.1052A > G; c.1421T > G, c.1424C > T
Muscular dystrophy	001081–9685	DMD	900 bp del M promoter -exon 1
Myotonia congenital	000698–9685	CLCN1	c.1930+1G > T
Niemann-Pick C1	000725–9685	NPC1	c.2864G > C, c.1322A > C
Niemann-Pick C2	002065–9685	NPC2	c.82+5G > A

(continued on next page)

Table 2
(continued)

Disease	OMIA Entry	Gene	Mutation[b]
Neuronal ceroid lipofuscinosis (NCL7)	001962–9685	MFSD8	c.19G > C, c.780delT
Porphyria (congenital erythropoietic)[c]	001175–9685	*UROS*	c.140 C > T, c.331 G > A
Porphyria (acute intermittent)[c]	001493–9685	*HMBS*	c.842_844delGAG, c.189dupT, c.250G > A, c.445C > T, c.107_110delACAG, c.826-1G > A
Rickets – Type IB	002221–9685	CYP2R1	c.1386delT
Testicular hypoplasia persistent primary dentition	002219–9685	TAC3	c.220G > A
Vitamin D–resistant rickets	000837–9685	CYP27B1	c.731delG; c.637G > T

[a] The presented conditions are not prevalent in breeds or populations but may have been established into research colonies.

[b] Not all transcripts for a given gene may have been discovered or well documented in the cat, mutations presented as interpreted from original publication. Confirm variant positions if designing assays.

[c] A variety of DNA variants have been identified, yet unpublished, for porphyrias in domestic cats. Contact PennGen at the University of Pennsylvania for additional information. OMIA: Online Mendelian Inheritance in Animals (http://omia.angis.org.au/home/) entries provides links to citations and clinical descriptions of the phenotypes and the diseases.

technologies, known as NextGeneration (NextGen) sequencing, has provided an alternative to the tedious sequencing of genes with many and or large exons.

Whole Genome and Whole Exome Sequencing

With the significant reduction of the cost of whole genome sequencing (WGS) (<$1000 per cat) and whole exome sequencing (WES) (<$250 per cat), the exploration for novel, causative DNA variants can be more cost-effective using WGS/WES than by sequencing one or more specific candidate genes one at a time (see "Precision/Genomic Medicine for Domestic Cats" by Buckley and Lyons, elsewhere in this issue). For example, if the patient had a suspected retinal degeneration or hypertrophic cardiomyopathy, WGS/WES would be a more cost-effective approach than attempting to directly sequence each of the dozens of genes known to cause either of these conditions. The candidate gene scanning approach is valid in particular cases when clinical data are highly indicative of a gene, but increasingly, the WGS/WES approach is supplanting historical techniques. Although genetic testing and candidate gene screening are aspects of P/GM, WGS/WES are the newest techniques to advance the concept. A veterinarian can now ask for WGS/WES to support the clinical diagnosis of a cat with a suspected heritable disease. Any of the mentioned genetic testing laboratories can help find researchers that can conduct WGS/WES to find novel disease mutations, or, in the near future, these laboratories may be offering the technique themselves.

Direct-to-Consumer DNA Testing in Cats

Animal genetic testing has been performed using a mixture of nondirect and DTC submissions. Historically, if a blood sample was required, or if blood or urine-based metabolites were assayed to support a clinical diagnosis, requests for genetic testing were usually submitted to university-based veterinary teaching hospitals, such as the Scott-Ritchey Research Center at Auburn University, (for gangliosidosis), or PennGen at the University of Pennsylvania (for lysosomal storage and other diseases). The advent of the polymerase chain reaction (PCR) and fluorescence-based direct Sanger sequencing indirectly supported the introduction of DTC genetic testing as these techniques allowed for smaller amounts of DNA to conduct a test. The release of the cat *PKD1* test was one of the first, large-scale DTC tests because DNA collected on buccal swabs could be submitted by owners directly to various testing laboratories around the world to get a direct DNA test for the variant causing polycystic kidney disease (PKD) in cats; no veterinarian needed to be involved. The test for PKD was first offered in 2005, which allowed cat owners, particularly owners of Persian or Persian-related cats, to determine which cats would develop cystic kidneys,[2] and hence, which cats may progress to early renal failure. Hopefully, the owner would relay this information to their veterinarian. Armed with these genetic test results, veterinarians could make dietary and other recommendations for affected cats and establish more diligent screening and wellness visits for *PKD1*-positive cats. Recent studies on dietary management in cats have suggested that interval feeding may slow cystic progression in PKD cats.[4,5]

Because veterinarians could now be circumvented in genetic testing, some laboratories invoked DNA profiling as a companion to the PKD test.[6] One outcome was if a cat's identity came into question, the DNA profile would link the *PKD1* test result with the correct animal. However, not all genetic laboratories perform this additional test. This lack of rigor is hidden from consumers and is a weakness in some DTC tests. Importantly, some cat registries still require samples to be collected and submitted by veterinarians, allowing the cat identity to be correlated with a microchip. *To improve accountability, DTC laboratories usually indicate on the test reports whether the sample was submitted by a veterinarian.*

Direct-to-Consumer Genetic Testing Panels

Because breeders show a strong interest in, and use aesthetic traits to support mating selections, a plethora of genetic testing in cats is available DTC. Commercial laboratories offering cat genetic testing have flourished to meet the demand of cat breeders to test for aesthetic traits and to support health care. To be competitive and to lower costs, commercial services have attempted to group several DNA tests into a variety of small "packages" of appropriate genetic tests for a breed. For example, common DNA variants in Abyssinians/Somalis are the known mutations for blood type, pyruvate kinase deficiency, and the 2 forms of progressive retinal atrophy (see **Table 1**). Alternatively, genetic testing in Persians and related breeds would instead include *PKD*, progressive retinal atrophy, folded ears, and most of the more than 15 variants affecting coat colors, as Persians need a different package of tests than Abyssinians/Somalis. The DNA testing "packages" or "panels" will expand and become more complex as research for genetic diseases and traits continues to be successful. Because different cat registries around the world have different breed standards and allow different outcrossing programs, the selection of appropriate tests for any one breed becomes very complex and also less efficient. Therefore, many DTC companies are offering all DNA tests to all cats, regardless of breed, for the sake of efficiency and to lower costs.

Limitations of Direct-to-Consumer Testing

Correct interpretation of results from DTC tests requires a solid understanding of the limits of the specific assay and the type of variant being tested. DNA variant types can range between single nucleotide variants/polymorphisms (SNV/SNP), small insertions or deletions (indel), or complex genetic structural variants (SV). The specific type of variant being tested dictates the best technologies that can be used to assay that given variant. In addition, DNA sequence composition and neutral DNA polymorphisms surrounding the disease mutation can also affect the design and results of an assay.[7] A single all-encompassing genetic technology capable of accurately and efficiently genotyping all types of disease-causing DNA variants is currently not available. Current technologies can assay many DNA variants, including DNA arrays, mass spectroscopy, quantitative (real-time, digital) PCR, and targeted genotyping-by-sequencing (GBS). These technologies are often used to develop genetic testing panels that may incorporate 10 or more disease/trait-causing DNA variants into one assay. Although one technology is used to assay a given genetic panel, each test may have a different error rate, due to the DNA variation surrounding the individual variants or to the nature of the variant itself (a small indel, SNP, or an SV). Therefore, reputable laboratories often use different technologies to validate, retest and support their main testing technology.

As DTC testing has become more competitive, the response by many commercial laboratories is to go "bigger and better," which usually compromises testing accuracy. Stochastically, some tests will fail. When DNA testing is conducted by targeted GBS or large DNA arrays (ie, large panels of tests), the accuracy of the genotype "call" will be reduced as compared with a well-established direct Sanger sequencing test (the Gold Standard), PCR-based allele-specific assays, or fragment analysis (ie, single assay tests). Every type of method to assay a specific DNA variant has its strengths and weaknesses. Testing for one DNA variant at a time provides more control over potential errors. Therefore, large-panel testing, where dozens of DNA variants are tested in one assay, are typically not recommended for diagnostic purposes for health care, as the error rates are higher and more difficult to control.[8,9] Many DTC laboratories often have a qualifying statement regarding "the non-use for health care decisions" within their disclaimer information, which is generally not carefully read by the consumer. Often, a second evaluation is recommended, particularly from a laboratory that either specializes and conducts research on the given disease, or by using a laboratory that has a variety of technologies for DNA variant genotyping. These laboratories are less directed to cost savings and high throughput and more directed toward accuracy and health care. In addition, laboratories using large panels usually require a bolus of samples to run their assays cost-effectively, therefore results may not be obtained for 4 to 10 weeks, potentially. Laboratories running single assays strive to report results within a few days. Hence, if a DNA panel has indicated a cat may be a carrier of a disease mutation, the same testing facility should have a second technology to support that finding. The breeder and/or veterinarian should be able to request a single-test assay for validation and to have a very specific and sensitive result before making a health decision.

Genetic Counseling

An additional concern for DTC panel testing is the reporting of disease-causing DNA variants that are not common to cats in general or are not common to the breed of cat being tested. Without proper genetic counseling and education, cat owners and veterinarians may experience undue concern and panic. For example, the mucopolysaccharidosis MPS VI variant causes a mild presentation for disease when in conjunction with a more severe variant. The mild variant is more prevalent in cat populations and can appear in genetic test results without the other severe MPS VI variant being present.[10] Here, inadequate education can lead some breeders to think they have cats carrying a disease-causing allele, which is not the case, and, which may lead them to eliminate a healthy cat from a breeding program. In addition, a DTC company may list dozens of disease-causing variants as a marketing strategy. Consumers may choose the company that provides the most tests for the lowest price. As mentioned, the more tests in a panel, the higher the error rate and the higher the chance for stochastic "drop-out" of a result. Second, more than 55 disease-causing variants have been found in random bred cats. These variants are very likely novel, sporadic and "one-off" DNA variants and will not be found in other cats. What may look like "bang-for-your-buck" is actually a large number of tests with an extremely high likelihood of being negative and ultimately unnecessary. Plus, education and genetic counseling should be provided for each disease, which is often not the case. Third, because many mutations are specific to a particular random bred cat, control samples for these variants are not likely acquired by all the different DTC companies, making test validation during development questionable. Synthetic DNA sequences can be used as positive controls, but this technique falls well short of working with natural DNA from cats, and may have other DNA polymorphisms surrounding the causal mutation. Therefore, several companies may be offering genetic tests that have never been robustly validated because positive control samples are not available.

Another concern for DTC testing is an owner or veterinarian may not realize that a given disease or phenotype has multiple DNA variants (alleles) that can cause the same presentation (see **Tables 1** and **2**). For example, if a DNA panel does not include all 4 DNA variants for taillessness in the cat, or the plethora of variants for cystinuria, porphyria, and blood type, improper result interpretation may occur. Owners and veterinarians are unfamiliar with the number of variants known or involved with diseases, and laboratories generally do not mention what they DO NOT test. This lack of education can lead to false assumptions and incorrect interpretations. Along the same vein, many laboratories do not provide adequate genetic counseling. If there is a concern for hypertrophic cardiomyopathy and DTC test results for the Maine Coon and the Ragdoll known variants are negative, the risk for hypertrophic cardiomyophathy is still relatively unknown but remains a concern. The cat just does not have the 2 *known* variants. In addition, although some laboratories offer testing for a variety of animals, a given laboratory may not have the same depth of expertise for all species, particularly as a means to reduce costs, thus, limiting genetic counseling and customer service.

General weaknesses of some large-panel DTC providers include the following:

1. Not using positive control samples to establish the accuracy of their developed tests
2. Incomplete transparency as to how tests are conducted and error rates determined
3. Slow reporting time, often 4 to 10 weeks
4. Some ignore patent rights and do not support the investigators who conducted the research to identify the variants from which they make profits
5. Poor customer service
   a. Poor knowledge of a breed/population – they don't know cats!
   b. Poor knowledge of the disease or trait
   c. Poor knowledge of the specifics of the variant
   d. Poor knowledge of surrounding DNA variation that can affect accuracy
   e. Poor response times

Many services post information regarding the scientific publication that documents the DNA variant, but good customer care has either genetic and or veterinary expertise to answer questions regarding interpretation of results. Also, many companies do not realize the consumer, be it the veterinarian or owner, may not know the proper questions to ask in the first place. For instance, if a genetic diversity test states that 2 cats are compatible for breeding, based on relatedness, this statement may not consider other DNA information that may indicate both cats in a breeding pair may carry a disease. In these cases, there is a risk of producing affected offspring or a blood type incompatibility in the kittens. All the results from the large panel need to be taken into consideration to make proper breeding recommendations.

The complexity of understanding cats and genetic tests is highlighted when considering coat color genetics. Tests for aesthetic traits really need strong support from staff who are quite familiar with cats. Breeders will make breeding decisions on the provided information, which, if not accurate or incorrectly interpreted, could lead to the production of unwanted kittens with less desired phenotypes.

FUTURE OF DIRECT-TO-CONSUMER GENETIC TESTING IN CATS

DTC genetic testing will likely grow and become a staple for cat breeders and cat owners. When conducted with rigor, DTC can be very useful and efficient, provided appropriate genetic counseling and customer service is available. Professionally educated genetic counselors provide information and guidance in human medicine, both prepartum and postpartum, supporting the role of the physician in health care. Veterinary medicine currently lacks professional genetic counselors, placing the burden on the veterinarian to understand all aspects of genetic testing. Perhaps a new profession, the veterinary genetic counselor, could fill the void in this newly developing area. Veterinary genetic counselors could provide the expertise regarding what tests are appropriate, the genetic aspects of a disease, the mode of inheritance, provide counseling for mating decisions, support the submission of genetic material, and, importantly, be able to decipher the technology and resulting sensitivities and specificities of DTC genetic tests for health care decisions.

REFERENCES

1. Jaffey JA, Reading NS, Giger U, et al. Clinical, metabolic, and genetic characterization of hereditary methemoglobinemia caused by cytochrome b5 reductase deficiency in cats. J Vet Intern Med 2019;33:2725–31.
2. Lyons LA, Biller DS, Erdman CA, et al. Feline polycystic kidney disease mutation identified in *PKD1*. J Am Soc Nephrol 2004;15:2548–55.
3. Sakharkar MK, Chow VT, Kangueane P. Distributions of exons and introns in the human genome. In Silico Biol 2004;4:387–93.
4. Yu Y, Shumway KL, Matheson JS, et al. Kidney and cystic volume imaging for disease presentation and progression in the cat autosomal dominant polycystic kidney disease large animal model. BMC Nephrol 2019;20:259.
5. Torres JA, Kruger SL, Broderick C, et al. Ketosis ameliorates renal cyst growth in polycystic kidney disease. Cell Metab 2019;30:1007–23.
6. Lipinski MJ, Amigues Y, Blasi M, et al. An international parentage and identification panel for the domestic cat (*Felis catus*). Anim Genet 2007;38:371–7.
7. Turba ME, Loechel R, Rombola E, et al. Evidence of a genomic insertion in intron 2 of *SOD1* causing allelic drop-out during routine diagnostic testing for canine degenerative myelopathy. Anim Genet 2017;48:365–8.
8. Longeri M, Chiodi A, Brilli M, et al. Targeted genotyping by sequencing: a new way to genome profile the cat. Anim Genet 2019;50(6):718–25.
9. Gandolfi B, Alhaddad H, Abdi M, et al. Applications and efficiencies of the first cat 63K DNA array. Sci Rep 2018;8:7024.
10. Lyons LA, Grahn RA, Genova F, et al. Mucopolysaccharidosis VI in cats - clarification regarding genetic testing. BMC Vet Res 2016;12:136.

Feline Infectious Peritonitis
Update on Pathogenesis, Diagnostics, and Treatment

Melissa A. Kennedy, DVM, PhD

KEYWORDS

- Feline infectious peritonitis • Feline coronavirus • Pathogenesis • Diagnostics
- Treatment

KEY POINTS

- Mutations lead to enhanced virulence of the feline coronavirus.
- Diagnosis requires multiple factors, including virus detection.
- Current developments in treatment of feline infectious peritonitis are ongoing and involve inhibition of virus replication and modification of the cat's immune response.

Feline infectious peritonitis (FIP) remains a frustrating and enigmatic disease for practitioners, and a heartbreaking diagnosis for the cat owner. There has been a great deal of research into not only understanding this disease but also improving diagnostics and developing treatment. This article summarizes new insights into this puzzling disease.

FIP is distinctive in that infection with the causative agent, feline coronavirus (FCoV), is common, but life-threatening FIP is not. FIP is most common in cats less than 2 years of age. Diagnosis is challenging, because identification of the FCoV, or the antibody response to this virus, is virtually useless in identifying FIP. There has been a great deal of research into the viral mutations responsible for disease development, but discovery of the changes that convert the relatively innocuous "good twin," which causes only mild to asymptomatic, self-resolving infection into the virulent "evil twin" causing lethal disease, have remained elusive.

SIGNALMENT, HISTORY, AND CLINICAL SIGNS

As already noted, FIP occurs most commonly in the young, often less than 1 year of age. Breed predisposition has been postulated, but susceptibility to FIP seems to occur primarily along familial lineages, with afflicted cats connected genetically through breeding lines.[1–3] Disease may occur in unrelated cats as well, such as shelter

Department of Biomedical and Diagnostic Sciences, College of Veterinary Medicine, University of Tennessee, Room A205 VMC, 2407 River Drive, Knoxville, TN 37996-4543, USA
E-mail address: mkenned2@utk.edu

Vet Clin Small Anim 50 (2020) 1001–1011
https://doi.org/10.1016/j.cvsm.2020.05.002
0195-5616/20/© 2020 Elsevier Inc. All rights reserved.

cats. Host factors known to contribute to the incidence of FIP include major histocompatibility complex (MHC) characteristics, quality of cytokine responses, and features of the cell-mediated immune (CMI) response.[4] It is known that cats that develop FIP mount a significant humoral response to the virus rather than a more effective CMI response. However, the identity of the precise molecular properties that predispose to disease development remains speculative.

History of a recent stressful event or condition, such as shelter housing and adoption, surgery (eg, spay or neuter), or even more subtle events (eg, changes in social hierarchy), is commonly noted.[5] Most afflicted cats originate in a high-density multicat setting, such as a breeding cattery or rescue facility,[6] increasing both the chance of exposure to FCoV and the quantity of FCoV being shed (through stress). Stress may also contribute to predisposition for development of FIP disease.

Clinical signs of FIP vary depending on the humoral response to the virus. It is known that the underlying pathologic condition is immune mediated involving at least in part antibody-dependent cytotoxicity and immune complex deposition[5] due to the robust, yet ineffective, antibody response to the virus and virus-infected cells. A relatively rapid course and widespread vasculitis is seen with the effusive or "wet" form, which manifests as fluid accumulation in the body cavities, particularly the abdomen. A more protracted, insidious course is observed with the noneffusive or "dry" form, and signs are referable to the organ or tissues involved. Examples include enteritis, renal disease, central nervous system disease, or anterior uveitis of one or both eyes. In most cats, illness includes vague signs of lethargy, decreased or absent appetite, weight loss, and fever often of a waxing-waning nature.

PATHOGENESIS UPDATE

How does this inevitably fatal disease follow infection in a small proportion of cats infected with a relatively innocuous and common virus? The agent, host properties, and environment play a role. Much investigation has gone into the agent itself, and what converts the "good twin," or avirulent FCoV, to the "evil twin," or virulent FIP virus (FIPV).

FCoV is a group I coronavirus, related to canine enteric coronavirus and transmissible gastroenteritis virus of pigs. Most field strains are type I FCoV, whereas type II FCoVs are more closely related antigenically to canine enteric coronavirus. Coronaviruses have a large RNA genome, which predisposes to a high mutation rate within a single isolate as well as the ability to undergo recombination between viruses when more than 1 virus isolate infects a cell.[7] It is thought that type II FCoVs are a result of a recombination event between a type I FCoV and a canine enteric coronavirus in the Spike envelope glycoprotein gene.[7,8] This resulted in a FCoV antigenically related to group I canine coronavirus.

Although infection with FCoV initially occurs in intestinal epithelial cells, the virus mutates and acquires the ability to enter and replicate in monocytes and macrophages. FIPV, the "evil twin," replicates with high efficiency in monocytes and macrophages.[7,9] This allows systemic spread of FIPV. Interestingly, as the efficiency of replication in monocytes and macrophages increases, the ability to replicate in enterocytes decreases.[10] Thus, FIPV is not shed or is shed at very low levels, which may be 1 reason FIP epidemics, unlike those observed with other pathogens (eg, panleukopenia virus or feline calicivirus), are uncommon.

Mutations occur as (corona)viruses replicate and copy their genome. RNA viruses are inherently mutable because their viral polymerase is prone to mistakes and lacks proofreading ability. Thus, the more a virus replicates, the more likely it is that mutations will arise. Chronic infections with ongoing virus replication are the perfect scenario for mutations to occur. FCoV is known to cause persistent infections with chronic, often intermittent shedding in feces.[5,10]

To understand the mutations, one has to have some familiarity with the genome of FCoV (**Fig. 1**). The first open reading frame (ORF) encodes more than 10 individual proteins used in replication of the virus. Next is the gene encoding the major envelope protein, the Spike protein (S). This protein is used in attachment of the virus to its target cell after which it enters the cell. This is followed by several ORFs encoding nonstructural proteins of unknown function, including the 3a-c ORFs. The M gene encodes the membrane protein, a small structural protein that interacts with the envelope as well as the core of the virus. The E gene produces a minor envelope protein, whereas the N gene encodes the capsomer protein, which covers the nucleic acid in a helical core. Finally, the 7a-b ORFs also encode nonstructural proteins of unknown function. Candidates for mutation, which leads to an FIP phenotype, are the Spike gene, 3a-c genes, the membrane gene, and the 7a-b ORFs.[11,12]

The viral genomic mutation that leads to the change in cellular tropism may contribute to a change in virulence and development of FIP. This change is due at least in part to a mutation in Spike envelope glycoprotein gene. Because this surface protein of the virus is needed for attachment of the virus to its target cell, it plays a major role in cellular tropism. The mutations seen in the Spike protein gene include 2 alternative codons identified by Chang and colleagues[13] that correlate with the FIP phenotype in greater than 95% of the isolates out of 183 FIPV isolates characterized at this genomic region. These nucleotide changes result in the alterations of amino acids in 2 positions within the region responsible for fusion between the viral envelope and the cell membrane. The investigators speculated that these changes lead to efficient replication of the virus in monocytes and macrophages. This change in cellular tropism is thought to play a role in development of FIP.

Licitra and colleagues[14] investigated the cleavage site within the Spike protein gene for changes that correlated with acquisition of the virulent nature. The investigators concluded that changes within this genomic region, which lead to modulation of the proteolytic enzyme furin family recognition site of the Spike protein, are critical for development of FIP. Furin proteolytic enzymes are calcium-dependent serine proteases that are commonly used by viruses to cleave precursor proteins into their active forms. Cleavage of the coronavirus Spike protein into its subunits uses this enzyme family.

At least 1 diagnostic polymerase chain reaction (PCR) for detection of the virus in biologic samples looks for the Spike gene mutation.[15,16] Whether this mutation is the only mutation associated with change in tropism or development of FIP is unknown. Although required for FIP, this change in tropism does not appear to be sufficient to cause FIP in all cats, because many cats have viruses present in the blood but are otherwise healthy.

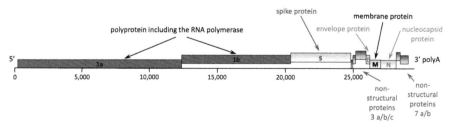

Fig. 1. FCoV genome with base number; bars indicate ORFs for FCoV proteins. (*Courtesy of* E. Barker, BSc(RVC), BVSc(Bristol), PhD(Bristol), DipECVIM-CA, Bristol, UK.)

In addition, the change in tropism is speculated to involve mutations in the 3c protein gene.[11,12] The 3c protein is a nonstructural viral protein of unknown function. In 1 study, all fecal isolates of FCoV had an intact 3c gene; those with deletions in the 3c gene were not shed in feces.[11] The investigators concluded that an intact 3c gene was required for intestinal replication. The change in cellular tropism may result in loss of the ability to replicate in intestinal epithelia, which may additionally explain why outbreaks of FIP in multiple cats are rarely seen.

Other mutations speculated to affect the virulence of the virus include those occurring in the genes encoding the nonstructural proteins 7a and 7b ORFs. The protein products are of unknown function, but mutations in these genes have been found in the virus detected in cases of FIP.[12,17] These mutations include deletional mutations of 7a ORF as well as multiple mutations in the 7b protein gene. However, mutations in these ORFs are not consistently occurring in viruses of FIP, limiting usefulness of tests directed at identifying these ORFs.

Mutations in the gene encoding the membrane protein of FCoV have been studied. Brown and colleagues[18] identified mutations in the M gene of FIPV, which correlated with the virulent biotype. However, other studies have not found consistent changes in the M gene to be associated with the FIP phenotype.[12] In fact, it may be that more than 1 mutation is required and may not be identical in all FIP viruses. This contributes to the frustration of developing a single, noninvasive diagnostic test for FIP.

Host factors are also important in development of FIP. These factors include genetic characteristics, age, and concurrent disease, especially immunosuppressive diseases and can all affect the cat's immune system status, including MHC diversity, cytokine production, and lymphocyte apoptosis. For example, aspects of MHC II may affect the ability and quality of the immune response to clear the virus or affect the predisposition to a humoral response to FCoV.[4] Production of cytokines, such as interferon-γ (which enhances the cellular immune response), may be altered.[19] T lymphocytes, which do not support viral infection and replication and remain free from infection, are known to undergo apoptosis in cats with FIP.[20] This lymphocyte apoptosis may result from the increased tumor necrosis factor-α (TNF-α) production found in cats with FIP.[21,22]

The precise role that genetics plays is unknown and depends on observed occurrences in different epidemiologic studies. FIP attacks certain familial lines of cats, and certain breeds appear to be more susceptible. Heritability to susceptibility is known to occur. In at least 1 study, the heterozygosity of an individual appears to be an important role such that loss of heterozygosity correlates with increased susceptibility and decreased resistance to FIP.[2,3] Inbreeding and using the sire or queen of cats that developed FIP should be avoided.

Environmental factors, including stressors, also seem to influence FIP development. Cats originating from, or living in, multicat settings are more likely to develop FIP. This development may be because the likelihood of FCoV infection is higher where multiple cats live together.[6,23] Other factors leading to FCoV exposure include high density of cats, frequent introductions, reintroductions, mingling of cats from different sources (eg, shelters, breeding facilities, at cat shows), presence of chronic FCoV shedders, and inadequate disinfection. In addition, stress can increase glucocorticoid production, which can negatively impact T lymphocytes, directly resulting in decreased CMI and lack of virus clearance.

DIAGNOSTICS UPDATE

Diagnosis of FIP remains a combination of signalment, history, and clinical signs along with a variety of clinical assays. One can think of it as building the diagnostic wall, brick by brick. Unfortunately, the best test remains histopathology using immunohisto-chemical staining (IHC) of affected tissues for FCoV, often only done post mortem.

Complete blood count findings include nonspecific leukocytosis with a lymphopenia in the terminal stages, and a normocytic normochromic anemia. Flow cytometry for immunophenotyping can aid in diagnosis: a study published in 2003 showed a selective decrease in T lymphocytes even in cats with normal total lymphocyte counts.[24] Although the investigators found that this alteration in lymphocyte distribution was not specific for FIP, they did identify a negative predictive value of 100% for a normal lymphocyte distribution on flow cytometry of whole blood. In addition, Pedersen and colleagues[20] found that lymphopenia characterized disease progression. In fact, the degree and time of onset of lymphopenia were predictors for terminal disease development: the greater the degree and earlier the onset were associated with increased severity and speed of disease progression. This effect on lymphocytes is puzzling given that the virus does not replicate in them. It has been speculated that the effect of the virus on monocytes and macrophages, important cytokine producers, may lead to lymphocyte apoptosis. Specifically, secretion of TNF-α may result in this phenomenon.[21]

Serum biochemistry changes reflect the organ or organs involved. Usually there is an elevated total protein and, almost always, a decreased albumin-to-globulin ratio (A:G) reflecting the increase in γ-globulins.[25] A study by Jeffery and colleagues[26] found that an A:G greater than 0.6 to 0.8 has a high negative predictive value for FIP. Thus, although specificity of a low A:G is poor, finding a higher A:G is helpful in ruling out FIP when prevalence in the population is low. A decreased A:G may be accompanied by a polyclonal gammopathy on serum protein electrophoresis. Most cats with FIP have bilirubinemia and bilirubinuria. This increase in bilirubin levels is due to destruction of red blood cells and accumulation of hemoglobin that often accompanies FIP, rather than hepatic involvement.[27] None of these findings are pathognomonic on their own.

Analysis of effusion fluid is extremely helpful. Typically, it is a cellular-, protein-, and fibrin-rich modified transudate. A recent study showed an elevation in acute phase proteins (APP), such as haptoglobin, serum amyloid A, and α-1 acid glycoprotein (AGP).[28] In this study, AGP was identified as the best APP to distinguish between cats with and without FIP in effusion, and a cutoff value of 1550 μg/mL had a sensitivity and specificity of 93% each for diagnosing FIP. However, the effusive form is not as challenging to diagnose as the noneffusive form, which may often manifest with vague signs and nonspecific blood parameters. Ultrasound may identify small amounts of fluid in the abdomen or pleural cavity to harvest for diagnostic evaluation.[29]

FCoV-specific testing involves virus-specific antibody testing and identification of FCoV infection through antigen or genetic detection. Serology for FCoV-specific antibody is known to be of little value. The presence of antibody regardless of magnitude only indicates exposure to FCoV.[30] The variability that exists among diagnostic laboratories in terms of cutoff values for FIP diagnosis as well as the strain of the virus used in the assay affects results of serologic assays and must also be considered. Although an elevated antibody titer is consistent with FIP, it is also seen in healthy FCoV-infected cats. In addition, cats with FIP may have low or negative FCoV antibody titers. This decrease in antibody levels may reflect binding of antibody by abundant virus, or immune exhaustion. Thus, antibody testing for FIP diagnosis is of dubious value. Even elevated antibody levels to virus-specific 7b protein, which had been speculated to be expressed only by the evil twin, have been shown to be nonspecific.[31] In neurologic disease, assessment of cerebrospinal fluid (CSF) antibody levels may be helpful: 1 study reported that a titer of greater than 640 in CSF was indicative of FIP.[32]

That leaves detection of the virus itself. This virus detection may be done through antigen detection, which for antemortem diagnosis often involves immunofluorescence (IF) of virus-infected cells. The highest sensitivity of this test is on macrophages from an effusion.[32] This study showed a sensitivity of 100% and a specificity of 71.4% for FCoV IF. The sample size in this investigation was small (10 cats with confirmed FIP, 7 cats without FIP). In addition, this test again requires effusive fluid, which is present only in the wet form of FIP. IF may be done on tissue samples from cases of the dry form, usually not sampled ante mortem. A study by Rissi[33] found that IF on fresh tissue samples was far inferior to IHC for FCoV detection in cases of neurologic FIP. Thus, the investigators concluded that IHC was more sensitive and reliable for FIP diagnosis than IF.

Alternatively, PCR used for genetic detection is likely the most common mode of virus identification currently. However, how to tell the "evil twin" from the "good twin" via PCR has remained problematic. It was first thought that detection of virus in the blood would be diagnostic for FIPV. However, FCoV may often be detected in blood of unaffected cats,[34] and conversely, especially in the dry form, detection of virus in the blood may be difficult.[16] Virus load is also of dubious helpfulness because cats from households where FCoV infection is occurring may have high-level viremia.

At least 1 commercial assay quantifies the amount of messenger RNA (mRNA) of the virus, specifically of the Membrane protein. The amount or copy numbers of viral mRNA correlates with degree of virus replication. Thus, its presence in samples from extraintestinal sites indicates viral replication in this tissue/fluid. FIPV is known to replicate efficiently in monocytes and macrophages, whereas the enteric form of the virus does not. Finding significant quantities of the viral mRNA in blood, effusion, or tissue indicates the presence of the virus of FIP. This assay, according to the laboratory data, identifies the virus of FIP with high specificity, and its absence indicates that replicating FIPV is not present.[35]

Several mutations have been found to be associated with FIP development. These mutations include point mutations in the Membrane protein gene, as well as in the gene encoding the nonstructural protein 3c; deletional mutations in the 7b nonstructural protein gene; and dual nucleotide changes in the Spike protein gene. Brown and colleagues[18] identified mutations in the Membrane protein gene that correlated with development of FIP. The investigators speculate that superinfection with the mutated virus occurs as opposed to mutations of an internal isolate. Hora and colleagues[36] concluded that the mutations in the M gene and homology of enteric and systemic FCoV supported the theory that in vivo mutation of the infecting isolate leads to FIP.

Much attention has been given to the nonstructural protein genes 3c and 7b. Deletional mutations leading to truncation of the 3c protein have been associated with systemic spread of the virus and loss of the ability to replicate in intestinal epithelial cells. Pedersen and colleagues[10] found that an intact 3c gene characterized all intestinal isolates of FCoV in their study and were the only FCoV isolates shed in the feces. They concluded that an intact 3c gene is required for intestinal replication. Bank-Wolf and colleagues[12] found that mutations in 3c along with changes in the spike protein gene were correlated with the FIP phenotype, whereas there were no changes in the Membrane protein or the 7a and 7b proteins that were associated with FIP. These seemingly conflicting results emphasize the difficulty in understanding of FIP pathogenesis as well as the mutability of the FCoV genome.

The presence of point mutations in the Spike protein gene has led to the availability of PCR assays, which identify the presence of these mutations. Although these assays may be helpful, it is not clear that these mutations are present in every case of FIP nor if these mutations may be present in asymptomatic virus-infected cats. In addition, effusive fluid remains the substrate of choice, which is absent in the noneffusive form of the disease.[37] In a study by Felten and colleagues[16] of 127 cats, of which 63 had FIP, the researchers found a specificity of 100% but a low sensitivity of 6.5% (serum or plasma) to 65% (effusion). The investigators concluded that although a positive PCR assay for the Spike mutation was good evidence for FIP, a negative result could not rule out this diagnosis, especially when testing serum or plasma. Another study by Barker and colleagues[38] found that of 102 cats, 57 with FIP, identification of mutations within the Spike protein gene does not significantly enhance the diagnosis of FIP compared with detection of FCoV alone by reverse transcription PCR.

Nevertheless, PCR is a useful assay regardless of the methodology used because it reveals the systemic spread and presence of the virus in extraintestinal sites. However, one must always remember that false negative and positive results are possible, meaning that although one more brick in that diagnostic wall, it is not possible to confirm a diagnosis of FIP with PCR alone. If the mutated or replicating virus is found in the blood, effusion, or tissue sample, along with the other indicators of FIP described here, it is good evidence of a diagnosis of FIP.

The gold standard remains histopathology with IHC for FCoV on affected tissue.[33,39] The distribution of lesions are vascular and perivascular and are usually pyogranulomatous in nature. Unfortunately, this involves invasive collection of samples, which is often not possible in a sick and debilitated cat. There was hope that testing of fine needle aspirates (FNA) of affected organs/tissue would be diagnostic. However, an investigation by Felten and colleagues[40] found that FNA used for IHC could neither confirm nor rule out FIP. Thus, the diagnosis of FIP ante mortem still requires construction of a diagnostic wall by identifying host factors and detecting the virus.

TREATMENT UPDATE

There are 2 approaches to the treatment of FIP: (1) modification of the cat's immune response to the FCoV, and (2) direct inhibition of FCoV replication.

Because FIP is an immune-mediated disease, the use of corticosteroids to suppress negative aspects of the immune response, including the humoral response, has long been the only option in treating this disease. This corticosteroid administration may provide some palliative relief, but does not affect the outcome. Corticosteroids may be most useful when the lesions are focal and restricted to a single tissue, such as anterior uveitis. Depending on the severity of disease and host factors, cats with FIP may survive for weeks or months.

Cytokines have been used for immune response modification with limited success. Interferon, both feline and human recombinant, has not shown any positive effect on cats with FIP.[41] The use of polyprenyl immunostimulant to enhance the T-lymphocyte response in an effort to promote CMI in the cat has variable success. The mechanism of action of this drug remains unclear. Some success has been documented with the dry form of FIP, enhancing survival of affected cats. However, this same success has not been seen in cats with the wet form of FIP.[42] In a field study using this compound, 8 cats out of 60 with FIP survived greater than 200 days, and 4 survived beyond 300 days. All had the dry form of FIP.[43]

Treatments targeting FCoV replication hold great hope. Antiviral drugs ideally target the pathogen specifically without affecting uninfected cells. Viral enzymes necessary for replication are good targets for intervention. In particular, viral proteases responsible for protein processing are often required for maturation of virus structure and may be excellent candidates for impacting virus replication. As mentioned earlier, coronaviruses are known to encode proteases necessary for viral protein cleavage that are viable targets for antiviral drugs. Such compounds have been synthesized and tested for efficacy against the coronaviral agents of severe acute respiratory syndrome and FIP with some success. Compounds have been identified that inhibit virus protease activity both in vitro and in vivo.[44] One, GC376, was found to inhibit disease development and led to remission in cats infected with FIPV.[45] The minimum course of therapy with GC376 was found to be 12 weeks. Thirteen of 20 cats with naturally occurring FIP in the trial ultimately succumbed to recurrence of disease, but 7 survived. Side effects included pain and subcutaneous inflammation at the injection site and delayed loss or retention of deciduous teeth and delayed development of adult teeth. Development of viral resistance to the drug was not noted. This drug requires further research but holds promise in treating FIP.

A nucleoside analogue, GS5734, and its parent drug, GS441524, developed to treat human viral infections, were tested for efficacy against FIPV. GS441524 was evaluated in vitro in feline cells and subsequently in vivo in laboratory cats.[46] A field trial in cats with naturally acquired FIP followed.[47] Twenty-six cats were tested with the drug for a 12-week period. Eighteen cats remained healthy, whereas 5 cats that relapsed were treated a second time at a higher dosage and went into remission. Two cats were treated for 2 relapses also responded well; thus, 25 cats were long-term survivors.

Currently, these drugs are not commercially available. They are available illegally through the black market. According to Dr Neils Pedersen, one of the coinvestigators of these drugs as therapeutics," A number of entities, largely in China, are manufacturing GS-441524 (GS) and GC376 (GC) for sale mainly to desperate owners of cats with FIP. Although the first effort was centered on GC, the emphasis of this black-market has rapidly shifted to GS. Although this sort of marketing and use of GS and GC is technically illegal and it could be considered unethical for veterinarians to assist in treating cats with such drugs, the companies holding patents on GC and GS have no effective means to halt this black-market use."[48] Therefore, use of these products is currently not advised except for research purposes.

Experimentally, a process using small interfering RNA has shown efficacy in limiting virus replication in vitro. It does this by inducing posttranscriptional gene silencing: small pieces of RNA duplexes corresponding to genomic sequences of FCoV are introduced and lead to sequence-specific targeting of viral mRNA for endonuclease destruction. This treatment has been effective in vitro for FCoV.[42,49,50] It remains to be seen whether this technology can be used in vivo for FCoV. Several obstacles remain, including drug delivery and eliminating off-target effects. However, this technology holds promise for therapeutic applications.

SUMMARY

FIP remains a feared and heartbreaking diagnosis. Because of its high mortality and the high prevalence of FCoV infection, not only is it a serious disease but also it can be frustrating to diagnose, and even more frustrating to treat. Diagnosis remains a combination of indicators, including detection of the virus. The future holds much promise for effective treatment regimens for FIP involving both modification of the host's immune response and inhibition of viral replication.

REFERENCES

1. Pesteanu-Somogyi LD, Radzai C, Pressler BM. Prevalence of feline infectious peritonitis in specific cat breeds. J Feline Med Surg 2006;8(1):1–5.

2. Pedersen NC, Liu H, Gandolfi B, et al. The influence of age and genetics on natural resistance to experimentally induced feline infectious peritonitis. Vet Immunol Immunopathol 2014;162(1–2):33–40.

3. Pedersen NC, Liu H, Durden M, et al. Natural resistance to experimental feline infectious peritonitis virus infection is decreased rather than increased by positive genetic selection. Vet Immunol Immunopathol 2016;171:17–20.

4. Addie DD, Kennedy LJ, Ryvar R, et al. Feline leucocyte antigen class II polymorphism and susceptibility to feline infectious peritonitis. J Feline Med Surg 2004; 6(2):59–62.

5. Hartmann K. Feline infectious peritonitis. Vet Clin North Am Small Anim Pract 2005;35(1):39–79, vi.

6. Drechsler Y, Alcaraz A, Bossong FJ, et al. Feline coronavirus in multicat environments. Vet Clin North Am Small Anim Pract 2011;41(6):1133–69.

7. Herrewegh A, Smeenk I, Horzinek MC, et al. Feline coronavirus type II strains 79-1683 and 79-1146 originate from a double recombination between feline coronavirus type I and canine coronavirus. J Virol 1998;72(5):4508–14.

8. Tekes G, Hofmann-Lehmann R, Bank-Wolf B, et al. Chimeric feline coronaviruses that encode type II spike protein on type I genetic background display accelerated viral growth and altered receptor usage. J Virol 2010;84(3):1326–33.

9. Pedersen NC. An update on feline infectious peritonitis: virology and immunopathogenesis. Vet J 2014;201(2):123–32.

10. Pedersen NC, Liu H, Scarlett J, et al. Feline infectious peritonitis: role of the feline coronavirus 3c gene in intestinal tropism and pathogenicity based upon isolates from resident and adopted shelter cats. Virus Res 2012;165(1):17–28.

11. Borschensky CM, Reinacher M. Mutations in the 3c and 7b genes of feline coronavirus in spontaneously affected FIP cats. Res Vet Sci 2014;97(2):333–40.

12. Bank-Wolf BR, Stallkamp I, Wiese S, et al. Mutations of 3c and spike protein genes correlate with the occurrence of feline infectious peritonitis. Vet Microbiol 2014;173(3–4):177–88.

13. Chang HW, Egberink HF, Halpin R, et al. Spike protein fusion peptide and feline coronavirus virulence. Emerg Infect Dis 2012;18(7):1089–95.

14. Licitra BN, Millet JK, Regan AD, et al. Mutation in spike protein cleavage site and pathogenesis of feline coronavirus. Emerg Infect Dis 2013;19(7):1066–73.

15. Felten S, Weider K, Doenges S, et al. Detection of feline coronavirus spike gene mutations as a tool to diagnose feline infectious peritonitis. J Feline Med Surg 2017;19(4):321–35.

16. Felten S, Leutenegger CM, Balzer HJ, et al. Sensitivity and specificity of a real-time reverse transcriptase polymerase chain reaction detecting feline coronavirus mutations in effusion and serum/plasma of cats to diagnose feline infectious peritonitis. BMC Vet Res 2017;13(1):228.

17. Kennedy M, Boedeker N, Gibbs P, et al. Deletions in the 7a ORF of feline coronavirus associated with an epidemic of feline infectious peritonitis. Vet Microbiol 2001;81:227–34.

18. Brown MA, Troyer JL, Pecon-Slattery J, et al. Genetics and pathogenesis of feline infectious peritonitis virus. Emerg Infect Dis 2009;15(9):1445–52.

19. Giordano A, Paltrinieri S. Interferon-gamma in the serum and effusions of cats with feline coronavirus infection. Vet J 2009;180(3):396–8.

20. Pedersen NC, Eckstrand C, Liu H, et al. Levels of feline infectious peritonitis virus in blood, effusions, and various tissues and the role of lymphopenia in disease outcome following experimental infection. Vet Microbiol 2015;175(2–4):157–66.

21. Takano T, Hohdatsu T, Hashida Y, et al. A "possible" involvement of TNF-alpha in apoptosis induction in peripheral blood lymphocytes of cats with feline infectious peritonitis. Vet Microbiol 2007;119(2–4):121–31.

22. Takano T, Hohdatsu T, Toda A, et al. TNF-alpha, produced by feline infectious peritonitis virus (FIPV)-infected macrophages, upregulates expression of type II FIPV receptor feline aminopeptidase N in feline macrophages. Virology 2007; 364(1):64–72.

23. Addie DD, Belak S, Boucrat-Baralon C, et al. Feline infectious peritonitis: ABCD guidelines on prevention and management. J Feline Med Surg 2009;11:594–604.

24. Paltrinieri S, Ponti W, Comazzi S, et al. Shifts in circulating lymphocyte subsets in cats with feline infectious peritonitis (FIP): pathogenic role and diagnostic relevance. Vet Immunol Immunopathol 2003;96(3–4):141–8.

25. Riemer F, Kuehner KA, Ritz S, et al. Clinical and laboratory features of cats with feline infectious peritonitis–a retrospective study of 231 confirmed cases (2000-2010). J Feline Med Surg 2016;18(4):348–56.

26. Jeffery U, Deitz K, Hostetter S. Positive predictive value of albumin: globulin ratio for feline infectious peritonitis in a mid-western referral hospital population. J Feline Med Surg 2012;14(12):903–5.

27. Pedersen NC. An update on feline infectious peritonitis: diagnostics and therapeutics. Vet J 2014;201(2):133–41.

28. Hazuchova K, Held S, Neiger R. Usefulness of acute phase proteins in differentiating between feline infectious peritonitis and other diseases in cats with body cavity effusions. J Feline Med Surg 2017;19(8):809–16.

29. Tasker S. Diagnosis of feline infectious peritonitis. J Feline Med Surg 2018;20: 228–43.

30. Paltrinieri S, Paroda Cammarata M, Comazzi S. Some aspects of humoral and cellular immunity in naturally occurring feline infectious peritonitis. Vet Immunol Immunopathol 1998;65:205–20.

31. Kennedy MA, Abd-Eldaim M, Zika SE, et al. Evaluation of antibodies against feline coronavirus 7b protein for diagnosis of feline infectious peritonitis in cats. Am J Vet Res 2008;69(9):1179–82.

32. Litster AL, Pogranichniy R, Lin TL. Diagnostic utility of a direct immunofluorescence test to detect feline coronavirus antigen in macrophages in effusive feline infectious peritonitis. Vet J 2013;198(2):362–6.

33. Rissi DR. A retrospective study of the neuropathology and diagnosis of naturally occurring feline infectious peritonitis. J Vet Diagn Invest 2018;30(3):392–9.

34. Meli M, Kipar A, Muller C, et al. High viral loads despite absence of clinical and pathological findings in cats experimentally infected with feline coronavirus (FCoV) type I and in naturally FCoV-infected cats. J Feline Med Surg 2004;6(2): 69–81.

35. Simons FA, Vennema H, Rofina JE, et al. A mRNA PCR for the diagnosis of feline infectious peritonitis. J Virol Methods 2005;124(1–2):111–6.

36. Hora AS, Asano KM, Guerra JM, et al. Intrahost diversity of feline coronavirus: a consensus between the circulating virulent/avirulent strains and the internal mutation hypotheses? ScientificWorldJournal 2013;2013:572325.

37. Longstaff L, Porter E, Crossley VJ, et al. Feline coronavirus quantitative reverse transcriptase polymerase chain reaction on effusion samples in cats with and without feline infectious peritonitis. J Feline Med Surg 2017;19(2):240–5.

38. Barker EN, Stranieri A, Helps CR, et al. Limitations of using feline coronavirus spike protein gene mutations to diagnose feline infectious peritonitis. Vet Res 2017;48(1):60.

39. Ziolkowska N, Pazdzior-Czapula K, Lewczuk B, et al. Feline infectious peritonitis: immunohistochemical features of ocular inflammation and the distribution of viral antigens in structures of the eye. Vet Pathol 2017;54(6):933–44.
40. Felten S, Hartmann K, Doerfelt S, et al. Immunocytochemistry of mesenteric lymph node fine-needle aspirates in the diagnosis of feline infectious peritonitis. J Vet Diagn Invest 2019;31(2):210–6.
41. Ritz S, Egberink H, Hartmann K. Effect of feline interferon-omega on the survival time and quality of life of cats with feline infectious peritonitis. J Vet Intern Med 2007;21(6):1193–7.
42. Anis EA, Wilkes RP, Kania SA, et al. Effect of small interfering RNAs on in vitro replication and expression of feline coronavirus. Am J Vet Res 2014;75(9): 828–34.
43. Legendre AM, Kuritz T, Galyon G, et al. Polyprenyl immunostimulant treatment of cats with presumptive non-effusive feline infectious peritonitis in a field study. Front Vet Sci 2017;4:7.
44. Kim Y, Shivanna V, Narayanan S, et al. Broad-spectrum inhibitors against 3C-like proteases of feline coronaviruses and feline caliciviruses. J Virol 2015;89(9): 4942–50.
45. Pedersen NC, Kim Y, Liu H, et al. Efficacy of a 3C-like protease inhibitor in treating various forms of acquired feline infectious peritonitis. J Feline Med Surg 2018; 20(4):378–92.
46. Murphy BG, Perron M, Murakami E, et al. The nucleoside analog GS-441524 strongly inhibits feline infectious peritonitis (FIP) virus in tissue culture and experimental cat infection studies. Vet Microbiol 2018;219:226–33.
47. Pedersen NC, Perron M, Bannasch M, et al. Efficacy and safety of the nucleoside analog GS-441524 for treatment of cats with naturally occurring feline infectious peritonitis. J Feline Med Surg 2019;21(4):271–81.
48. Pedersen NC. Fifty years' fascination with FIP culminates in a promising new antiviral. J Feline Med Surg 2019;21(4):269–70.
49. McDonagh P, Sheehy PA, Norris JM. Combination siRNA therapy against feline coronavirus can delay the emergence of antiviral resistance in vitro. Vet Microbiol 2015;176(1–2):10–8.
50. McDonagh P, Sheehy PA, Norris JM. In vitro inhibition of feline coronavirus replication by small interfering RNAs. Vet Microbiol 2011;150(3–4):220–9.

What's New in Feline Leukemia Virus Infection

Katrin Hartmann, Prof Dr med vet, Dr habil[a],*,
Regina Hofmann-Lehmann, Prof Dr med vet, FVH[b]

KEYWORDS

- FeLV • Regressive infection • Latent infection • PCR • Pathogenesis • Risk factors
- FeLV-associated diseases • Veterinary sciences

KEY POINTS

- Understanding the *pathogenesis of feline leukemia virus (FeLV) infection* is important to control and to further decrease prevalence of FeLV infection.
- Some factors influence the prevalence of FeLV, whereas other factors influence the course of infection and development of disease by altering the unstable balance between the immune system and the virus.
- There are 4 different courses of FeLV infection: progressive, regressive, abortive, and focal atypical infection, that can be distinguished by consecutive use of different diagnostic tests.
- Regressive FeLV infection rarely leads to clinical syndromes, but sometimes bone marrow disorders or lymphomas can be caused by integrated provirus without active virus replication.
- Regressively FeLV-infected cats do not shed the virus, but proviral DNA can be transmitted via blood transfusion leading to infection of the recipient.

INTRODUCTION

Feline leukemia virus (FeLV) is one of the most common infectious agents in cats worldwide. Prevalence and importance of FeLV have been decreasing over the past decades, primarily because of effective testing and eradication programs as well as routine use of FeLV vaccines. However, recent studies indicate that the decrease in prevalence has stagnated in many countries; therefore, awareness of this important infection and its prevention should not be neglected because this could allow resurgence in prevalence. There are different courses of FeLV infection: progressive,

[a] Clinic of Small Animal Medicine, Centre for Clinical Veterinary Medicine LMU Munich, Veterinaerstrasse 13, Munich 80539, Germany; [b] Clinical Laboratory, Department for Clinical Diagnostics and Services, Vetsuisse Faculty, University of Zurich, Winterthurerstrasse 260, Zurich 8057, Switzerland
* Corresponding author.
E-mail address: hartmann@uni-muenchen.de

Vet Clin Small Anim 50 (2020) 1013–1036
https://doi.org/10.1016/j.cvsm.2020.05.006
0195-5616/20/© 2020 Elsevier Inc. All rights reserved.

vetsmall.theclinics.com

regressive, abortive, and focal atypical infection, that have been characterized experimentally. However, field cats do not always follow the predefined courses and can present with confusing and contradictory test results.

The outcome of FeLV infection is determined by a battle between the cat's immune system and the virus; this is true particularly in the early phase of infection, usually over the first 12 weeks after exposure, when the course the infection will take is determined. In a few cats, the balance between virus and immune system will be unstable lifelong. The balance between host and virus can be altered by different factors, such as immunosuppression, coinfections, or change in environment, leading to a change in the outcome of FeLV infection and prognosis for the cat. These different courses and infection outcomes, along with the different meanings of the various diagnostic tests, pose significant challenges to the veterinarian needing to make decisions on management and judgments on the prognosis in a specific cat at any given point in time. Regressive infections and their implications especially are still poorly understood, and their impact on the health of cats is likely underestimated.

PATHOGENESIS OF FELINE LEUKEMIA VIRUS INFECTION

FeLV is a gammaretrovirus of domestic cats that belongs to the oncornavirus subfamily of retroviruses. Exogenous (foreign, "pathogenic") and endogenous (inherited, "nonpathogenic") retroviruses occur in cats.[1] The endogenous retroviruses (enFeLVs) are integrated into the genome of all domestic cats, in every cell line.[1] EnFeLVs might increase pathogenicity of exogenous FeLV, for example, as counterparts for recombination with exogenous FeLV (FeLV A) and subsequent development of other more pathogenic FeLV subgroups.[2] Interestingly, however, a recent study found that enFeLV copy numbers were inversely related to FeLV viral load and were associated with a better FeLV outcome.[3,4]

FeLV was first described in 1964 by Jarrett and coworkers,[5] when virus particles were seen budding from the membrane of malignant lymphoblasts from a cat with lymphoma.[6,7]

FeLV contains a protein core with single-stranded RNA protected by an envelope (**Fig. 1**). It replicates within many tissues, including bone marrow, salivary glands, and respiratory epithelium.[8] If the cat's immune response does not intervene after initial infection, FeLV spreads to the bone marrow and infects hematopoietic precursor cells.[9]

All retroviruses, including FeLV, rely on a DNA intermediate for replication. The single-stranded RNA genome is reversely transcribed into DNA, which, via an integrase, is integrated into the host's cell genome (the integrated DNA is called "provirus").[10] After reverse transcription, synthesis of viral proteins occurs with assembly of the virions near the cell membrane and budding from the cell. Infection of a cell by a retrovirus does not usually lead to cell death (**Fig. 2**). Once the provirus is integrated, cell division results in daughter cells that also contain viral DNA. The ability of the virus to become part of the host's own DNA is crucial for the lifelong persistence of the virus after bone marrow infection.[11–13]

Transmission

FeLV is contagious and spreads through close contact between virus-shedding cats and susceptible cats. Transmission of FeLV occurs primarily via saliva. Progressively infected cats shed millions of virus particles in saliva, and shedding through saliva occurs relatively consistently throughout the life of these cats.[14,15] FeLV is passed effectively horizontally among communal cats that have close contact. Fighting and biting

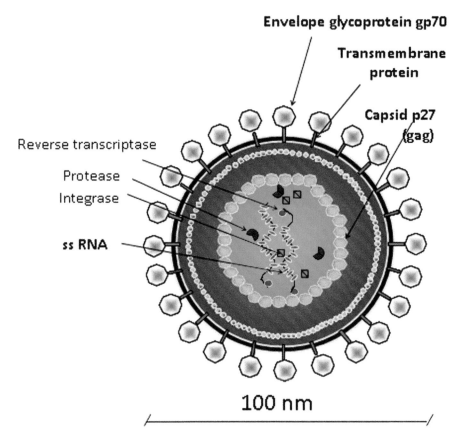

Fig. 1. FeLV particle. FeLV is an enveloped virus, which makes it rather unstable in the environment. FeLV is an RNA virus; thus to detect the viral genome a reverse transcriptase PCR is necessary (RT-PCR). The virus carries an enzyme (reverse transcriptase) that converts the viral RNA into DNA, once the virus has entered the host cell. The virus contains a viral capsid made of protein with a molecular weight of 27 kDa and called p27. This protein is detected in the virus antigen tests (point-of-care test [POCT], laboratory ELISA). ssRNA, single-stranded RNA. (*Courtesy of* R. Hofmann-Lehmann, Prof. Dr. med. vet., FVH, Zurich, Switzerland.)

behavior,[16,17] as well as affiliative social behavior, such as sharing food and water dishes and mutual grooming, are the most effective means of transmission. FeLV is less frequently spread in urine and feces and at lower concentrations.[18,19] Fleas have been considered a potential route of transmission because FeLV RNA has been detected in fleas and flea feces,[20,21] but flea transmission does not seem to play an important role in nature. Iatrogenic transmission can occur by contaminated needles, instruments, or blood transfusions.[13,22] Regressively infected cats do not shed the virus through saliva and other excretions (at least not after the potential initial viremic phase), but it has been shown that blood transfusions from regressively infected cats will transmit the virus effectively so that the recipients become infected.[22]

FeLV is readily and rapidly (within minutes) inactivated in the environment, because the viral envelope is lipid-soluble and inactivated by disinfectants, soaps, heating, and drying. Single cats kept strictly indoors are not at risk for acquiring infection,[23] and a waiting period is not needed before introducing a new cat into a household after

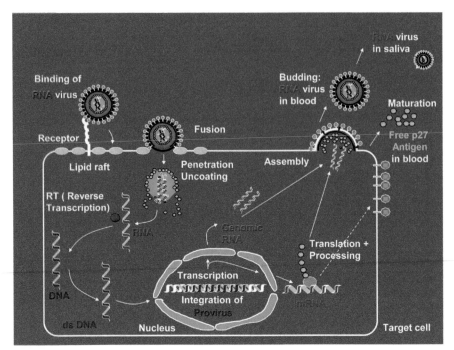

Fig. 2. FeLV replication. Once FeLV has attached to and fused with the host cell, the viral RNA is freed and converted into viral DNA. The viral DNA is transferred to the cell nucleus during cell division, where it is integrated into the host genomic DNA with the help of an integrase and then is called proviral DNA and can be detected using proviral DNA PCR. When the cell is activated, new viral RNA and proteins are produced and assembled at the host cell membrane to build new viral particles that are shed into the blood and saliva. In addition to viral particles, also soluble FeLV p27 capsid antigen is shed into the blood and can be detected by POCT and laboratory ELISA. BM, bone marrow. (*Courtesy of* R. Hofmann-Lehmann, Prof. Dr. med. vet., FVH, Zurich, Switzerland.)

removal of an FeLV-infected cat. FeLV is not a hazard in a veterinary hospital or boarding kennel as long as cats are housed in separate cages,[24] and routine cage disinfection and hand washing between handling cats are performed.[25]

Vertical transmission from queen to kitten commonly occurs in *progressively infected* cats. Neonatal kittens can be infected transplacentally or when the queen licks and nurses the kittens. Transmission can also occur in queens that are *regressively infected* (with negative results on p27 antigen tests) or have a *focal atypical FeLV infection*. If in utero infection occurs, reproductive failure, for example, fetal resorption, abortion, and neonatal death, is common, but up to 20% of vertically infected kittens can survive the neonatal period and become progressively infected adults. It is possible that newborn kittens from infected queens have negative p27 antigen test results initially at the time of birth but can become positive weeks to months after birth, once the virus starts replicating. Thus, if the queen or any kitten in a litter is infected, the entire family should be treated as if infected and should be isolated as a group.

Prevalence

FeLV infection exists in domestic cats worldwide, but FeLV prevalence varies considerably between geographic areas. Studies report a prevalence of progressive FeLV infection of 2.3% to 3.3% in the United States, 0.7% to 15.6% in Europe, 3.0% to

28.4% in South America, and 0.5% to 24.5% in Asia and Australia/New Zealand.[26–32] Newer prevalence studies have mainly focused on the detection of FeLV especially in third-world countries or on remote islands, where the prevalence of FeLV infections was previously unknown. FeLV has been detected almost everywhere. Only cats on some remote islands, such as Grenada, West Indies, Isabela, and Galapagos, were free of FeLV infection.[24]

The prevalence of FeLV has decreased over the last decades.[26,27,29,32,33] For example, in Germany, a steady decrease in FeLV prevalence from 6% to 1% was observed when investigating the FeLV infection rate from 1993 to 2002.[17] The decrease in prevalence was most likely the result of testing and removal programs, and the widespread use of vaccination. However, more recently, studies indicate that the decrease in prevalence has now stagnated in many countries, and thus, awareness of this important infection and its prevention should not be neglected.[32]

FACTORS INFLUENCING PREVALENCE, COURSE OF INFECTION, AND DEVELOPMENT OF DISEASE

Risk factors for FeLV infection influencing FeLV prevalence have been relatively well characterized, but the exact mechanisms for the different clinical responses are poorly understood.

Factors Influencing Feline Leukemia Virus Prevalence

Certain risk factors contribute to a higher prevalence (**Table 1**). The true prevalence of FeLV is difficult to ascertain because it depends on the population of cats being sampled.[34]

Table 1	
Risk factors influencing prevalence of feline leukemia virus infection	
Signalment	• Gender: male cats • Reproductive status: intact cats • Age: adult cats
Behavior	• Aggressive (cat fights, bites) or social (eg, grooming, sharing food bowls) behavior
Health status	• Presence of clinical signs, for example, bite wounds, abscesses, secondary infections, lymphoma, anemia, neuropathies, reproductive disorders, fading kitten syndrome
Vaccination status	• FeLV-unvaccinated cats
Lifestyle	• Outdoor access • Direct cat contact
Housing conditions	• Multicat household
Background	• Cats in households with FeLV infection • Stray cats (especially cats from regions without trap-neuter-return program) • Cats from shelters (especially from shelters with inadequate testing programs and hygiene strategies) • Cats from animal hoarders • Cats with inadequate nutrition, sanitation, medical care
Origin	• Cats from countries with higher prevalence • Cats from areas of a low PPP per capita and income

Health status

The prevalence is higher within a population of sick cats because FeLV predisposes cats to certain diseases and secondary infections. This bias becomes especially evident when cats with clinical problems that are associated with FeLV, such as bite wounds and abscesses, are examined.[16] If only sick cats were included in the surveys, FeLV prevalence was as high as 38%. In contrast, in healthy cats, the FeLV infection rate has been reported from 1% to 8% in Europe and the United States.[26,27] Originally, certain diseases, such as lymphoma, were associated with very high FeLV infection rates (up to 75%); however, prevalence of FeLV in cats with lymphoma has decreased as FeLV prevalence has decreased overall.[35,36]

Behavior

Prevalence is also higher in cats allowed to roam outside,[26,27] because direct contact is required for transmission. Although fighting, free-roaming, intact male cats are still considered mainly at risk for acquiring feline immunodeficiency virus (FIV) infection, the same factors also facilitate FeLV infection.[17,32] However, it was shown that being male (neutered or not) and having access to outdoor environments had a stronger impact on FIV prevalence than on FeLV prevalence, whereas presence of clinical illness was a stronger predictor for FeLV infection. Still, FeLV can no longer be considered primarily an infection of "social/friendly cats."

Sex

In earlier studies, FeLV infection rate was found to be almost equal in male and female cats.[37] However, in more recent studies (eg, in the United States, Brazil, and Germany), a significantly higher risk of FeLV infection among male cats was found.[17,26] Although FeLV transmission commonly occurs between infected queens and kittens and among cats living in prolonged close contact, it seems that aggressive behavior, a common male trait, plays a greater role than previously reported.[16] This finding is also supported by the fact that sexually intact cats are more frequently infected,[32] that cats exhibiting aggressive behavior have a higher risk of FeLV infection,[17] and that more than 8% of cats examined by veterinarians for fighting injuries were infected, a prevalence considerably higher than that in the healthy cat population.[16]

Age

In older studies, young age also was considered to be associated with a higher prevalence of FeLV, but this statement has to be revised. In a study of 18,038 cats in the United States, adult cats were more likely to be progressively FeLV infected than juveniles[26]; this was also reported in a recent shelter study in the United Kingdom,[38] and in a German study, the median age of FeLV-infected cats was not significantly lower than that of non-FeLV-infected cats.[17] This finding is unexpected because the susceptibility of cats to progressive FeLV infection is age-dependent.[39] However, because of increasing awareness, more cats are tested for FeLV, and medical care is provided earlier leading to a longer lifespan.

Breed

Although there is no breed predisposition, FeLV infection is less commonly found in purebred cats, possibly because they are commonly kept indoors, and awareness in the cat-breeder community leads to frequent testing.

Environment

Generally, environmental factors play an important role. Prevalence can significantly vary among shelters, depending on their testing and hygiene strategies.[38] Living in households of animal hoarders is a risk factor for FeLV (as well as other infectious agents). Animal hoarders accumulate animals in overcrowded conditions without adequate nutrition, sanitation, and veterinary care.[40] Being a stray cat was identified as risk factor. However, trap-and-neuter programs have a positive influence on prevalence. FeLV prevalence decreased significantly by 0.18% per year in a trap-neuter-return program operating for more than 2 decades.[41] Interestingly, supplemental feeding and cat caretaker activities in stray cats were recently detected as being associated with a higher FeLV prevalence, likely through increased aggregation of cats and/or altered foraging strategies.[42] One study looked into risk of disasters on FeLV infection rates among cats exported from the 2005 Gulf Coast hurricane disaster area, but could not demonstrate an increase in infection rates in this situation.[43]

Purchasing power parity

Interestingly, 1 study evaluated the association of FeLV prevalence with the purchasing power parity per capita (PPP). Information on FeLV prevalence in specific locations around the world was analyzed from 47 published articles and showed that the highest percentage of FeLV infection was found in cats living in areas of lower PPP with a decreasing rate of FeLV infection with increasing income. Reasons for this could be that lower PPP locations are also areas of higher stray cat populations with less emphasis on animal control programs and vaccination.[44] Alternatively, it could only be an indirect link, because in a recent Europe-wide study, no direct association between income and FeLV prevalence was found, but higher incomes were associated with higher FeLV vaccination rates and vice versa; higher FeLV vaccination rates can lead to lower FeLV prevalence. However, additional factors other than the FeLV vaccination rate and the PPP appeared to have an impact on the FeLV prevalence.[33]

Factors Influencing Outcome of Feline Leukemia Virus Infection

The clinical outcome in each individual cat is determined by a combination of viral and host factors. Infectious pressure is very important to determine the course of infection, but outcome also reflects genetic variation in both the virus and the naturally outbreeding host population. Properties of the virus include the subgroup that determines differences in the clinical picture. Also, mutational changes identified in FeLV strains were shown to significantly increase efficiency of receptor binding. Probably the most important host factor that determines the outcome is the age of the cat at the time of infection (**Table 2**).[39] Although most cats follow 1 of the 4 described courses a few weeks to months after infection, varying and discrepant FeLV test results can be observed during the early phase of FeLV infection, during which the interplay of the cat's immune system and the virus is at its peak and the host-virus balance

Table 2	
Risk factors influencing courses of feline leukemia virus infection	
Signalment	• Young age at time of infection
Immune system	• Insufficient virus-specific humoral and cell-mediated immunity (eg, absence of anti-FeLV antibodies) • Lack of FeLV vaccination
Infectious pressure	• High FeLV viral load in the cat population • Chronic contact with FeLV-shedding cats (multicat households with FeLV)
Virus virulence	• Emergence of more virulent FeLV subgroups within the cat (eg, FeLV-B, FeLV-C) • Mutations in the FeLV genome or integration of the FeLV genome near proto-oncogenes, both leading to activation of proto-oncogenes

has not yet been definitively set.[31] However, even later on during the infection, the host-virus balance is not fixed and might tip to the advantage of either party and, in turn, change the course of FeLV infection.[45] These changes include cats that have been positive for free FeLV p27 antigen for a long period of time (which would be classified as progressive infection) and then suddenly become antigen-negative.[45] On the other hand, in some regressively infected cats, FeLV infection might be reactivated.[8] Therefore, FeLV kinetics is not stable, and the course of infection is determined by a battle between immune system and virus, not only during initial infection but also lifelong in some cats.

Infection pressure
The outcome of FeLV infection will be different based on the infection pressure; for example, a cat that has a one-time short contact with an FeLV-shedding cat will have a different infection course than a cat living together with many FeLV-shedding cats in the same household over months to years sharing the same food and water bowls. It was suggested that in a cat with a first-time single contact with an FeLV-shedding cat, the risk to develop progressive infection is only about 3%. However, if an FeLV-shedding cat is introduced into a naïve group of cats, and the cats are housed together for an extended period, the risk for developing progressive infection increases to an average of 30%.[46] The importance of infectious pressure on the course of infection was also demonstrated in an experiment, in which naïve cats exposed to virus-containing feces developed anti-FeLV antibodies, representing a low-grade challenge, became infected, without direct cat-to-cat contact. These cats remained negative for FeLV antigen and provirus in blood, and only antibodies were present as an indicator of infection (ie, abortive infection; see later).[19]

Feline leukemia virus subgroups
FeLV isolates are classified into different subgroups that determine outcome of FeLV infection and prognosis. Today, FeLV classification, transmission, and disease-inducing potential of different subgroups have been defined sequentially by viral interference assays, Sanger sequencing, polymerase chain reaction (PCR), and next-generation sequencing.[47] FeLV subgroups are immunologically closely related but use different cellular receptors.[48] The 3 best and longest known FeLV subgroups are FeLV-A, FeLV-B, and FeLV-C. FeLV-A is contagious and passed horizontally from cat to cat in nature. The other subgroups evolve de novo in an FeLV-A-infected cat by mutation or recombination between FeLV-A and cellular or endogenous retroviral sequences contained in feline genomic DNA. Pathogenicity of FeLV-B and FeLV-C is higher than that of FeLV-A alone.[49] Different properties of the envelope proteins of the subgroups are the major pathogenic determinant, but the mechanisms by which envelope differences influence pathogenesis are not well understood.[50] FeLV-B is commonly associated with malignancies; it is particularly frequently associated with mediastinal lymphoma, but also occurs in multicentric lymphoma.[51] In experimental infections, an FeLV-B strain caused lymphoma in nearly 100% of kittens within 1 year of infection. Pure red cell aplasia can be caused by subgroup FeLV-C because FeLV-C FLVCR receptor interaction blocks the differentiation of erythroid progenitors between burst-forming units and colony-forming units by interfering with signal transduction pathways essential for erythropoiesis.[52,53] Bone marrow examination of FeLV-C-infected cats shows an almost complete lack of erythroid precursors (at least of the late forms) with normal myeloid and megakaryocytic precursors and an increased myeloid-erythroid ratio. These cats typically have severe anemia and macrocytosis without reticulocytes.[54]

Other FeLV subgroups have been described more recently. FeLV-D arose from recombination of FeLV-A and the *env* gene of a feline endogenous gammaretrovirus and was detected in the blood or tumor tissues of 1.1% FeLV-infected cats, but it is not clear whether FeLV-D is infectious or pathogenic. FeLV-T was identified experimentally but is likely not important in nature. Another experimental subgroup, "FeLV feline acquired immunodeficiency syndrome," is highly immunopathogenic and infects CD4[+] and CD8[+] T lymphocytes and B lymphocytes in blood, lymph nodes, and myeloid cells.[55] In addition, it was suggested that selection pressure in cats can cause novel FeLV subgroups to emerge, and further new strains, not belonging to a known subgroup have been detected.[56,57] Besides the influence of the different subgroups, outcome of FeLV infection is also determined by genetic variation within subgroups.

Age
One important host factor that determines the courses of infection and the clinical outcome is the cat's age at the time of infection because susceptibility of cats to FeLV is age-dependent.[39] As cats mature, they acquire an increasing resistance. Age resistance is independent of immunity from previous contact or vaccination. When older cats become infected, they tend to have abortive or regressive infections or, if they develop progressive infection, have milder signs and a more protracted period of apparent good health. Thus, likelihood of becoming progressively infected is highest in young kittens. In a household of FeLV-infected cats, 70% of kittens adopted at 3 months of age became antigen-positive within 5 months.[58] Neonatal kittens develop marked thymic atrophy after infection ("fading kitten syndrome"), resulting in severe immunosuppression, wasting, and early death. Experimental infection gets more difficult when cats become adult. To overcome the higher resistance of older cats to FeLV, immunosuppressive doses of glucocorticoids were used in some studies before challenge to reach a sufficient number of progressively infected cats. However, resistance depends on the challenge model; for example, the FeLV strains used. In 1 study, experimental infection was even difficult to achieve in kittens older than 16 weeks of age.[39] However, in another study, cats were experimentally infected with FeLV at the age of 14 months, and 80% of naïve cats developed progressive infection. The virus challenge was performed intraperitoneally but without immunosuppressive drugs.[59] Thus, the age resistance in adult cats might not be absolute and could be overcome if a large dose of virus is transmitted, for example, through bites of an infected cat. An explanation for the age resistance might be that the number of cellular receptors necessary for FeLV-A to enter target cells might decrease in older cats, and thus, establishment of infection might become more difficult. Age resistance also could be related to maturation of macrophage function.[46] Thus, age-related resistance is not absolute, but the risk of an adult cat becoming progressively infected after a single short contact with an FeLV-shedding cat is certainly very low.

Host genetic factors
It has been proposed that a genetic predisposition might contribute to a susceptibility of a cat for FeLV. Analysis of genetic single-nucleotide polymorphisms (SNP) showed that a certain SNPs were significantly correlated with the susceptibility to FeLV infections, whereas another combination was positively correlated with absence of FeLV infections.[60] Also the level of immune response might play a role in the course of FeLV infection, because silencing of virus-specific humoral and cell-mediated immunity host effector mechanisms was associated with progressive infection.[61]

Table 3
Different courses of feline leukemia virus infection and expected test results and consequences

Parameter	Progressive Infection	Regressive Infection	Abortive Infection	Focal Infection (Rare)	No Infection
Infection and immune response	Persistent viremia (poor immune response)	Undetectable or transient viremia (good immune response)	Virus undetectable (very good immune response)	Discordant FeLV results (good immune response)	No FeLV infection
Free FeLV p27 antigen (p27 ELISA or immunomigration) on whole blood or serum/plasma	Positive	Negative (only positive during transient viremia or after reactivation)	Negative	Alternating or low positive	Negative
Intracellular FeLV p27 antigen (IFA) on blood smear	Positive (~3 wk after free p27 antigen tests)	Negative (only positive during transient viremia or after reactivation)	Negative	Negative	Negative
Proviral FeLV DNA (PCR) on whole blood	Positive	Positive	Negative	Negative or low positive	Negative
Anti-FeLV antibodies (different tests) on serum/plasma	Negative (or low titers)	Positive (high titers)	Positive (variable titers)	Positive (high titers)	Negative (only possibly positive if vaccinated)
Replicating virus (virus isolation) on whole blood	Positive	Negative (only positive during transient viremia or after reactivation)	Negative	Negative	Negative
Viral RNA (RT-PCR) on whole blood	Positive	Usually negative	Negative	Usually negative	Negative
Viral shedding	Yes	No (only during transient viremia or after reactivation)	No	Usually no shedding	No
Consequences	FeLV-associated disease common, poor prognosis	Disease uncommon (rarely lymphoma or bone marrow suppression), after reactivation common	None	Disease unlikely	None
Usefulness of vaccination	No	No	Presumptively no	Probably no	Yes

Table 4
Tests available to diagnose the different courses of feline leukemia virus infection

Structure	Test	Detection Method	Material	Characteristics
Free (soluble) FeLV p27 antigen (virus core protein)	POCT or laboratory tests (plate ELISA)	Direct	Blood (whole blood or serum/plasma)	• Indicate antigenemia (viremia) • Good diagnostic value of POC tests • Slightly varying diagnostic sensitivities and specificities • False-positive results more common (because of the low FeLV prevalence) • Negative results very reliable • Not yet positive in the early phase of infection (3–6 wk) • Not reliable with saliva
Intracellular p27 antigen	IFA	Direct	Blood (blood smear, in neutrophils and platelets)	• Indicate antigenemia (viremia) • Become positive about 3 wk later (only after the bone marrow is infected) than tests for free p27 antigen • Not recommended as a screening test • Require special processing, fluorescent microscopy, and highly experienced staff • Only results of experienced reference laboratories valuable • False-negative results due to neutropenia and thrombocytopenia • False-positive results due to unspecific staining or interference when using anticoagulated blood

(continued on next page)

Table 4
(continued)

Structure	Test	Detection Method	Material	Characteristics
Replicating virus	Virus isolation (cell culture)	Direct	Blood (whole blood)	• Indicate replication of infectious virus (viremia) • Positive already in early infection (even before p27 antigen tests) • Not practicable for routine diagnosis (difficult and time-consuming) • Not recommended as screening test • Only in few specialized laboratories available • Can be used as confirmatory test
Proviral DNA (DNA copy of the viral RNA integrated into the cat's genome)	PCR	Direct	Blood (whole blood)	• Indicate presence of provirus • Variable diagnostic value because not standardized • Only results of laboratories with adequate quality control valuable • Very sensitive • Highly specific • Test of choice to detect regressive infection • Recommended confirmatory tests for positive antigen test result • Can help resolve cases with discordant antigen test results

Target	Method	Sample	Type	Comments
Viral RNA (RNA of replicating virus, free or cell-associated virus)	RT-PCR	Blood (whole blood) or saliva	Direct	• Indicate virus replication (viremia) in blood in most cases • Indicate virus shedding in saliva and thus antigenemia (viremia) • Variable diagnostic value because not standardized • Only results of laboratories with adequate quality control valuable • Highly specific • Highly sensitive (and positive in blood already 1 wk after infection) • In blood mainly useful to detect very early infection • In saliva mainly useful to rule out presence of FeLV-shedding cats in a multicat environment
Antibodies	Different tests (IFA, ELISA)	Blood (serum/plasma)	Indirect	• Indicate (previous) exposure to the virus (or certain FeLV vaccines) • Currently only performed in specialized laboratories • Available as POCT but not evaluated yet for the field • Positive in cats with regressive and abortive infection • Only tests to identify abortive infection • Enable quantification of the immune response

DIFFERENT COURSES OF FELINE LEUKEMIA VIRUS INFECTION

Cats with FeLV infection follow different courses (**Table 3**) that can be distinguished by the consecutive use of different diagnostic tests (**Table 4**). These courses include progressive infection, regressive infection, abortive infection, and rarely, focal atypical infection. The 4 courses have been well characterized in experimental infection,[62–64] but the outcomes following natural infection can be different and confusing. The outcome of FeLV infection is a battle between immune system and virus, especially in the early phase of FeLV infection (generally the first 12 weeks of infection will define the course in most cats), but for some cats, lifelong. In those cats, the balance can be altered by factors, such as immunosuppression, coinfections, or change in environment, leading to a switch in FeLV infection outcome and prognosis for the cat.

Older studies suggested that approximately 1/3 of cats in multicat households became persistently viremic (progressive infection), and up to 2/3 of cats would eventually "clear the infection."[46] However, newer research suggested that all infected cats remain infected for life after exposure but can revert to an aviremic state in which no antigen or culturable virus is present in the blood but FeLV proviral DNA still can be detected in the blood by PCR (*regressive infection*) or in which neither antigen or culturable virus nor proviral DNA, but only antibodies are detected (*abortive infection*).[64–66] Most infected cats will be abortively infected, followed by regressive infection, and only a small proportion will be *progressively infected* (see **Table 3**).

Progressive Infection

In cats with progressive FeLV infection, virus is not contained early in the infection, and extensive replication occurs, first in the lymphoid tissues and then in the bone marrow and in mucosal and glandular epithelial tissues (**Fig. 3**).[9] Mucosal and glandular infection is associated with excretion of infectious virus. Progressive infection is characterized by insufficient FeLV-specific immunity, and cats have low levels or undetectable neutralizing antibodies.[29,67] Viremia persists longer than 12 weeks, and these cats usually remain persistently viremic and infectious to other cats for the remainder of their lives. This condition of "persistent viremia" is the typical feature of progressive infection. Virus persistently replicates in bone marrow, spleen, lymph nodes, and salivary glands. These cats are lifelong virus shedders and usually develop FeLV-associated diseases after years that can be fatal.

Regressive Infection

It has been suggested that in multicat environments with FeLV-shedding cats (high infectious pressure), approximately one-third of cats develop regressive infection. Regressive infection is accompanied by an effective immune response, and virus replication and viremia are contained before (or shortly after) the time of bone marrow infection. These cats never develop or eventually clear viremia.[64–66] In regressively infected cats, FeLV provirus is integrated into the cat's genome, and cats remain infected for life (FeLV provirus carrier).[8,10] Although proviral DNA remains integrated, virus is not actively produced; thus, these cats have negative results on routine tests (such as enzyme-linked immunosorbent assay [ELISA] or immunofluorescence assay [IFA]) that detect FeLV p27 antigen. The continuous presence of provirus explains the long persistence of virus-neutralizing antibodies in these regressively infected cats.[65] Before the development of PCR, regressive infections were described as "latent" infections in which the absence of antigenemia was accompanied by persistence of culturable virus in bone marrow or other tissues, but not in blood. Latency was at that

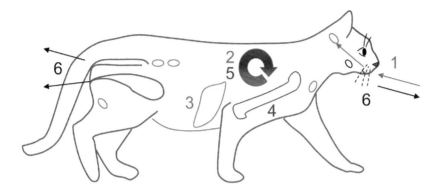

1. Oropharynx, local lymphoid tissue   Starting time
2. Primary cell-associated viremia (<u>lymphocytes, monocytes</u>) point
3. Lymphoid tissue throughout body   up to 2 weeks
---
4. Bone marrow (neutrophils, platelet precursors), intestine   1-3 weeks
5. Secondary viremia (<u>neutrophils, platelets</u>, high loads)   2-4 weeks
6. Shedding (mucosal and glandular tissue)   3-8 weeks

Fig. 3. Pathogenesis of progressive FeLV infection. Cats are mostly infected via the oral-nasal route. The virus reaches the local lymphoid tissue and infects lymphocytes and monocytes spread the infection throughout the body (primary viremia). In some of the cats, those with weak immunity to FeLV, the virus can reach the bone marrow and infect precursor cells, which results in the release of FeLV-infected neutrophils and platelets into the bloodstream (second viremia). Subsequently, mucosal and glandular tissues are infected (gastrointestinal tract, salivary glands), and the virus is shed mainly by saliva, but also by feces, urine, and milk. DsRNA, double-stranded RNA; mRNA, messenger RNA. (*Courtesy of* R. Hofmann-Lehmann, Dr. med. vet., FVH, Zurich, Switzerland.)

time detected by culturing bone marrow cells in the presence of glucocorticoids resulting in active virus replication in cell culture.[62,68–70]

Regressively infected cats do not shed infectious virus in saliva, but proviral DNA can be transmitted via blood transfusion.[22] In cats with regressive infection, FeLV infection can be reactivated and viremia can reoccur particularly if the cats are immunosuppressed, when they as a consequence will shed virus in saliva and can develop FeLV-associated disease.[68] The risk of reactivation of viremia decreases over time,[65,68–71] but it has been shown that the integrated provirus retains its replication capacity lifelong, and reactivation is possible even many years after the initial exposure to FeLV.[8,72] Regressive infections can also reactivate during pregnancy as a result of immunosuppression from endogenous progesterone. During lactation, mammary glands of regressively infected queens can begin to produce infectious viral particles.[73] In some cats, regressive infection itself (without reactivation) can be responsible for lymphoma[35] or bone marrow suppression.[74]

Regressive and progressive infections can be distinguished by repeated testing for free p27 antigen in blood.[64] Either regressively infected cats never go through an episode of viremia (and thus, are never positive on p27 antigen tests) or they develop an initial antigenemia/viremia (usually within 3 up to 6 weeks after virus exposure) during which free FeLV p27 antigen is detectable and cats might shed virus through saliva. However, a regressively infected cat will then test negative for viral antigen 1 to 6 (sometimes 12) weeks later or, in rare cases, even after months.[45] During early infection, blood proviral DNA and viral RNA loads of cats with progressive and regressive infections are not significantly different. However, subsequently, both are associated with different viral loads.[66]

Abortive Infection

Approximately one-third of cats likely will develop low-grade infection with subsequent immunity. In these cats, viral replication can be stopped after initial replication in the local lymphoid tissue in the oropharynx by an effective humoral and cell-mediated immune response; these cats never become viremic.[62,68–70] Thus, in these abortively infected cats, direct virus detection methods will always be negative, and the only signs of FeLV exposure will be the presence of FeLV-specific antibodies. Abortive infection has been observed sometimes following experimental FeLV inoculation and is characterized by negative test results for culturable virus, antigen, viral RNA, and proviral DNA.[64,75] Abortive infection likely is caused by low-dose exposure to FeLV.[76] Although not common after experimental infection, abortive infection seems to be more common in the field as cats possessing antibodies but that are antigen- and provirus-negative are commonly detected.[29,31] The envelope transmembrane protein p15E is considered a promising candidate for detection of FeLV antibodies.[76,77] Abortively infected cats have the same life expectancy as cats that have never been exposed to FeLV.[13] They build a very effective immunity and are protected against new viral challenges, probably for several years if not lifelong.

Focal (Atypical) Infection

Focal infections, also called atypical infections, have been reported in early experimental studies in up to 10% of infected cats. They are considered rare under natural circumstances. In these cats, FeLV infection is restricted to certain tissues, such as mammary glands, bladder, eyes, spleen, lymph nodes, or small intestine, in which persistent atypical local viral replication occurs.[46,73,78] A queen with atypical infection of their mammary glands was reported to have transmitted FeLV to her kittens via milk even when negative in p27 antigen tests in the blood.[73] The production of p27 antigen and release into the blood can be intermittent or low grade in atypically infected cats. Therefore, cats can have weakly positive or discordant results in p27 antigen tests, or positive and negative results can alternate. Some of these cats test positive for free p27 antigen but are negative in virus isolation or even provirus PCR depending on the sensitivity of the assay.[48,79] Focal infections can be the reason for unclear and confusion test results.

CLINICAL SYNDROMES ASSOCIATED WITH REGRESSIVE FELINE LEUKEMIA VIRUS INFECTION

Active virus replication occurs in cats with progressive FeLV infection and is generally responsible for the development of clinical signs.[80] However, certain diseases (such as lymphoma and bone marrow suppression) have also been described in regressively infected cats. Even progressively infected cats can be clinically healthy for many years, however, their life expectancy is generally reduced.[17,27,81,82] A variety of disease conditions can be associated with progressive FeLV infection, including bone marrow disorders (mainly anemia), neoplasia (mainly lymphoma), immunosuppression leading to susceptibility to secondary infections, and some other clinical syndromes, such as immune-mediated diseases, FeLV-associated neuropathies, reproductive disorders, and fading kitten syndrome.[46,83,84] Thus, although progressive FeLV infection increases the risk for a wide variety of conditions, it is not always possible to determine whether concurrent diseases are a consequence of FeLV infection or independent events.

In contrast to progressive infection, regressive FeLV infection does not have an impact on life expectancy, unless infection is reactivated and cats become viremic, at which point they are at risk for the same diseases as those with progressive infection. In addition, there are a few clinical syndromes that can be caused by regressive infection even without reactivation, such as bone marrow suppression or lymphoma. In these conditions, the provirus itself can disturb cellular mechanisms or act as an oncogenic substance leading to tumor development without necessity of replicating virus. One study found a high prevalence of regressive infection in older cats at necropsy and suggested an association with hematologic changes and inflammatory processes.[85]

Bone Marrow Disorders

Bone marrow suppression, especially anemia, is the most common clinical syndrome associated with FeLV infection and results from infection of both hematopoietic stem cells and bone marrow stromal cells that constitute the supporting environment for blood precursor cells. Anemia at time of FeLV diagnosis had a negative impact on the longevity of the FeLV-infected cats in a recent study.[82] Usually, bone marrow suppression is caused by progressive infection in FeLV-infected cats but in rare cases, regressive infection can be associated with myelosuppression.[67,74] In 1 study, 5.4% of cats with nonregenerative cytopenias and negative FeLV antigen test had positive results in bone marrow PCR indicating regressive infection.[74]

Lymphoma

Progressive FeLV infection causes various tumors in cats, most commonly lymphoma and less commonly leukemia and other hematopoietic tumors as well as some unusual tumors, such as neurolymphomatosis, osteochondromas, olfactory neuroblastoma, uterine adenocarcinoma, and cutaneous horns. Progressively FeLV-infected cats have an about 60-fold increased risk of developing lymphoma compared with noninfected cats, and lymphoma can affect up to one-quarter of cats with progressive FeLV infection. Mediastinal (thymic) lymphoma is the most common form of FeLV-associated lymphoma, followed by multicentric lymphoma, although spinal, renal, ocular, and other forms of lymphomas are occasionally reported in progressively FeLV-infected cats.[86] Because the prevalence of FeLV decreased since its discovery, so has the incidence of FeLV-associated lymphoma.[36,87] A study in Germany showed a decrease of progressive FeLV infection in cats with lymphomas from 59% in 1980 to 1995 to 20% in 1996 to 1999.[36] Other studies worldwide confirmed a decrease of progressive FeLV infection in cats with lymphoma with current prevalence of 0% to 21%[74,87–90] In a study in the Netherlands, only 5.6% of cats with lymphoma were progressively FeLV infected, although 31.0% of these cats had mediastinal lymphoma, which has the strongest association with FeLV infection.[88] In contrast, in countries with high general FeLV prevalence, such as Brazil, progressive FeLV infection is still very common in cats with lymphoma, for example, with prevalence of 52.0%[91] and 56.6% in cats with lymphoma[92] and 78.4% in cats with leukemia.[93]

If FeLV is the cause of lymphoma, it is usually through progressive infection; however, regressive FeLV infection can also be involved in tumor formation. Cats from FeLV cluster households had a 40-fold higher rate of development of FeLV antigen-negative lymphomas than cats from the general population. FeLV proviral DNA has been detected in lymphomas of FeLV antigen-negative cats,[94] and lymphomas have also occurred in FeLV antigen-negative laboratory cats previously infected with FeLV.[95] Results of different studies concerning the prevalence of regressive FeLV infection in cats with lymphoma vary significantly,[35,67,94,96,97] but more recent studies found evidence of provirus in only 10.0%[67] and in 0% (0/50) of FeLV antigen-negative lymphomas,[35] suggesting that regressive infection is only rarely involved in tumor development today.

The mechanism by which regressive FeLV infection causes lymphomas is through insertion of the provirus at many different sites in the host's genome, and integrated FeLV provirus can interrupt or inactivate cellular genes in the infected cells. Alternately, regulatory features of viral DNA might alter expression of neighboring genes. In addition, because bone marrow microenvironment cells (eg, myelomonocytic progenitor cells and stromal fibroblasts) provide a reservoir for regressive FeLV infections, it is possible that integrated provirus can alter cellular functions and contribute to the pathogenesis. Finally, FeLV can appropriate cellular genes, and several such transduced genes also present in regressively infected cells have been implicated in viral oncogenesis.[95,98,99] The most important oncogenetic mechanism seems to be insertion of the FeLV genome into the cellular genome near a cellular oncogene (most commonly *myc*),[100–102] resulting in activation and overexpression of that gene. These effects lead to uncontrolled proliferation of these cells. FeLV can also incorporate the oncogene to form a recombinant virus (eg, FeLV-B, FeSV) containing cellular oncogene sequences that are then rearranged and activated. When they enter a new cell, these recombinant viruses are oncogenic.

SUMMARY

Today, FeLV is still an important infection affecting many cats worldwide. Courses of infections differ between individual cats, are not always clearly defined, and can vary over time. The complex pathogenesis, variety in outcome, as well as availability of many different tests make FeLV one of the most complicated infections in cats and a challenge for veterinarians. This complex pathogenesis is especially true for cats with regressive FeLV infection that are not detected by routine diagnostic methods measuring free FeLV p27 antigen, but that can still transmit FeLV through blood transfusions and can reactivate viremia at any time and develop clinical signs.

DISCLOSURE

The authors declare that they have no conflict of interest. The authors received no specific grant from any funding agency in the public, commercial, or not-for profit sectors for the preparation of this article.

REFERENCES

1. Polani S, Roca AL, Rosensteel BB, et al. Evolutionary dynamics of endogenous feline leukemia virus proliferation among species of the domestic cat lineage. Virology 2010;405:397–407.

2. Kawasaki J, Nishigaki K. Tracking the continuous evolutionary processes of an endogenous retrovirus of the domestic cat: ERV-DC. Viruses 2018;10:179.

3. Powers JA, Chiu ES, Kraberger SJ, et al. Feline leukemia virus (FeLV) disease outcomes in a domestic cat breeding colony: relationship to endogenous FeLV and other chronic viral infections. J Virol 2018;92: e00649-18.

4. Tandon R, Cattori V, Pepin AC, et al. Association between endogenous feline leukemia virus loads and exogenous feline leukemia virus infection in domestic cats. Virus Res 2008;135:136–43.

5. Jarrett WF, Martin WB, Crighton GW, et al. Transmission experiments with leukemia (lymphosarcoma). Nature 1964;202:566–7.

6. Russell PH, Jarrett O. The specificity of neutralizing antibodies to feline leukaemia viruses. Int J Cancer 1978;21:768–78.

7. Willett BJ, Hosie MJ. Feline leukaemia virus: half a century since its discovery. Vet J 2013;195:16–23.

8. Helfer-Hungerbuehler AK, Widmer S, Kessler Y, et al. Long-term follow up of feline leukemia virus infection and characterization of viral RNA loads using molecular methods in tissues of cats with different infection outcomes. Virus Res 2015;197:137–50.

9. Rojko JL, Hoover EA, Mathes LE, et al. Pathogenesis of experimental feline leukemia virus infection. J Natl Cancer Inst 1979;63:759–68.

10. Cattori V, Tandon R, Pepin A, et al. Rapid detection of feline leukemia virus provirus integration into feline genomic DNA. Mol Cell Probes 2006;20:172–81.

11. Cattori V, Pepin AC, Tandon R, et al. Real-time PCR investigation of feline leukemia virus proviral and viral RNA loads in leukocyte subsets. Vet Immunol Immunopathol 2008;123:124–8.

12. Cattori V, Hofmann-Lehmann R. Absolute quantitation of feline leukemia virus proviral DNA and viral RNA loads by TaqMan real-time PCR and RT-PCR. Methods Mol Biol 2008;429:73–87.

13. Lutz H, Addie D, Belak S, et al. Feline leukaemia. ABCD guidelines on prevention and management. J Feline Med Surg 2009;11:565–74.

14. Gomes-Keller MA, Tandon R, Gonczi E, et al. Shedding of feline leukemia virus RNA in saliva is a consistent feature in viremic cats. Vet Microbiol 2006;112: 11–21.

15. Gomes-Keller MA, Gonczi E, Tandon R, et al. Detection of feline leukemia virus RNA in saliva from naturally infected cats and correlation of PCR results with those of current diagnostic methods. J Clin Microbiol 2006;44:916–22.

16. Goldkamp CE, Levy JK, Edinboro CH, et al. Seroprevalences of feline leukemia virus and feline immunodeficiency virus in cats with abscesses or bite wounds and rate of veterinarian compliance with current guidelines for retrovirus testing. J Am Vet Med Assoc 2008;232:1152–8.

17. Gleich SE, Krieger S, Hartmann K. Prevalence of feline immunodeficiency virus and feline leukaemia virus among client-owned cats and risk factors for infection in Germany. J Feline Med Surg 2009;11:985–92.

18. Cattori V, Tandon R, Riond B, et al. The kinetics of feline leukaemia virus shedding in experimentally infected cats are associated with infection outcome. Vet Microbiol 2009;133:292–6.

19. Gomes-Keller MA, Gonczi E, Grenacher B, et al. Fecal shedding of infectious feline leukemia virus and its nucleic acids: a transmission potential. Vet Microbiol 2009;134:208–17.

20. Vobis M, D'Haese J, Mehlhorn H, et al. The feline leukemia virus (FeLV) and the cat flea (Ctenocephalides felis). Parasitol Res 2003;90(Suppl 3):S132–4.

21. Vobis M, D'Haese J, Mehlhorn H, et al. Evidence of horizontal transmission of feline leukemia virus by the cat flea (Ctenocephalides felis). Parasitol Res 2003;91:467–70.

22. Nesina S, Katrin Helfer-Hungerbuehler A, Riond B, et al. Retroviral DNA–the silent winner: blood transfusion containing latent feline leukemia provirus causes infection and disease in naive recipient cats. Retrovirology 2015;12:105.

23. Mostl K, Addie DD, Boucraut-Baralon C, et al. Something old, something new: update of the 2009 and 2013 ABCD guidelines on prevention and management of feline infectious diseases. J Feline Med Surg 2015;17:570–82.

24. Little S, Levy J, Hartmann K, et al. 2020 AAFP Feline Retrovirus Testing and Management Guidelines. J Feline Med Surg 2020;22(1):5–30.

25. Addie DD, Boucraut-Baralon C, Egberink H, et al. Disinfectant choices in veterinary practices, shelters and households: ABCD guidelines on safe and effective disinfection for feline environments. J Feline Med Surg 2015;17:594–605.

26. Levy JK, Scott HM, Lachtara JL, et al. Seroprevalence of feline leukemia virus and feline immunodeficiency virus infection among cats in North America and risk factors for seropositivity. J Am Vet Med Assoc 2006;228:371–6.

27. Gleich S, Hartmann K. Hematology and serum biochemistry of feline immunodeficiency virus-infected and feline leukemia virus-infected cats. J Vet Intern Med 2009;23:552–8.

28. Hellard E, Fouchet D, Santin-Janin H, et al. When cats' ways of life interact with their viruses: a study in 15 natural populations of owned and unowned cats (Felis silvestris catus). Prev Vet Med 2011;101:250–64.

29. Englert T, Lutz H, Sauter-Louis C, et al. Survey of the feline leukemia virus infection status of cats in Southern Germany. J Feline Med Surg 2012;14:392–8.

30. Spada E, Proverbio D, della Pepa A, et al. Seroprevalence of feline immunodeficiency virus, feline leukaemia virus and Toxoplasma gondii in stray cat colonies in northern Italy and correlation with clinical and laboratory data. J Feline Med Surg 2012;14:369–77.

31. Westman M, Norris J, Malik R, et al. The diagnosis of feline leukaemia virus (FeLV) infection in owned and group-housed rescue cats in Australia. Viruses 2019;11. https://doi.org/10.3390/v11060503.

32. Hofmann-Lehmann R, Gonczi E, Riond B, et al. Feline leukemia virus infection: importance and current situation in Switzerland. Schweiz Arch Tierheilkd 2018; 160:95–105.

33. Studer N, Lutz H, Saegerman C, et al. Pan-European study on the prevalence of the feline leukaemia virus infection - reported by the European Advisory Board on Cat Diseases (ABCD Europe). Viruses 2019;11. https://doi.org/10.3390/v11110993.

34. Westman ME, Paul A, Malik R, et al. Seroprevalence of feline immunodeficiency virus and feline leukaemia virus in Australia: risk factors for infection and geographical influences (2011-2013). JFMS Open Rep 2016;2. https://doi.org/10.1177/2055116916646388.

35. Stutzer B, Simon K, Lutz H, et al. Incidence of persistent viraemia and latent feline leukaemia virus infection in cats with lymphoma. J Feline Med Surg 2011; 13:81–7.

36. Meichner K, Kruse DB, Hirschberger J, et al. Changes in prevalence of progressive feline leukaemia virus infection in cats with lymphoma in Germany. Vet Rec 2012;171:348.

37. Lee IT, Levy JK, Gorman SP, et al. Prevalence of feline leukemia virus infection and serum antibodies against feline immunodeficiency virus in unowned free-roaming cats. J Am Vet Med Assoc 2002;220:620–2.

38. Stavisky J, Dean RS, Molloy MH. Prevalence of and risk factors for FIV and FeLV infection in two shelters in the United Kingdom (2011-2012). Vet Rec 2017; 181:451.
39. Hoover EA, Olsen RG, Hardy WD Jr, et al. Feline leukemia virus infection: age-related variation in response of cats to experimental infection. J Natl Cancer Inst 1976;57:365–9.
40. Polak KC, Levy JK, Crawford PC, et al. Infectious diseases in large-scale cat hoarding investigations. Vet J 2014;201:189–95.
41. Kreisler RE, Cornell HN, Levy JK. Decrease in population and increase in welfare of community cats in a twenty-three year trap-neuter-return program in Key Largo, FL: the ORCAT Program. Front Vet Sci 2019;6:7.
42. Hwang J, Gottdenker NL, Oh DH, et al. Disentangling the link between supplemental feeding, population density, and the prevalence of pathogens in urban stray cats. PeerJ 2018;6:e4988.
43. Levy JK, Edinboro CH, Glotfelty CS, et al. Seroprevalence of Dirofilaria immitis, feline leukemia virus, and feline immunodeficiency virus infection among dogs and cats exported from the 2005 Gulf Coast hurricane disaster area. J Am Vet Med Assoc 2007;231:218–25.
44. Ludwick K, Clymer JW. Comparative meta-analysis of feline leukemia virus and feline immunodeficiency virus seroprevalence correlated with GDP per capita around the globe. Res Vet Sci 2019;125:89–93.
45. Hofmann-Lehmann R, Holznagel E, Aubert A, et al. Recombinant FeLV vaccine: long-term protection and effect on course and outcome of FIV infection. Vet Immunol Immunopathol 1995;46:127–37.
46. Hoover EA, Mullins JI. Feline leukemia virus infection and diseases. J Am Vet Med Assoc 1991;199:1287–97.
47. Chiu ES, Hoover EA, VandeWoude S. A retrospective examination of feline leukemia subgroup characterization: viral interference assays to deep sequencing. Viruses 2018. https://doi.org/10.3390/v10010029.
48. Miyazawa T, Jarrett O. Feline leukaemia virus proviral DNA detected by polymerase chain reaction in antigenaemic but non-viraemic ('discordant') cats. Arch Virol 1997;142:323–32.
49. Rojko J, Essex M, Trainin Z. Feline leukemia/sarcoma viruses and immunodeficiency. Adv Vet Sci Comp Med 1988;32:57–96.
50. Moser M, Burns CC, Boomer S, et al. The host range and interference properties of two closely related feline leukemia variants suggest that they use distinct receptors. Virology 1998;242:366–77.
51. Ahmad S, Levy LS. The frequency of occurrence and nature of recombinant feline leukemia viruses in the induction of multicentric lymphoma by infection of the domestic cat with FeLV-945. Virology 2010;403:103–10.
52. Quackenbush SL, Donahue PR, Dean GA, et al. Lymphocyte subset alterations and viral determinants of immunodeficiency disease induction by the feline leukemia virus FeLV-FAIDS. J Virol 1990;64:5465–74.
53. Shelton GH, Linenberger ML. Hematologic abnormalities associated with retroviral infections in the cat. Semin Vet Med Surg (Small Anim) 1995;10:220–33.
54. Hardy WD Jr, McClelland AJ, Zuckerman EE, et al. Prevention of the contagious spread of feline leukaemia virus and the development of leukaemia in pet cats. Nature 1976;263:326–8.
55. Quackenbush SL, Dean GA, Mullins JI, et al. Analysis of FeLV-FAIDS provirus burden and productive infection in lymphocyte subsets in vivo. Virology 1996; 223:1–9.

56. Miyake A, Watanabe S, Hiratsuka T, et al. Novel feline leukemia virus interference group based on the env gene. J Virol 2016;90:4832–7.

57. Miyake A, Kawasaki J, Ngo H, et al. Reduced folate carrier: an entry receptor for a novel feline leukemia virus variant. J Virol 2019;93. https://doi.org/10.1128/JVI.00269-19.

58. Cotter SM. Management of healthy feline leukemia virus-positive cats. J Am Vet Med Assoc 1991;199:1470–3.

59. Lehmann R, Franchini M, Aubert A, et al. Vaccination of cats experimentally infected with feline immunodeficiency virus, using a recombinant feline leukemia virus vaccine. J Am Vet Med Assoc 1991;199:1446–52.

60. de Castro FL, Junqueira DM, de Medeiros RM, et al. Analysis of single-nucleotide polymorphisms in the APOBEC3H gene of domestic cats (Felis catus) and their association with the susceptibility to feline immunodeficiency virus and feline leukemia virus infections. Infect Genet Evol 2014;27:389–94.

61. Flynn JN, Dunham SP, Watson V, et al. Longitudinal analysis of feline leukemia virus-specific cytotoxic T lymphocytes: correlation with recovery from infection. J Virol 2002;76:2306–15.

62. Hofmann-Lehmann R, Cattori V, Tandon R, et al. Vaccination against the feline leukaemia virus: outcome and response categories and long-term follow-up. Vaccine 2007;25:5531–9.

63. Hofmann-Lehmann R, Cattori V, Tandon R, et al. How molecular methods change our views of FeLV infection and vaccination. Vet Immunol Immunopathol 2008;123:119–23.

64. Torres AN, Mathiason CK, Hoover EA. Re-examination of feline leukemia virus: host relationships using real-time PCR. Virology 2005;332:272–83.

65. Hofmann-Lehmann R, Huder JB, Gruber S, et al. Feline leukaemia provirus load during the course of experimental infection and in naturally infected cats. J Gen Virol 2001;82:1589–96.

66. Pepin AC, Tandon R, Cattori V, et al. Cellular segregation of feline leukemia provirus and viral RNA in leukocyte subsets of long-term experimentally infected cats. Virus Res 2007;127:9–16.

67. Beatty JA, Tasker S, Jarrett O, et al. Markers of feline leukaemia virus infection or exposure in cats from a region of low seroprevalence. J Feline Med Surg 2011;13:927–33.

68. Rojko JL, Hoover EA, Quackenbush SL, et al. Reactivation of latent feline leukaemia virus infection. Nature 1982;298:385–8.

69. Madewell BR, Jarrett O. Recovery of feline leukaemia virus from non-viraemic cats. Vet Rec 1983;112:339–42.

70. Pacitti AM, Jarrett O. Duration of the latent state in feline leukaemia virus infections. Vet Rec 1985;117:472–4.

71. Hayes KA, Rojko JL, Mathes LE. Incidence of localized feline leukemia virus infection in cats. Am J Vet Res 1992;53:604–7.

72. Helfer-Hungerbuehler AK, Cattori V, Boretti FS, et al. Dominance of highly divergent feline leukemia virus A progeny variants in a cat with recurrent viremia and fatal lymphoma. Retrovirology 2010;7:14.

73. Pacitti AM, Jarrett O, Hay D. Transmission of feline leukaemia virus in the milk of a non-viraemic cat. Vet Rec 1986;118:381–4.

74. Stutzer B, Muller F, Majzoub M, et al. Role of latent feline leukemia virus infection in nonregenerative cytopenias of cats. J Vet Intern Med 2010;24:192–7.

75. Torres A, Larson L, Schultz RD, et al. Insight into FeLV:host relationships using real-time DNA and RNA qPCR. In: 8th International Feline Retrovirus Research Symposium. Washington, DC, October 8-11, 2006.
76. Major A, Cattori V, Boenzli E, et al. Exposure of cats to low doses of FeLV: seroconversion as the sole parameter of infection. Vet Res 2010;41:17.
77. Boenzli E, Hadorn M, Hartnack S, et al. Detection of antibodies to the feline leukemia virus (FeLV) transmembrane protein p15E: an alternative approach for serological FeLV detection based on antibodies to p15E. J Clin Microbiol 2014;52:2046–52.
78. Hayes KA, Rojko JL, Tarr MJ, et al. Atypical localised viral expression in a cat with feline leukaemia. Vet Rec 1989;124:344–6.
79. Jarrett O, Pacitti AM, Hosie MJ, et al. Comparison of diagnostic methods for feline leukemia virus and feline immunodeficiency virus. J Am Vet Med Assoc 1991;199:1362–4.
80. Hartmann K, Levy JK. Feline leukemia virus infection. In: Ettinger SJ, Feldmann EC, Cote E, editors. Textbook of veterinary internal medicine. 8th edition. St Louis (MO): Saunders Elsevier; 2017. p. 978–91.
81. Addie DD, Dennis JM, Toth S, et al. Long-term impact on a closed household of pet cats of natural infection with feline coronavirus, feline leukaemia virus and feline immunodeficiency virus. Vet Rec 2000;146:419–24.
82. Spada E, Perego R, Sgamma EA, et al. Survival time and effect of selected predictor variables on survival in owned pet cats seropositive for feline immunodeficiency and leukemia virus attending a referral clinic in northern Italy. Prev Vet Med 2018;150:38–46.
83. Hartmann K. Clinical aspects of feline immunodeficiency and feline leukemia virus infection. Vet Immunol Immunopathol 2011;143:190–201.
84. Hartmann K. Clinical aspects of feline retroviruses: a review. Viruses 2012;4:2684–710.
85. Suntz M, Failing K, Hecht W, et al. High prevalence of non-productive FeLV infection in necropsied cats and significant association with pathological findings. Vet Immunol Immunopathol 2010;136:71–80.
86. Hartmann K. Management of feline retrovirus-infected cats. In: Bonagura JD, Twedt DC, editors. Kirk's current veterinary therapy XVI. St Louis (MO): Saunders Elsevier; 2015. p. 1275–83.
87. Louwerens M, London CA, Pedersen NC, et al. Feline lymphoma in the post-feline leukemia virus era. J Vet Intern Med 2005;19:329–35.
88. Teske E, van Straten G, van Noort R, et al. Chemotherapy with cyclophosphamide, vincristine, and prednisolone (COP) in cats with malignant lymphoma: new results with an old protocol. J Vet Intern Med 2002;16:179–86.
89. Simon D, Eberle N, Laacke-Singer L, et al. Combination chemotherapy in feline lymphoma: treatment outcome, tolerability, and duration in 23 cats. J Vet Intern Med 2008;22:394–400.
90. Fabrizio F, Calam AE, Dobson JM, et al. Feline mediastinal lymphoma: a retrospective study of signalment, retroviral status, response to chemotherapy and prognostic indicators. J Feline Med Surg 2014;16:637–44.
91. Leite-Filho RV, Panziera W, Bandinelli MB, et al. Epidemiological, pathological, and immunohistochemical aspects of 125 cases of feline lymphoma in southern brazil. Vet Comp Oncol 2019. https://doi.org/10.1111/vco.12535.
92. Cristo TG, Biezus G, Noronha LF, et al. Feline lymphoma and a high correlation with feline leukaemia virus infection in Brazil. J Comp Pathol 2019;166:20–8.

93. Cristo TG, Biezus G, Noronha LF, et al. Feline leukaemia virus associated with leukaemia in cats in Santa Catarina, Brazil. J Comp Pathol 2019;170:10–21.

94. Jackson ML, Haines DM, Meric SM, et al. Feline leukemia virus detection by immunohistochemistry and polymerase chain reaction in formalin-fixed, paraffin-embedded tumor tissue from cats with lymphosarcoma. Can J Vet Res 1993;57:269–76.

95. Rohn JL, Linenberger ML, Hoover EA, et al. Evolution of feline leukemia virus variant genomes with insertions, deletions, and defective envelope genes in infected cats with tumors. J Virol 1994;68:2458–67.

96. Gabor LJ, Jackson ML, Trask B, et al. Feline leukaemia virus status of Australian cats with lymphosarcoma. Aust Vet J 2001;79:476–81.

97. Wang J, Kyaw-Tanner M, Lee C, et al. Characterisation of lymphosarcomas in Australian cats using polymerase chain reaction and immunohistochemical examination. Aust Vet J 2001;79:41–6.

98. Rezanka LJ, Rojko JL, Neil JC. Feline leukemia virus: pathogenesis of neoplastic disease. Cancer Invest 1992;10:371–89.

99. Sheets RL, Pandey R, Jen WC, et al. Recombinant feline leukemia virus genes detected in naturally occurring feline lymphosarcomas. J Virol 1993;67:3118–25.

100. Tsatsanis C, Fulton R, Nishigaki K, et al. Genetic determinants of feline leukemia virus-induced lymphoid tumors: patterns of proviral insertion and gene rearrangement. J Virol 1994;68:8296–303.

101. Fujino Y, Ohno K, Tsujimoto H. Molecular pathogenesis of feline leukemia virus-induced malignancies: insertional mutagenesis. Vet Immunol Immunopathol 2008;123:138–43.

102. Sumi R, Miyake A, Endo T, et al. Polymerase chain reaction-based detection of myc transduction in feline leukemia virus-infected cats. Arch Virol 2018;163:1073–7.

Hypertension: Why Is It Critical?

Rebecca F. Geddes, MA, VetMB, MVetMed, PhD, FHEA, MRCVS

KEYWORDS

- Hypertension • Cat • Feline • Target organ • TOD • Blood pressure

KEY POINTS

- Hypertension is common, particularly in older cats and those with comorbidities, such as chronic kidney disease, acute kidney injury, and hyperthyroidism.
- Blood pressure measurement should be considered in at-risk cats: those with comorbidities, cats exposed to pharmacologic agents or toxins associated with hypertension, and those older than 9 years.
- Target organ damage (TOD) affecting the eyes, brain, heart/vasculature, and kidneys have all been documented in cats and the rationale for treatment is to prevent TOD occurring.
- Treatment should always be administered even if TOD has already been documented, as there is evidence that treatment can ameliorate TOD, including retinal reattachment and restoration of vision.

INTRODUCTION

It is vital to think about the possibility of hypertension in cats that may be at risk of this condition, because patients rarely have overt warning clinical signs. It is devastating for your patient (and the patient's owner) if the animal loses its sight due to a condition that was not checked for, but so easily could have been (**Fig. 1**). Untreated hypertension also puts the other target organs at risk of damage, resulting in increased morbidity and mortality. This condition is common; a recent epidemiologic study of cats in the United Kingdom found an incidence risk of 19.5%.[1] This article discusses how we define hypertension, which cats are at risk, when to monitor blood pressure (BP), and how we can apply evidence-based medicine to treat this condition.

DEFINING HYPERTENSION

Although it is possible to measure systolic arterial BP (SBP), diastolic arterial blood pressure, and to calculate mean arterial blood pressure, measurements of SBP are considered to be the most reliable in cats and are therefore used for recommendations of when to treat and how to monitor for treatment response. Studies that have tried to establish what a "normal" SBP is in healthy cats have had varied results, but one study

Queen Mother Hospital for Animals, Royal Veterinary College, Hawkshead Lane, North Mymms, Hertfordshire AL9 7TA, UK
E-mail address: rgeddes@rvc.ac.uk

Vet Clin Small Anim 50 (2020) 1037–1052
https://doi.org/10.1016/j.cvsm.2020.04.001
0195-5616/20/© 2020 Elsevier Inc. All rights reserved.
vetsmall.theclinics.com

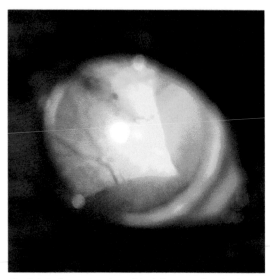

Fig. 1. Complete retinal detachment and mydriasis in a cat that had never previously had BP measurement performed.

that measured blood pressure in almost 780 healthy cats in a rehoming center found the median SBP was 120 mmHg (interquartile range 110–132 mmHg).[2] This study also found that median SBP increased with age in healthy cats, with cats ≥9 years of age having significantly higher SBP than cats aged 3 to 9 years, although the difference between the median measurements was only approximately 10 mmHg. The proportion of cats that developed hypertension also increased with advancing age in a study of healthy cats and cats with chronic kidney disease (CKD).[3] However, not all studies have found consistent results regarding age and increasing blood pressure.[4,5]

The latest American College of Veterinary Internal Medicine (ACVIM) guidelines[4] on hypertension define the following categories for SBP:

- Normotensive: lower than 140 mmHg; risk of target organ damage (TOD) is minimal
- Prehypertensive: 140 to 159 mmHg; risk of TOD is low
- Hypertensive: 160 to 179 mmHg; risk of TOD is moderate
- Severely hypertensive: >180 mmHg; risk of TOD is high

These categories can be guidelines only, as blood pressure will inevitably vary day-to-day and depending on circumstances. Care must be taken when measuring SBP to try to minimize the effect of situational hypertension (discussed in the next section); however, these categories help provide a framework for the diagnosis and treatment of hypertension.

TYPES OF HYPERTENSION

There are generally 3 categories of hypertension: situational (or white coat) hypertension, idiopathic (or primary) hypertension, and secondary hypertension.

Situational Hypertension

Cats can be prone to situational hypertension, in which stress increases SBP through autonomic nervous system alterations on higher centers of the central nervous system. It is difficult to quantify exactly how much stress can increase SBP. In the previously mentioned study of 780 healthy cats in a rehoming center, SBP was lowest in cats that appeared calm during the measurement (median 112.8 mmHg), increased significantly in cats deemed "cooperative but anxious" (median 123.2 mmHg), and was significantly higher again in cats that were "nervous, excited, or aggressive" during BP measurement (median 131.6 mmHg).[2] The main concern is that situational hypertension could lead to a false diagnosis of true hypertension and unnecessary treatment. If you obtain a high BP reading, this should prompt fundic examination to look for supportive evidence that true hypertension is present (discussed further later in this article); however, a normal fundic examination cannot definitively rule out hypertension, and at present the search for biomarkers that can confirm the presence of hypertension has been unrewarding.[6] Measurement of elevated BP on one occasion, without evidence of hypertensive retinopathy should be confirmed at another consultation within 1 to 2 weeks. It appears that cats adapt quickly to having BP measurement performed, and a repeated measurement on a subsequent visit can often be lower; in 3 recent randomized, placebo-controlled studies for treatment of hypertension, 18% to 28% of cats in the placebo arm achieved a reduction in SBP of ≥15% or to less than 150 mmHg by 28 days.[7–9] There is no evidence to suggest situational hypertension should be treated in cats; however, the consequences of not treating true hypertension can be severe. Therefore, if a cat demonstrates persistently elevated SBP (>160 mmHg) on repeated measurements on different occasions, antihypertensive medication should be initiated.

Another consideration is which cats should have BP measurement performed. It has been suggested that BP measurements should be initiated in cats from 3 years of age every 12 months, to start obtaining baseline readings for the individual animal.[10] However, as with any test, the likelihood of a type 1 error (ie, a false positive) is increased with a lower prevalence of disease. Therefore, measurement of BP in young healthy cats in which the prevalence of hypertension is very low will inevitably produce false positive results that provide a clinical conundrum for the clinician: to treat, or not to treat? One study of 137 healthy cats aged 0.7 to 16.6 years found 21.9% of the cats had an SBP measurement that would assign them to the ACVIM "Hypertensive" category with moderate risk of TOD, and no association was found between SBP and age[5]; however, none of the cats had fundic examination and repeat measurements were not performed to help rule out situational hypertension. In addition, 4 cats had an SBP higher than 180 mmHg, but 3 of these were younger than 3 years of age and were subsequently removed from the analysis, highlighting the difficulty of deciding what to do with young cats that are seemingly hypertensive. As a result, the ACVIM consensus statement argues that screening for hypertension is reasonable on an annual basis from 9 years of age, but should not be performed in younger animals,[4] although consideration could be given to performing a fundic examination on a regular basis in cats of all ages as part of a complete physical examination.

Steps should be taken to minimize stress and to reduce the type I error rate of diagnosing hypertension by considering the following points:

- Measure BP only in patients considered to have a possibility of having hypertension due to the following[4]:
  - The presence of clinical abnormalities consistent with hypertensive TOD
  - A diagnosis of a condition known to be associated with hypertension
  - Treatment with a pharmacologic agent (eg, erythropoietin, darbepoetin alfa) or ingestion of a toxin known to be associated with hypertension

(eg, cocaine, methamphetamine, 5-hydroxytryptophan; although hypertension associated ingestion of these toxins has only been reported in dogs to date)
  ○ An older cat (≥9 years of age) with possible occult disease
- Reduce stress factors as much as possible (eg, having a quieter and calmer environment for monitoring BP or allowing more time for acclimatization before measuring).

A summary of which cats should have BP measurement performed is shown in **Box 1**.

Idiopathic Hypertension

Idiopathic hypertension seemingly accounts for approximately 13% to 24% of feline hypertension[11-13]; however, this is a diagnosis of exclusion and it is possible these percentages are overestimates. If hypertension is diagnosed in a patient without a known underlying cause, this should prompt diagnostics to ensure there are no concurrent conditions resulting in secondary hypertension.

Secondary Hypertension

Secondary hypertension occurs in conjunction with another disease process or due to a medication or toxin that elevates BP. This is the most common type of hypertension in cats.[4,10] The exact etiology of hypertension in association with concurrent disease is incompletely understood. In other species, chronic activation of the renin-angiotensin-aldosterone system (RAAS) is known to play a role; however, studies have failed to identify increased plasma renin activity in either hypertensive cats with CKD[14] or in hypertensive hyperthyroid cats.[15] A recent study found polymorphisms in the uromodulin gene to be associated with SBP, but not with renal function or CKD; further work is required to explore the impact of these specific polymorphisms; however, they may affect water and sodium handling in the thick ascending limb of the loop of Henle.[16]

  Diagnosis of any of the following conditions should prompt measurement of SBP, and if hypertension is present, the cat requires antihypertensive treatment in addition to treatment of the underlying condition. Conditions associated with secondary hypertension include the following:

Box 1
Which cats should undergo blood pressure (BP) measurement?

- Cats with sudden-onset blindness or central neurologic signs
- Cats newly diagnosed with chronic kidney disease (CKD), acute kidney injury, hyperthyroidism, diabetes mellitus, hyperaldosteronism, Cushing's disease, or pheochromocytoma
- Cats already diagnosed with CKD: BP should be checked at diagnosis and at regular intervals (eg, every 3–6 months)
- Cats at diagnosis of hyperthyroidism, at the point they become euthyroid and at subsequent reexaminations
- Cats already receiving medication for hypertension, at all reexaminations
- Cats receiving other pharmaceutical agents (eg, darbepoetin alfa) or that have had toxin ingestion known to affect blood pressure (eg, cocaine)

- CKD: this is the most common cause of secondary hypertension in cats,[1,12,13,17] and the prevalence of hypertension with CKD has been documented at 19% to 61%.[18,19] The cause-and-effect relationship of CKD and hypertension is complex and discussed in further detail later in this article under TOD.
- Acute kidney injury (AKI): hypertension also has been documented in 58.7% of cats with community-acquired AKI, and was not related to the grade of AKI or serum creatinine.[20]
- Hyperthyroidism: prevalence of hypertension varies from approximately a quarter of cases,[1,12] up to 87% of cats having systolic or diastolic hypertension in one study.[19] Other studies have documented increasing prevalence (approximately twofold) within 6 months of restoration of euthyroidism, although a proportion of these cats also developed azotemic CKD.[15,21] There is no association between the prevalence of hypertension and the severity of hyperthyroidism.[22] Therefore, documentation and treatment of hypertension in all hyperthyroid cats at diagnosis and at reexaminations once euthyroid is paramount.
- Diabetes mellitus: an association between diabetes mellitus and hypertension has been made in cats, although prevalence appears to be low. One study of 14 diabetic cats found a zero prevalence of hypertension,[23] whereas another study including 66 diabetic cats found 15% to have hypertension, although this was not a significantly higher proportion than in the control cats.[24] A large epidemiologic study of cats with hypertension found 2.1% had a concurrent diagnosis of diabetes mellitus,[1] although additional concurrent diseases may not have been thoroughly excluded. Two cats in a study of hypertensive cats with hypertensive retinopathy had diabetes mellitus, although one also had concurrent CKD.[13] However, it would still be prudent to periodically check for hypertension in the diabetic feline patient.
- Hyperaldosteronism (see also Primary Hyperaldosteronism in Cats: An Underdiagnosed Disorder by Kooistra in Part II, elsewhere in this issue): this is not common but should be suspected particularly if hypertension is documented in combination with hypokalemia or signs of hindlimb weakness and/or cervical ventroflexion.[25]
- Pheochromocytoma[26] and Cushing's syndrome[27] both can cause hypertension, but are uncommon conditions in the cat.

THE IMPACT OF HYPERTENSION

Regardless of the underlying cause, sustained increases in BP cause tissue injury, and the aim of treatment is to prevent this damage from occurring. The so-called "target organs" are at risk due to the presence of a rich arteriolar blood supply, or via sustained increases in systemic vascular resistance. Damage occurs with loss of autoregulatory mechanisms in arterial blood flow in these organs, which include the eyes, brain, kidney, and myocardium.

Target Organ Damage: the Eyes

The retinal vessels share similar physiologic characteristics to the encephalic and cardiac microcirculations; therefore, examination of the retinal vessels is important to detect changes that may compromise vision as early as possible and also to provide an indication of how hypertension may also be affecting other organs. Lesions that may be apparent with hypertensive retinopathy include hemorrhages, bullous detachments, vessel narrowing and/or tortuosity, and retinal edema. Occasionally, hyphema and vitreal hemorrhage can occur, and hyphema can lead to secondary glaucoma. For review of feline hypertensive retinopathy lesions, readers are referred elsewhere.[28] Cats may present with blindness and complete mydriasis, and historically, restoration of vision has been considered unlikely,[4] with documentation of some vision being regained in only 13% of blind eyes in one feline study.[13] However, a very recent study found that vision, as assessed by menace response, was regained in 76 (57.6%) of 132 blind eyes in cats with hypertensive chorioretinopathy following treatment of their hypertension.[29] Initial treatment was amlodipine monotherapy in 94% of the cats. Complete retinal reattachment took longer than 60 days in some cases, and persistence of vision at last reexamination was actually higher in cats in which reattachment had taken more than 60 days, compared to within 3 weeks.

The vulnerability of the eye to TOD appears variable; BP was significantly higher in cats with retinal lesions in one study of 58 cats (SBP 262 ± 34 mm Hg) when compared with other hypertensive cats without retinal lesions (SBP 221 ± 34 mmHg),[30] but lesions have been reported in other studies to occur at SBP elevations as low as 168 to 170 mmHg.[13,17] In humans, choroidal vascular changes appear more common with an acute elevation in BP, whereas retinal vascular changes appear more likely with chronic hypertension.[31] In addition, hypertension due to renal diseases, particularly glomerular pathologies in humans, results in more severe retinopathies than in those with essential (ie, idiopathic) hypertension.[32] Hypertensive changes in the eye are seen in approximately 40% to 60% of geriatric cats with hypertension,[11,12] and appear most common with concurrent CKD.[13,33]

The eye is the quickest (and cheapest!) organ to evaluate for TOD, and fundic examination should be performed to help confirm all cases of suspected hypertension (eg, if SBP is >160 mmHg) so that treatment can be initiated as quickly as possible. One large epidemiologic study found that ocular examination was not performed in 38.6% of cats diagnosed with hypertension,[1] suggesting there is a barrier to performing this examination in first opinion practice. There are a number of methods available for performing fundic examination, which have been reviewed in detail elsewhere,[28] but indirect ophthalmoscopy is an inexpensive and rapid method of examining a large field of view and should be widely considered before use of a direct ophthalmoscope. For a guide to performing this technique, see **Box 2**, **Figs. 2** and **3**.

Retinal imaging software, such as VAMPIRE (Vascular Assay and Measurement Platform for Images of the Retina), is now starting to be used in cats to analyze vessel widths and arteriolar bifurcations.[35] Application of advanced technology such as this may help improve sensitivity of TOD detection in the future.

Target Organ Damage: the Brain

TOD in the brain can result in hypertensive encephalopathy and appears more likely with a sudden increase in BP, an SBP greater than 180 mmHg, or both.[36] Two of 4 cats that underwent surgical reduction of renal mass had an abrupt increase (40–50 mmHg) in SBP and developed severe neurologic signs of ataxia, blindness, stupor, and seizures within 12 to 18 hours.[37] Post mortem, these cats demonstrated diffuse brain edema with cerebral arteriosclerosis.

In studies of cats with spontaneous hypertension that have all had hypertensive retinopathy, 29% to 48% have had concurrent neurologic signs including disorientation, seizures, depression, ataxia, and vestibular signs.[13,38] Treatment of hypertensive encephalopathy can be successful if initiated early.[36,39] Hypertension accounted for 8.1% of reactive seizures in feline patients in another study, with SBP measurements of 170 to 186 mmHg; satisfactory seizure control was achieved with amlodipine in 3 of 5 cases.[40]

Box 2
How to perform indirect ophthalmoscopy

- Ask an assistant to help hold the patient and to keep the head still and if needed, to gently open the eyelids.
- Hold a light source against the side of your head and look for a tapetal reflection.
- Once the reflection can be seen, place a 20-diopter or 2.2 pan retinal lens in front of the eye.
- Obtaining an image of the fundus in the lens requires your eye and the light source, the lens, and the cat's eye to be in line with each other. Tilting the lens slightly and moving it toward and away from the patient can be tried to improve the image obtained.
- Resting your third or fourth finger on the cat's head or on your assistant's hand can be helpful to improve stability.

Tip:
- Pupil dilation allows a more thorough examination of the fundus and is extremely helpful when less experienced with this technique.
- Placing the cat in a dark room can help to achieve mydriasis, but if this is not sufficient, then applying 1 drop of 1% tropicamide to each eye will usually achieve mydriasis within 15 minutes.[34]

Target Organ Damage: the Kidneys

Hypertension and CKD are common comorbidities; azotemia is seen in approximately 70% of hypertensive cats[11] and, conversely, approximately 60% cats with CKD are hypertensive.[3,19] In addition, cats that are normotensive at diagnosis of CKD are significantly more likely to develop hypertension over time compared with healthy older cats, although the prevalence of hypertension increases over time in this group as well (see **Fig. 3**).[3] One study has suggested that cats with later-stage CKD may be more likely to have severe hypertension than cats in International Renal Interest Society (IRIS) stage 2,[41] but other studies have found no relationship between severity of CKD and severity of hypertension.[3,18,19]

Hypertension contributes to kidney damage; increasing SBP is associated with increasing proteinuria[42] and a higher time-averaged blood pressure is associated with glomerulosclerosis and hyperplastic arteiolosclerosis,[43] that is, renal injury. Progressive CKD, defined by an increase in plasma creatinine greater than 25% over

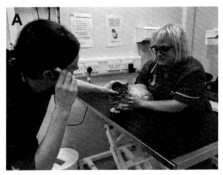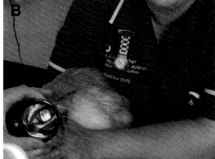

Fig. 2. (*A*) To perform indirect ophthalmoscopy, ask an assistant to gently restrain your patient, hold a light source next to your head and stand nearly an arm's length away from your patient. (*B*) Look for a tapetal reflection and then place your lens between you and the cat's eye, moving it slowly until you see the fundus. In the correct position the fundus will fill the lens.

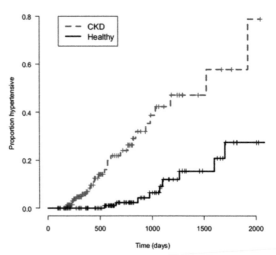

Fig. 3. Kaplan-Meier curve of probability to become hypertensive. Time is in days from first visit. Cats with CKD have a greater probability to be hypertensive at each time point than healthy cats (*P*<.001). Censored cases are represented by ticks. (*From* Bijsmans ES, Jepson RE, Chang YM, et al. Changes in Systolic Blood Pressure over Time in Healthy Cats and Cats with Chronic Kidney Disease. J Vet Intern Med. 2015; 29(3); 855-861; with permission.)

12 months, was also associated with proteinuria and with a higher prevalence of hypertension (40%) compared with cats with stable CKD over the same timeframe (29%).[44] Severity of proteinuria is highly correlated with survival time,[42] and antihypertensive treatment can reduce proteinuria,[11] even with amlodipine monotherapy, despite the action of amlodipine to dilate the afferent arteriole, which should increase glomerular pressure. The glomerular pressure change is presumably offset by the larger decrease in systemic BP, although at present it is not clear if the subsequent drop in proteinuria represents a reduction in kidney injury or is a surrogate marker for the changes in glomerular filtration rate induced by both the systemic and glomerular pressure changes.[11,45]

Target Organ Damage: the Heart and Vasculature

On clinical examination, 42% to 74% hypertensive cats have a systolic cardiac murmur[30,38,46] and 13% to 16% of hypertensive cats have a gallop rhythm.[30,38] Left ventricular hypertrophy (LVH), or an abnormal left ventricular geometric pattern, is a common finding in hypertensive cats, affecting 74% to 85% of cases[30,46]; however, the degree of hypertrophy does not correlate with the severity of the hypertension[46] and cause and effect remain uncertain.[47] Treatment with amlodipine reduced the number of cats deemed to have LVH in one study, but no significant difference in any echocardiographic measurements were found before and after treatment.[46] The effect of telmisartan on LVH in hypertensive cats has not yet been evaluated; however, studies in both humans and rodent models have revealed that telmisartan can directly inhibit cardiomyocyte hypertrophy via its actions on the cardiac angiotensin II receptor.[48] It is therefore possible that in addition to reducing SBP and therefore cardiac afterload, treatment of hypertensive cats with telmisartan may have additional impact on the heart.

The great vessels also can be affected by hypertension. Calculating the ratio of the diameters of the proximal ascending aorta relative to the aortic annulus can be helpful for differentiating hypertensive from nonhypertensive cats.[49] In addition, severe hypertension (SBP 260 mm Hg) was thought to be the cause of a dissecting aortic aneurysm in a recent case report of a 10-year-old domestic short-hair; however, investigations into possible causes of the hypertension were not performed.[50] Furthermore, a recent study demonstrated the presence of vasa vasorum arteriopathy in cats with hypertension.[51] The vasa vasorum is the delicate network of arterioles that supplies blood to the walls of the great vessels. This study included 24 cats, with 46% having a diagnosis of hypertension; however, this was largely based on clinical and/or pathologic evaluation, as only 6 cats (4 hypertensive) had had their BP measured. Nevertheless, vasa vasorum arteriopathy correlated with hypertension status, the presence of renal arteriosclerosis, and degenerative lesions within the great vessels.

Effect on Survival Time

Counterintuitively, numerous studies have failed to find an association between how well controlled hypertension is with treatment and survival time.[11,12,38,42] In addition, there was no significant difference in survival between hypertensive cats with normal and abnormal echocardiographic findings.[30] However, cats that present for monitoring of concurrent disease have better survival rates than cats diagnosed due to the presence of clinical signs, which presumably reflects owner motivation for monitoring and treating their cat.[1] A major confounding factor to studying survival time is that the vast majority of cats in these studies have been treated for their hypertension. The impact of antihypertensive therapy may mask the effect of hypertension on morbidity and mortality; however, withholding treatment would not be ethically acceptable.

Survival times vary slightly between populations: cats still alive 7 days after diagnosis of hypertension in first-opinion practice had a median survival time of 400 days[1]; 24 cats with hypertensive retinopathy had a median survival time of 18 months[38]; whereas another study of 141 hypertensive cats had an overall survival time of only 260 days.[11] In that last study, survival was strongly associated with severity of proteinuria at diagnosis of hypertension. Proteinuric cats with urine protein-to-creatinine ratio (UPC) >0.4 survived a median of only 162 days, whereas survival time for borderline proteinuric cats (UPC 0.2–0.4) was 313 days, and for nonproteinuric cats (UPC <0.2) it was 490 days. Importantly, UPC was shown to significantly decrease with amlodipine besylate treatment in this study.

THE GREATEST BARRIER TO DIAGNOSIS

The biggest reason that hypertension is not diagnosed is likely due to BP measurement not being performed. Only 4.4% of cats ≥9 years, had BP "assessed" during a 2-year period (2012–2013) in a recent study of 347,889 cats in first opinion practice in the United Kingdom.[1] In addition, in some cases the assessment was based on ocular changes (70 cats) or clinical signs alone (5 cats) and did not include BP measurement. The most common reason for BP assessment was presentation with clinical signs (63.1%), followed by monitoring of concurrent disease (31.2%). Unsurprisingly, given that most cats had to present with clinical signs before BP was measured, more than 90% of the cats diagnosed with hypertension were in the "severe" category. Owners of 535 cats were offered BP measurement, but declined.

Waiting for owners to report clinical signs of illness in cats is likely to result in underdiagnosis of a number of common conditions, including hypertension. A study of 100 apparently healthy cats aged 6 years and older, found 8 cats had SBP greater than 160 mmHg, of which 4 were borderline proteinuric and 1 had a heart murmur, although no fundic lesions were reported and repeat SBP measurements on a subsequent visit were not performed.[52]

Furthermore, in a recent online survey of owners of 1089 cats with CKD, only 3% were reported to have concurrent hypertension.[53] As this study was an owner survey, the results will have been subject to self-selection bias regarding participation and it is possible some owners did not realize their cats had been tested for and/or diagnosed with hypertension. However, because other studies suggest prevalence rates of hypertension in cats with CKD of more like 20% to 65%, either these were very unusual cats with CKD, or hypertension was being underdiagnosed in this cohort, which included cats in numerous countries. Creatinine concentration is an independent risk factor for becoming hypertensive,[3] and the frequency of severe hypertension increases as IRIS stage increases in cats with CKD.[41] However, 17% of cats that are normotensive at diagnosis of azotemic CKD can still go on to develop hypertension later.[3] It is therefore recommended that SBP should be measured at CKD diagnosis and if normal, every 3 to 6 months thereafter. Similarly, given the high prevalence of hypertension at diagnosis of hyperthyroidism (25%–87%)[1,12,19] and increasing prevalence following treatment,[15,21] it is recommended that SBP should be measured at diagnosis of hyperthyroidism, on restoration of euthyroidism, and every 3 to 6 months thereafter.

DIAGNOSING HYPERTENSION IN CATS

Tips for performing BP measurement:

- Let the cat acclimatize to the environment for 5 to 10 minutes, this could be during history taking. Ideally let the cat be in or out of the cat carrier as it prefers, but take the top of the carrier off if the cat is to be allowed to stay in there, so that the SBP measurement can be performed with the cat in the box.
- If the cat is already hospitalized, then BP could be taken in the kennel if the cat seems relaxed with you doing so.
- However, do not specifically hospitalize a cat for SBP measurement, as this may stress them more.
- Use Doppler or high-definition oscillometry (HDO),[54] as traditional oscillometry does not perform reliably in cats.[55] If using HDO, the tail may be the easiest place to place the cuff. The HDO needs to be coupled to a computer to confirm that the pulse waves produce an adequate trace. Further information on this is available elsewhere.[10]
- Try not to shave any fur off (if you have to because the pulse is difficult to find, then the cat needs time to relax again afterward), instead wet the fur and skin with surgical spirit but try not to get it on the cat's pads because it is cold and cats do not like it.
- Have the cat held by the owner if possible, or by someone comfortable and familiar with cats. The restraint should be as light as possible. Place a cuff (width should be 30%–40% of the diameter of the leg) around one of the limbs or around the tail.
- Use plenty of gel with your probe to find the pulse and keep the volume of the Doppler machine low or use headphones.
- Inflate the sphygmomanometer to 20 to 40 mmHg above where the sound of the pulse vanishes and then slowly release the pressure. Ignore the first reading.
- Take 5 to 7 readings and record them all if possible. If the readings are all trending in one direction, then discount them and take another 5 readings. The aim is to have 5 similar readings and then take the mean of those 5 as your overall reading.

- Record what cuff size and which extremity used. Repeated measurements on other occasions should ideally have the same person performing the measurement and replicate the same cuff and the same leg or tail.
- An average SBP reading greater than 160 mmHg should prompt fundic examination to help differentiate true hypertension from situational hypertension.
- Treatment should be initiated immediately in cats with SBP greater than 160 mmHg and evidence of TOD.
- If there is no evidence of TOD, then BP measurement should be repeated, ideally within 2 weeks, and treatment recommended if SBP is still greater than 160 mmHg.

TREATMENT OF FELINE HYPERTENSION

There are 2 first-line treatment options for feline hypertension: the calcium channel antagonist amlodipine besylate, and the angiotensin II receptor blocker telmisartan. Both have been evaluated in prospective, randomized, placebo-controlled clinical trials of hypertensive cats with SBP 160 to 200 mmHg that did not have evidence of TOD.[7–9] Initial reductions of 20 to 30 mmHg can be expected with both medications.

Traditionally, the recommended starting dosage of amlodipine is 0.625 mg per cat every 24 hours by mouth. However, cats that require a dose increase to achieve adequate control of their hypertension have a higher SBP at baseline,[1,56] and recent evidence suggests that if baseline SBP is >200 mmHg, a starting dosage of 1.25 mg per cat every 24 hours by mouth should be considered.[56] If needed, amlodipine can be increased to a maximum of 2.5 mg per cat every 24 hours by mouth, but this is rarely necessary and should prompt a careful discussion with the owner to check compliance.

The recommended starting dosage of telmisartan is 2 mg/kg every 24 hours by mouth in Europe (http://www.noahcompendium.co.uk/?id=-4696560) and an initial 14 days of 1.5 mg/kg every 12 hours by mouth in the United States, then subsequent reduction to 2 mg/kg every 24 hours (http://www.semintra.com/pdf/MERL18201%20SEMINTRA%20US%201-page%20PI%20v1c.pdf). The dosage may need to be decreased at a later date depending on response. There are no current studies comparing amlodipine with telmisartan, and treatment choice is largely clinician dependent at present. However, data on the use of telmisartan for cats with SBP >200 mmHg or with TOD is currently lacking, excepting 1 case report of its use in a cat with amlodipine-induced gingival hyperplasia.[57] Treatment with amlodipine has been shown to ameliorate numerous types of TOD. Amlodipine treatment reduced the proportion of cats with ventricular hypertrophy from 11 of 14 to 6 of 14.[46] In 70% of cats, sole agent amlodipine reduced UPC by a median of 0.12.[11] Amlodipine treatment can result in resolution of reactive seizures[40] and reduction in other signs of hypertensive encephalopathy and retinopathy.[36] Treatment with amlodipine, when used as a sole agent in 94% of 88 cats with hypertensive chorioretinopathy, resulted in 57.6% cats with bilateral blindness regaining some vision as assessed by the menace response.[29]

Because antihypertensive treatment can reduce proteinuria,[11] the priority in cats that are both hypertensive and proteinuric (UPC >0.4) is to adequately control BP first and then to reassess UPC to see if additional antiproteinuric therapy is required. As noted in a small number of cats, the combination of amlodipine with telmisartan appears to be well tolerated,[58] therefore if required, a second agent can be added to the treatment regimen.

Interestingly, unlike in humans, dietary sodium chloride supplementation has not been found to affect renal function or BP in either healthy older cats[59] or in cats with nephrectomy models of CKD.[60] However, dietary sodium chloride restriction in feline nephrectomy models can activate the RAAS, reduce glomerular filtration rate, and result in urinary potassium wasting,[60] therefore it is prudent to avoid dietary salt restriction in hypertensive cats.

Although widely used as antihypertensive therapy in dogs, angiotensin-converting enzyme inhibitors are not recommended for monotherapy use in cats with hypertension because the reduction in SBP is typically only approximately 10 mmHg and is therefore unlikely to be sufficient for most cats. In addition, beta blockers (eg, atenolol) have limited effect on BP and are not therefore recommended for feline hypertension.

Following initiation of treatment, cats should be reassessed every 7 to 10 days for BP measurement and dosages tailored to achieve an SBP of less than 160 mmHg at a minimum and preferably less than 140 mmHg. However, SBP less than 110 mmHg or less than 120 mmHg in conjunction with lethargy/weakness should raise concern for hypotension and prompt a reduction in antihypertensive medication dosage. SBP should be rechecked on all future examinations if a cat is on antihypertensive medication.

Hypertensive Crises

Cats presenting with an acute hypertensive crisis, particularly those with SBP $\geq$180 mmHg with signs of intracranial TOD require emergency treatment and 24-hour care, therefore referral should be sought if 24-hour care cannot otherwise be provided.[4,10] Intravenous medications are likely to be required and BP needs to be carefully and gradually decreased. Evidence for medication selection is largely lacking, but a discussion of possible medications can be found elsewhere.[4]

SUMMARY

Hypertension is common in cats, particularly older cats and those with certain comorbidities. It is crucial that small animal clinicians identify at-risk patients and assess for hypertension before being presented with a patient already showing clinical signs. However, any patient already exhibiting TOD should have treatment initiated immediately, then be carefully reexamined to assess response and change treatment doses as needed. Hypertension that is detected and controlled produces excellent outcomes, with no effect on survival time.

DISCLOSURE

R.F. Geddes has a consultancy agreement with Boehringer Ingelheim.

REFERENCES

1. Conroy M, Chang YM, Brodbelt D, et al. Survival after diagnosis of hypertension in cats attending primary care practice in the United Kingdom. J Vet Intern Med 2018;32(6):1846–55.
2. Payne JR, Brodbelt DC, Luis Fuentes V. Blood pressure measurements in 780 apparently healthy cats. J Vet Intern Med 2017;31(1):15–21.
3. Bijsmans ES, Jepson RE, Chang YM, et al. Changes in systolic blood pressure over time in healthy cats and cats with chronic kidney disease. J Vet Intern Med 2015;29(3):855–61.

4. Acierno MJ, Brown S, Coleman AE, et al. ACVIM consensus statement: guidelines for the identification, evaluation, and management of systemic hypertension in dogs and cats. J Vet Intern Med 2018;32(6):1803–22.

5. Hori Y, Heishima Y, Yamashita Y, et al. Epidemiological study of indirect blood pressure measured using oscillometry in clinically healthy cats at initial evaluation. J Vet Med Sci 2019;81(4):513–6.

6. Bijsmans ES, Jepson RE, Wheeler C, et al. Plasma N-terminal probrain natriuretic peptide, vascular endothelial growth factor, and cardiac troponin i as novel biomarkers of hypertensive disease and target organ damage in cats. J Vet Intern Med 2017;31(3):650–60.

7. Glaus TM, Elliott J, Herberich E, et al. Efficacy of long-term oral telmisartan treatment in cats with hypertension: results of a prospective European clinical trial. J Vet Intern Med 2019;33(2):413–22.

8. Huhtinen M, Derré G, Renoldi HJ, et al. Randomized placebo-controlled clinical trial of a chewable formulation of amlodipine for the treatment of hypertension in client-owned cats. J Vet Intern Med 2015;29(3):786–93.

9. Coleman AE, Brown SA, Traas AM, et al. Safety and efficacy of orally administered telmisartan for the treatment of systemic hypertension in cats: results of a double-blind, placebo-controlled, randomized clinical trial. J Vet Intern Med 2019;33(2):478–88.

10. Taylor SS, Sparkes AH, Briscoe K, et al. ISFM consensus guidelines on the diagnosis and management of hypertension in cats. J Feline Med Surg 2017;19(3):288–303.

11. Jepson RE, Elliott J, Brodbelt D, et al. Effect of control of systolic blood pressure on survival in cats with systemic hypertension. J Vet Intern Med 2007;21(3):402–9.

12. Elliott J, Barber PJ, Syme HM, et al. Feline hypertension: clinical findings and response to antihypertensive treatment in 30 cases. J Small Anim Pract 2001;42(3):122–9.

13. Maggio F, DeFrancesco TC, Atkins CE, et al. Ocular lesions associated with systemic hypertension in cats: 69 cases (1985-1998). J Am Vet Med Assoc 2000;217(5):695–702.

14. Jepson RE, Syme HM, Elliott J. Plasma renin activity and aldosterone concentrations in hypertensive cats with and without azotemia and in response to treatment with amlodipine besylate. J Vet Intern Med 2014;28(1):144–53.

15. Williams TL, Elliott J, Syme HM. Renin-angiotensin-aldosterone system activity in hyperthyroid cats with and without concurrent hypertension. J Vet Intern Med 2013;27(3):522–9.

16. Jepson RE, Warren HR, Syme HM, et al. Uromodulin gene variants and their association with renal function and blood pressure in cats: a pilot study. J Small Anim Pract 2016;57(11):580–8.

17. Sansom J, Rogers K, Wood JL. Blood pressure assessment in healthy cats and cats with hypertensive retinopathy. Am J Vet Res 2004;65(2):245–52.

18. Syme HM, Barber PJ, Markwell PJ, et al. Prevalence of systolic hypertension in cats with chronic renal failure at initial evaluation. J Am Vet Med Assoc 2002;220(12):1799–804.

19. Kobayashi DL, Peterson ME, Graves TK, et al. Hypertension in cats with chronic renal failure or hyperthyroidism. J Vet Intern Med 1990;4(2):58–62.

20. Cole L, Jepson R, Humm K. Systemic hypertension in cats with acute kidney injury. J Small Anim Pract 2017;58(10):577–81.

21. Morrow L, Adams V, Elliott J, et al. Hypertension in hyperthyroid cats: prevalence, incidence and predictors of its development. J Vet Intern Med 2009;23:699 (abstract).
22. Watson N, Murray JK, Fonfara S, et al. Clinicopathological features and comorbidities of cats with mild, moderate or severe hyperthyroidism: a radioiodine referral population. J Feline Med Surg 2018;20(12):1130–7.
23. Sennello KA, Schulman RL, Prosek R, et al. Systolic blood pressure in cats with diabetes mellitus. J Am Vet Med Assoc 2003;223(2):198–201.
24. Al-Ghazlat SA, Langston CE, Greco DS, et al. The prevalence of microalbuminuria and proteinuria in cats with diabetes mellitus. Top Companion Anim Med 2011; 26(3):154–7.
25. Ash RA, Harvey AM, Tasker S. Primary hyperaldosteronism in the cat: a series of 13 cases. J Feline Med Surg 2005;7(3):173–82.
26. Henry CJ, Brewer WG, Montgomery RD, et al. Clinical vignette. Adrenal pheochromocytoma. J Vet Intern Med 1993;7(3):199–201.
27. Valentin SY, Cortright CC, Nelson RW, et al. Clinical findings, diagnostic test results, and treatment outcome in cats with spontaneous hyperadrenocorticism: 30 cases. J Vet Intern Med 2014;28(2):481–7.
28. Carter J. Hypertensive ocular disease in cats: a guide to fundic lesions to facilitate early diagnosis. J Feline Med Surg 2019;21(1):35–45.
29. Young WM, Zheng C, Davidson MG, et al. Visual outcome in cats with hypertensive chorioretinopathy. Vet Ophthalmol 2019;22(2):161–7.
30. Chetboul V, Lefebvre HP, Pinhas C, et al. Spontaneous feline hypertension: clinical and echocardiographic abnormalities, and survival rate. J Vet Intern Med 2003;17(1):89–95.
31. de Venecia G, Jampol LM. The eye in accelerated hypertension. II. Localized serous detachments of the retina in patients. Arch Ophthalmol 1984;102(1):68–73.
32. Heidbreder E, Hüller U, Schäfer B, et al. Severe hypertensive retinopathy. Increased incidence in renoparenchymal hypertension. Am J Nephrol 1987; 7(5):394–400.
33. Carter JM, Irving AC, Bridges JP, et al. The prevalence of ocular lesions associated with hypertension in a population of geriatric cats in Auckland, New Zealand. N Z Vet J 2014;62(1):21–9.
34. Stiles J, Kimmitt B. Eye examination in the cat: step-by-step approach and common findings. J Feline Med Surg 2016;18(9):702–11.
35. Cirla A, Drigo M, Ballerini L, et al. VAMPIRE. Vet Ophthalmol 2019;22(6):819–27.
36. Mathur S. Effects of the calcium channel antagonist amlodipine in cats with surgically induced hypertensive renal insufficiency. Am J Vet Res 2002;63(6):833.
37. Brown CA, Munday JS, Mathur S, et al. Hypertensive encephalopathy in cats with reduced renal function. Vet Pathol 2005;42(5):642–9.
38. Littman MP. Spontaneous systemic hypertension in 24 cats. J Vet Intern Med 1994;8(2):79–86.
39. Kyles AE, Gregory CR, Wooldridge JD, et al. Management of hypertension controls postoperative neurologic disorders after renal transplantation in cats. Vet Surg 1999;28(6):436–41.
40. Kwiatkowska M, Hoppe S, Pomianowski A, et al. Reactive seizures in cats: a retrospective study of 64 cases. Vet J 2019;244:1–6.
41. Hori Y, Heishima Y, Yamashita Y, et al. Relationship between indirect blood pressure and various stages of chronic kidney disease in cats. J Vet Med Sci 2018; 80(3):447–52.

42. Syme HM, Markwell PJ, Pfeiffer D, et al. Survival of cats with naturally occurring chronic renal failure is related to severity of proteinuria. J Vet Intern Med 2006; 20(3):528–35.
43. Chakrabarti S, Syme HM, Brown CA, et al. Histomorphometry of feline chronic kidney disease and correlation with markers of renal dysfunction. Vet Pathol 2013;50(1):147–55.
44. Chakrabarti S, Syme HM, Elliott J. Clinicopathological variables predicting progression of azotemia in cats with chronic kidney disease. J Vet Intern Med 2012;26(2):275–81.
45. King JN, Gunn-Moore DA, Tasker S, et al. Benazepril in Renal Insufficiency in Cats Study G. Tolerability and efficacy of benazepril in cats with chronic kidney disease. J Vet Intern Med 2006;20(5):1054–64.
46. Snyder PS, Sadek D, Jones GL. Effect of amlodipine on echocardiographic variables in cats with systemic hypertension. J Vet Intern Med 2001;15(1):52–6.
47. Lesser M, Fox PR, Bond BR. Assessment of hypertension in 40 cats with left ventricular hypertrophy by Doppler-shift sphygmomanometry. J Small Anim Pract 1992;33(2):55–8.
48. Li X, Lan Y, Wang Y, et al. Telmisartan suppresses cardiac hypertrophy by inhibiting cardiomyocyte apoptosis via the NFAT/ANP/BNP signaling pathway. Mol Med Rep 2017;15(5):2574–82.
49. Nelson L, Reidesel E, Ware WA, et al. Echocardiographic and radiographic changes associated with systemic hypertension in cats. J Vet Intern Med 2002; 16(4):418–25.
50. Gouni V, Papageorgiou S, Debeaupuits J, et al. Aortic dissecting aneurysm associated with systemic arterial hypertension in a cat. Schweiz Arch Tierheilkd 2018; 160(5):320–4.
51. Kohnken R, Scansen BA, Premanandan C. Vasa vasorum arteriopathy: relationship with systemic arterial hypertension and other vascular lesions in cats. Vet Pathol 2017;54(3):475–83.
52. Paepe D, Verjans G, Duchateau L, et al. Routine health screening: findings in apparently healthy middle-aged and old cats. J Feline Med Surg 2013; 15(1):8–19.
53. Markovich JE, Freeman LM, Labato MA, et al. Survey of dietary and medication practices of owners of cats with chronic kidney disease. J Feline Med Surg 2015; 17(12):979–83.
54. Martel E, Egner B, Brown SA, et al. Comparison of high-definition oscillometry – a non-invasive technology for arterial blood pressure measurement – with a direct invasive method using radio-telemetry in awake healthy cats. J Feline Med Surg 2013;15(12):1104–13.
55. Jepson RE, Hartley V, Mendl M, et al. A comparison of CAT Doppler and oscillometric Memoprint machines for non-invasive blood pressure measurement in conscious cats. J Feline Med Surg 2005;7(3):147–52.
56. Bijsmans ES, Doig M, Jepson RE, et al. Factors influencing the relationship between the dose of amlodipine required for blood pressure control and change in blood pressure in hypertensive cats. J Vet Intern Med 2016;30(5):1630–6.
57. Desmet L, van der Meer J. Antihypertensive treatment with telmisartan in a cat with amlodipine-induced gingival hyperplasia. JFMS Open Rep 2017;3(2). 2055116917745236.
58. Sent U, Gossl R, Elliott J, et al. Comparison of efficacy of long-term oral treatment with telmisartan and benazepril in cats with chronic kidney disease. J Vet Intern Med 2015;29(6):1479–87.

59. Reynolds BS, Chetboul V, Nguyen P, et al. Effects of dietary salt intake on renal function: a 2-year study in healthy aged cats. J Vet Intern Med 2013;27(3): 507–15.
60. Buranakarl C, Mathur S, Brown SA. Effects of dietary sodium chloride intake on renal function and blood pressure in cats with normal and reduced renal function. Am J Vet Res 2004;65(5):620–7.

Primary Hyperaldosteronism in Cats

An Underdiagnosed Disorder

Hans S. Kooistra, DVM, PhD

KEYWORDS

- Hyperaldosteronism • Conn's syndrome • Adrenal glands • Adrenalectomy
- Aldosterone

KEY POINTS

- Primary hyperaldosteronism, the most common adrenocortical disorder in cats, is caused by idiopathic (bilateral) nodular hyperplasia of the zona glomerulosa or a unilateral or bilateral adenoma or adenocarcinoma of the zona glomerulosa.
- Presenting physical features are usually dominated by signs caused by hypokalemia and/or signs of arterial hypertension.
- The ratio of plasma aldosterone concentration to plasma renin activity is the best screening test for feline primary hyperaldosteronism and must be followed by diagnostic imaging.
- Distinction between bilateral and unilateral primary hyperaldosteronism, and the detection of any vascular extension or distant metastases, are essential to determine the optimal therapeutic strategy.
- Unilateral adrenalectomy is the treatment of choice for confirmed unilateral primary hyperaldosteronism.

INTRODUCTION

Primary hyperaldosteronism, also referred to as Conn's syndrome, is an adrenocortical disorder characterized by excessive, autonomous secretion of mineralocorticoids, mainly aldosterone, leading to systemic arterial hypertension and/or hypokalemia.[1] After its first description in a woman in 1955,[2] Conn suggested that primary hyperaldosteronism is the underlying cause in as many as 20% of people with arterial hypertension.[3] A few years later, he changed this figure to 10%, which would still mean that primary hyperaldosteronism is a rather common disorder in humans. Nevertheless, primary hyperaldosteronism was considered rare for many decades. With improved screening methods, the disorder is diagnosed more often nowadays, and recent studies show that the prevalence of primary hyperaldosteronism is indeed

Department of Clinical Sciences of Companion Animals, Faculty of Veterinary Medicine, Utrecht University, Yalelaan 108, Utrecht 3508 TD, The Netherlands
E-mail address: H.S.Kooistra@uu.nl

Vet Clin Small Anim 50 (2020) 1053–1063
https://doi.org/10.1016/j.cvsm.2020.05.007   **vetsmall.theclinics.com**

much higher than previously thought. Primary hyperaldosteronism is found in about 6% of all human patients with arterial hypertension and in up to 11% of those with therapy-resistant arterial hypertension.[4]

Primary hyperaldosteronism is the most common adrenocortical disorder in cats and, as in humans, is associated with arterial hypertension. Although the cat is considered to be the domestic animal in which primary hyperaldosteronism is most prevalent, the disease is not often diagnosed in veterinary practice. It is underdiagnosed, as it is in humans, which excludes a potentially large number of cats from appropriate therapy and possibly a cure for the disease. This may in part be due to the frequent association of arterial hypertension and/or hypokalemia with chronic kidney disease. In many cases of arterial hypertension and/or hypokalemia, chronic kidney disease may be considered the causal disorder, thereby halting further diagnostic efforts, whereas in fact the chronic kidney disease may itself be a consequence of primary hyperaldosteronism.[5] Arterial hypertension and hypokalemia are often treated symptomatically only, without a thorough search for the underlying cause. Moreover, arterial blood pressure is not measured routinely, if at all, in many veterinary practices.

ALDOSTERONE SYNTHESIS

The adrenal cortex consists of 3 layers: the outer zona glomerulosa, the middle zona fasciculata, and the inner zona reticularis. The difference in hormone production between the 3 adrenocortical zones is due to differences in expression of cytochrome P-450 enzymes.[6] These cytochrome P-450 enzymes are responsible for most of the enzymatic conversions from cholesterol to steroid hormones (**Fig. 1**). The characteristic enzyme in the zona fasciculata and the zona reticularis is 17α-hydroxylase (17,20-lyase, CYP 17), which catalyzes the 17α-hydroxylation of pregnenolone and progesterone as well as the side-chain cleavage at C_{17} of 17-α-hydroxy C_{21} steroids.[6] In other words, the low expression of 17α-hydroxylase (CYP 17) in the zona glomerulosa is the main reason why cholesterol is converted into aldosterone instead of cortisol or androgens in the zona glomerulosa. The other steroidogenic enzymes are expressed in all 3 zones (see **Fig. 1**).

Aldosterone was historically considered to be a hormone produced exclusively in the adrenal cortex. However, recent research has revealed that aldosterone is also produced in tissues other than the adrenal cortex, including the heart, brain, and blood vessels.[7] In these extra-adrenal tissues, aldosterone is thought to act in a paracrine or autocrine mode. These new insights may contribute to the understanding of a number of long-term complications of primary hyperaldosteronism.

ALDOSTERONE METABOLISM

Little is known about the metabolism of aldosterone in cats. The liver is generally considered to be the most important site for inactivation and conjugation of steroid hormones. In cats, cortisol, estradiol, and progesterone are excreted mainly or almost exclusively via the bile into the feces[8] and, considering the structural similarities, it can be expected that this is the main excretion route for aldosterone, as well. This hypothesis is supported by a study by Syme and colleagues,[9] who found that urinary excretion of free aldosterone in cats was 77 times less than in humans and 7 times less than in dogs.

REGULATION OF ALDOSTERONE SECRETION

The production and release of glucocorticoids and androgens by the middle and inner zones of the adrenal cortex are almost exclusively regulated by the plasma

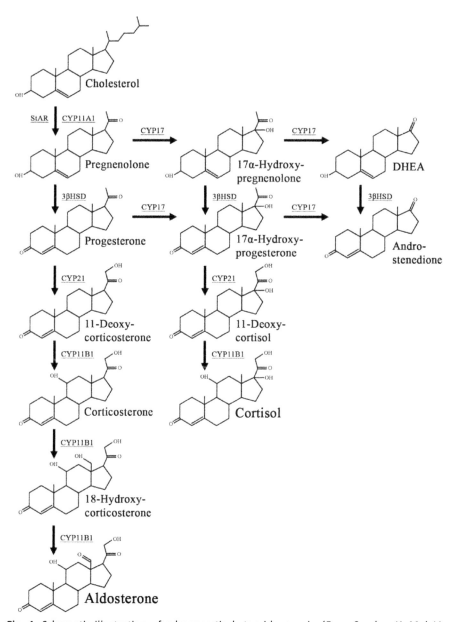

Fig. 1. Schematic illustration of adrenocortical steroidogenesis. (*From* Sanders K, Mol JA, Kooistra HS, et al. New insights in the functional zonation of the canine adrenal cortex. J Vet Intern Med. 2016; 30:741-750; with permission.)

adrenocorticotropic hormone (ACTH) concentration. In contrast, the 2 primary mechanisms controlling aldosterone release are the renin–angiotensin system and potassium. The renin–angiotensin system keeps the circulatory blood volume constant by promoting aldosterone-induced sodium retention during periods of hypovolemia and by decreasing aldosterone-dependent sodium retention during hypervolemia.

Potassium ions directly regulate aldosterone secretion, independent of the renin–angiotensin system. Thus, aldosterone secretion is regulated by negative feedback loops for both potassium and the renin-angiotensin system. In addition to these 2 regulatory mechanisms, aldosterone secretion is influenced by several other factors (ACTH, natriuretic peptides, and a variety of neurotransmitters), none of which is directly connected to a negative feedback loop. They have the common feature of usually responding to stress. ACTH is the classic representative of the group. Although ACTH is a very potent acute aldosterone secretagogue, its action is not sustained and it is not necessary to maintain normal glomerulosa cell function.[10]

PHYSIOLOGIC EFFECTS OF THE RENIN–ANGIOTENSIN SYSTEM

The proteolytic enzyme renin is synthesized in the juxtaglomerular apparatus of the kidney. Stimulation of renal baroreceptors is the most potent mechanism for renin release by the juxtaglomerular cells. These stretch receptors in the afferent arteriole stimulate renin release in response to decreased renal perfusion pressure caused, for example, by hypovolemia. Additional regulation is provided by macula densa cells, a group of modified cells of the distal tubule near the end of the loop of Henle and intimately associated with the juxtaglomerular cells. The sodium concentration in the tubular lumen is monitored by the cells of the macula densa and low sodium levels trigger communication between the macula densa and the juxtaglomerular cells, resulting in renin release.

Angiotensinogen, the precursor of several angiotensin peptides, is produced mainly in the liver from its precursor preproangiotensinogen. In the circulation angiotensinogen is cleaved by renin and other enzymes to release angiotensin I. The angiotensin-converting enzyme converts the inactive decapeptide angiotensin I to the active octapeptide angiotensin II. Angiotensin-converting enzyme-inhibiting compounds are used clinically to disrupt the renin–angiotensin system, as in the treatment of heart failure.

The vast majority of the physiologic actions of the renin-angiotensin system are mediated by angiotensin II and one of its receptors (AT_1-receptor). They include arteriolar vasoconstriction, cell growth, and aldosterone production. Angiotensin II increases vascular resistance and blood pressure. Angiotensin II also regulates the glomerular filtration rate and renal blood flow by constricting the efferent and afferent glomerular arterioles.

PHYSIOLOGIC EFFECTS OF ALDOSTERONE

Aldosterone has 2 important physiologic actions: (1) it regulates extracellular fluid volume and (2) it is a major determinant of potassium homeostasis. These effects are mediated by the binding of aldosterone to the mineralocorticoid receptor in the cytosol of epithelial cells. The epithelia of the kidneys, colon, and salivary glands are the classic target tissues for circulating aldosterone. Aldosterone easily passes through the plasma membrane of these epithelial cells and binds to the mineralocorticoid receptor in the cytoplasm. The aldosterone receptor has equal affinity for both aldosterone and cortisol. Circulating concentrations of cortisol are much higher than those of aldosterone. The mineralocorticoid receptor in the classic aldosterone target tissues is preferentially made available to aldosterone by the enzyme 11β-hydroxysteroid dehydrogenase type 2 (11β-HSD2). This enzyme converts cortisol to cortisone, which has little affinity for the receptor. The aldosterone receptor complex moves from the cytosol to the nucleus, where it modulates the expression of multiple genes.

In the distal convoluted tubule aldosterone, increases sodium reabsorption and potassium excretion. In these tubular cells, the aldosterone receptor complex initiates a sequence of events leading to activation of sodium channels in the apical membrane. Subsequently, increased sodium influx stimulates the Na^+,K^+-ATPase in the basolateral membrane. As aldosterone increases active sodium reabsorption, an electrochemical gradient is established that facilitates the passive transfer of potassium from tubular cells into the urine. Thus, potassium is not excreted in direct exchange for sodium, but rather in a manner that depends directly on the active reabsorption of sodium.

In addition to its endocrine effects on classic epithelial target tissues, aldosterone has major effects on other epithelial and nonepithelial tissues. The effects of aldosterone on endothelial cells and on cardiac tissue contribute to blood pressure homeostasis.[7] It seems that aldosterone may increase blood pressure through 2 main mechanisms: (1) expansion of plasma and extracellular fluid volume and (2) increased total peripheral resistance. With regard to the nonepithelial actions, it should be mentioned that long-term mineralocorticoid excess may lead to microangiopathies that contribute to fibrosis and proliferation of endothelial and smooth muscle cells in the heart, kidney, and other tissues.[7] In cats, primary hyperaldosteronism has been reported as a mediator of progressive renal disease.[5]

PRIMARY HYPERALDOSTERONISM

Two pathophysiologic mechanisms may lead to hypersecretion of aldosterone. A decrease in the effective arterial blood volume (eg, owing to heart failure or edema caused by hypoproteinemia), activates the renin–angiotensin system, which in turn stimulates aldosterone synthesis. This pathophysiologic response to hypovolemia is called secondary hyperaldosteronism or high renin hyperaldosteronism. In contrast, the autonomous and excessive aldosterone secretion in primary hyperaldosteronism is associated with suppressed plasma renin (activity) and is thus low renin hyperaldosteronism.

Primary hyperaldosteronism can be due to autonomous hypersecretion of aldosterone (and/or deoxycorticosterone) by an adrenocortical tumor or by nontumorous, hyperplastic zona glomerulosa tissue. In the majority of the reported cases, feline primary hyperaldosteronism was caused by a unilateral adrenocortical tumor of varying degrees of malignancy, ranging from well-capsulated adenomas to carcinomas with growth into the caudal vena cava and distant metastasis.[11] These reported figures seem to differ markedly from those in humans, where bilateral hyperplasia of the zona glomerulosa accounts for 60% to 65% of cases and aldosterone-producing adenomas for 30% to 35%.[12] However, the diagnosis of idiopathic primary hyperaldosteronism in humans can be established clinically, whereas in cats histopathologic examination of the adrenal glands is required. However, cats with hyperplasia of the zona glomerulosa are often treated medically, meaning that adrenal tissue is not examined histologically except in postmortem examinations. This practice probably means that idiopathic bilateral nodular hyperplasia of the zona glomerulosa occurs more often in cats than suggested by data based on histopathologic findings. In line with this hypothesis, Javadi and colleagues[5] reported 11 cats with "idiopathic" primary hyperaldosteronism in which diagnostic imaging failed to demonstrate an adrenal tumor, suggesting that the cause was adrenocortical hyperplasia (**Fig. 2**).

CLINICAL PRESENTATION OF PRIMARY HYPERALDOSTERONISM IN CATS

Primary hyperaldosteronism mainly occurs in middle-aged and older cats. The pathophysiologic consequences of excessive aldosterone secretion are a consequence

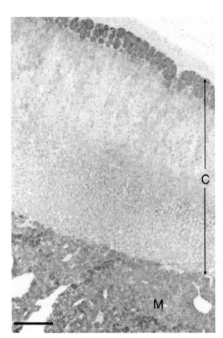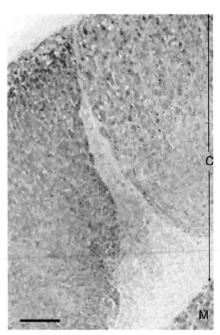

Fig. 2. Histologic sections of adrenals stained with neuron-specific enolase (NSE). In the healthy cat (*left*), the staining of the cortex (*C*) is mainly confined to the zona glomerulosa. In the cat with primary hyperaldosteronism (*right*), the cortex consists of multiple hyperplastic nodules, staining positively for NSE. Staining of the adrenal medulla (*M*) is similar in the 2 sections. Bar = 200 μm.[1]

of increased sodium and water retention and increased renal potassium excretion, which may result in systemic arterial hypertension and potassium depletion, respectively. The progressive depletion of potassium and the development of hypokalemia affect several organ systems, but become particularly manifest in the neuromuscular system by affecting the polarization of nerve and muscle membranes. Muscle weakness is likely to occur at a plasma potassium concentration of less than 2.5 mmol/L, although the severity of muscle weakness is not strictly correlated with the plasma potassium concentration. Affected cats may have (episodic) muscle weakness that results in a plantigrade stance in the hind limbs, difficulty in jumping, and/or a characteristic ventroflexion of the neck (**Fig. 3**). In some cases there is progression to flaccid paresis with hyporeflexia, muscle hypotonia, and difficulty in breathing. In other cats, the presenting physical features of excessive aldosterone secretion are dominated by the consequences of arterial hypertension, that is, loss of vision owing to retinal detachment and/or intraocular hemorrhages. Not all cats with primary hyperaldosteronism present with both signs of hypokalemia and with signs of arterial hypertension.

Primary hyperaldosteronism, especially when owing to micronodular hyperplasia of the zona glomerulosa, is associated with cardiovascular and renal complications in both humans[7] and cats.[5] It has been hypothesized that mild hyperaldosteronism with incomplete renin suppression associated with micronodular hyperplasia of the zona glomerulosa results in the combined deleterious, proinflammatory, and profibrotic effects of elevated aldosterone and angiotensin II levels.

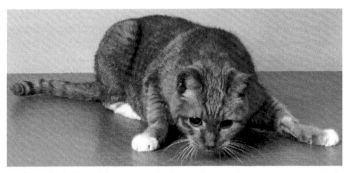

Fig. 3. Cat with typical clinical features of primary hyperaldosteronism: cervical ventroflex-ion (muscle weakness owing to hypokalemia) and mydriasis (owing to arterial hyperten-sion). (*From* Djajadiningrat-Laanen SC, Galac S, Kooistra HS. Primary hyperaldosteronism, expanding the diagnostic net. J Feline Med Surg. 2011; 13:641-650; with permission.)

The most consistent routine laboratory finding is hypokalemia. Aldosterone excess also favors increased acid secretion, which may lead to (usually mild) hypokalemic metabolic alkalosis. Either hypophosphatemia or hypomagnesemia or both may develop in affected cats. Some cats may have increased plasma creatine kinase con-centrations.[11] In cats, idiopathic hyperaldosteronism is frequently associated with (slowly progressing) renal insufficiency, probably owing to aldosterone-induced arte-riolar and glomerular sclerosis, tubular atrophy, and interstitial fibrosis and the delete-rious effects of arterial hypertension.

DIAGNOSIS OF FELINE PRIMARY HYPERALDOSTERONISM

In primary hyperaldosteronism owing to an adrenocortical tumor, the plasma aldo-sterone concentration is usually quite high as well as the plasma concentration of aldosterone precursors, such as progesterone.[13] In cats with idiopathic primary hyperaldosteronism, that is, owing to hyperplasia of zona glomerulosa tissue, the plasma aldosterone concentration is usually only slightly elevated or even within the (upper limit of the) reference range. Because hypokalemia is a predominant fac-tor in decreasing aldosterone secretion, the combination of hypokalemia and a moderately increased aldosterone value should be considered inappropriately high and abnormal.

In primary hyperaldosteronism, the classic characteristics are an increased plasma aldosterone concentration with concomitant decreased plasma renin (activ-ity). The combination of a high normal or elevated plasma aldosterone concentra-tion and low plasma renin (activity) indicates persistent (autonomous) aldosterone synthesis in the presence of little or no stimulation by the renin–angiotensin system. In humans the plasma aldosterone to renin ratio is considered to be a very useful aid in diagnosing primary hyperaldosteronism. This also seems to be true for cats with primary hyperaldosteronism.[5] The diagnostic value of the aldosterone to renin ratio is principally determined by the sensitivity of the renin assay. It is important to take into account that renin values should be interpreted in compari-son with an appropriate control population. The accuracy of the aldosterone to renin ratio also depends on preservation of renin (activity) during sample collection and storage: blood samples should be collected in ice-chilled tubes and centri-fuged in a chilled centrifuge, and the plasma should be kept in the refrigerator until assayed.

An alternative diagnostic approach may be measurement of the urinary aldosterone to creatinine ratio (UACR). Cats excrete smaller quantities of aldosterone and its 18-glucuronidated metabolite in urine than do humans or dogs,[9] but nevertheless the UACR can be determined.[14] It provides an integrated reflection of aldosterone secretion over time. It has the advantage that the urine sample for measurement of aldosterone does not have to be cooled and a urine sample can be collected quite easily by the owner. Unfortunately, the reference range for the UACR proved to be quite wide and did not easily facilitate differentiation between healthy cats and those with primary hyperaldosteronism, although a high UACR points to hyperaldosteronism.[15]

A dynamic test using a suppressive agent that reduces aldosterone secretion in healthy cats but has little or no effect in those with primary hyperaldosteronism would seem to be the best method to show the presence of hyperfunctioning zona glomerulosa tissue. Oral administration of fludrocortisone has been shown to suppress circulating aldosterone concentration in healthy adult cats.[15] In another study, it was shown that oral administration of sodium chloride (0.25 g/kg body weight, twice daily for 4 consecutive days) did not significantly lower the UACR in healthy cats, but oral administration of fludrocortisone acetate (0.05 mg/kg body weight, twice daily for 4 consecutive days) did reduce the UACR by more than 40% in healthy cats.[14]

This fludrocortisone suppression test, using the UACR, was also used in a study with 19 client-owned cats with arterial hypertension caused by primary hyperaldosteronism (n = 9) or other causes (n = 10).[16] The results of this study show that all cats with primary hyperaldosteronism had a basal UACR more than 7.5×10^{-9}. In all cats without primary hyperaldosteronism and a basal UACR of more than 7.5×10^{-9}, fludrocortisone administration induced more than 50% suppression of the UACR. In contrast, fludrocortisone administration resulted in less than 50% suppression in 6 of the 9 cats with primary hyperaldosteronism. The results suggest that measuring the UACR before and after 4 days of administering fludrocortisone is a practical method of confirming most cases of feline primary hyperaldosteronism, and especially of substantiating the absence of primary hyperaldosteronism in cats.[16]

A suppression test using telmisartan, an angiotensin II receptor blocker, may also have the potential to diagnose primary hyperaldosteronism in cats. Theoretically, suppression of aldosterone secretion would be expected in healthy cats, whereas cats with primary hyperaldosteronism, that is, cats with autonomous aldosterone secretion, are not expected to have a significant decrease in aldosterone secretion. The fludrocortisone or telmisartan suppression test may prove to be a practical noninvasive diagnostic tool to diagnose primary hyperaldosteronism in cats, but further evaluation of these tests is required, particularly with regard to its discriminatory power in diagnosing "idiopathic" primary hyperaldosteronism.

DIAGNOSTIC IMAGING

Differentiating between tumorous and nontumorous mineralocorticoid excess, requires diagnostic imaging. Diagnostic imaging techniques such as ultrasound examination, MRI, and computed tomography scan are used to identify adrenal abnormalities and, in case of neoplasia, to evaluate for possible extension into blood vessels as well as evidence of distant metastases. Although the presence of visible tumor tissue in the caudal vena cava indicates that surgical removal may be difficult, failure to detect it by diagnostic imaging is no guarantee of its absence and does not necessarily predict an uncomplicated adrenalectomy.

There are more limitations to conventional diagnostic imaging in determining the optimal treatment strategy for primary hyperaldosteronism. Functional neoplasms of the zona glomerulosa do not have to be large to cause clinically relevant hyperaldosteronism, and may therefore be well below the detection limit of ultrasound examination, computed tomography scan, or MRI. Similarly, clinically relevant hyperplasia of zona glomerulosa tissue may not be revealed by these conventional diagnostic imaging techniques. Failure to see an obvious mass for many endocrine tumors simply indicates that the tumor is small. Some nonfunctional adrenocortical neoplasms, that is, "incidentalomas," may become quite large and be readily visualized with ultrasound examination, computed tomography scan, or MRI, but may not cause clinical signs. Therefore, a visible adrenal mass may not be a functional neoplasm of the zona glomerulosa, which is causing the clinical signs of primary hyperaldosteronism, and if surgery is planned on the basis of conventional diagnostic imaging alone, the wrong adrenal gland may be removed or the patient may be inappropriately selected for, or excluded from, adrenalectomy. It can be concluded that whatever imaging technique is used, the findings should be interpreted in conjunction with those of biochemical studies.

Adrenal vein sampling was introduced in human medicine in the late 1960s and, despite potentially severe complications, it has become the gold standard to determine the laterality (left or right adrenal) of excessive aldosterone production in humans. Each adrenal vein is cannulated in turn and samples are collected while peripheral venous blood samples are collected simultaneously. The plasma aldosterone and cortisol concentrations in the adrenal and peripheral venous samples are compared to detect the source of excess aldosterone. Unfortunately, the much smaller vascular dimensions in cats preclude adrenal venous sampling and thus determination of the laterality of primary hyperaldosteronism continues to rely on diagnostic imaging.

TREATMENT OF FELINE PRIMARY HYPERALDOSTERONISM

Unilateral adrenalectomy is the treatment of choice for confirmed unilateral primary hyperaldosteronism, at least when diagnostic imaging has not revealed metastases. Adrenalectomy can be performed via a ventral midline celiotomy or via a paracostal approach. In some centers, adrenalectomy in cats is now routinely performed by laparoscopy, with lower perioperative morbidity and mortality than by open transabdominal surgery. Laparoscopic adrenalectomy may become the surgical procedure of choice in veterinary medicine, but most surgeons still prefer transabdominal access because it provides maximal exposure of the adrenal and blood vessels. There have been several reports of successful surgical interventions in cats,[17,18] including the excision of an adrenocortical carcinoma together with its extension into the vena cava.[19]

Preoperatively and perioperatively, hypokalemia should be controlled as well as possible, by oral or intravenous supplementation. During the first few weeks after surgery, a generous dietary intake of sodium can be provided to avoid the hyperkalemia that could develop from hypoaldosteronism as a consequence of chronic contralateral adrenocortical suppression. Analogous to the postoperative management of hypercortisolemia owing to an adrenocortical tumor, temporary fludrocortisone therapy could also be considered. However, in the reported cases such postsurgical measures have not been necessary and their omission does not seem to have had deleterious effects.

After complete removal of a unilateral, nonmetastasized, aldosterone-producing tumor, the prognosis is excellent, with no medication required in most cases. Most of the cats that survived the immediate postoperative period have continued to be clinically asymptomatic for 1 to several years. However, perioperative complications have been reported, including intraoperative or postoperative intra-abdominal hemorrhage. Hemorrhage was not specifically related to the type of neoplasia, intravenous tumor extension, or the presence or absence of arterial hypertension as a presenting clinical sign. Therefore, all owners considering the surgical management of primary hyperaldosteronism in their cat should be informed of this potential complication.

Surgery may be contraindicated when the cat is diagnosed with bilateral hyperplasia of the zona glomerulosa, a nonresectable unilateral adrenocortical neoplasm, distant metastases, financial limitations, or comorbid conditions. These cats can be treated medically with a mineralocorticoid receptor blocker, together with potassium supplementation and antihypertensive drugs if needed. The aldosterone receptor blocker most often used in cats is spironolactone. The initial dose is 2 mg/kg body weight orally, twice daily, increased as needed to control hypokalemia. Persistent arterial hypertension can be treated with the calcium blocker amlodipine, at an initial oral dose of 0.1 mg/kg body weight, once daily. Telmisartan, being an angiotensin II receptor blocker, is less effective as an antihypertensive agent, because it does not block the effects of aldosterone.

In cats, hyperaldosteronism owing to bilateral adrenocortical hyperplasia is usually somewhat milder than that owing to neoplasia and normokalemia may be sustained for long intervals with spironolactone alone or combined with low doses of potassium. However, the prognosis may not be as favorable as that after complete removal of an aldosterone-producing neoplasm, because medical treatment does not permanently abolish the mineralocorticoid excess.

DISCLOSURE

The author does not have any commercial or financial conflicts of interest and no funding sources to disclose.

REFERENCES

1. Galac S, Reusch CE, Kooistra HS, et al. Adrenals. In: Rijnberk A, Kooistra HS, editors. Clinical endocrinology of dogs and cats. 2nd edition. Hannover (Germany): Schlütersche; 2010. p. 93–154.
2. Conn JW. Primary aldosteronism, a new clinical syndrome. J Lab Clin Med 1955; 45:3–17.
3. Conn JW. The evolution of primary aldosteronism: 1954–1967. Harvey Lect 1966-1967;62:257–91.
4. Douma S, Petidis K, Doumas M, et al. Prevalence of primary hyperaldosteronism in resistant hypertension: a retrospective observational study. Lancet 2008;371: 1921–6.
5. Javadi S, Djajadiningrat-Laanen S, Kooistra HS, et al. Primary hyperaldosteronism, a mediator of progressive renal disease in cats. Domest Anim Endocrinol 2005;28:85–104.
6. Sanders K, Mol JA, Kooistra HS, et al. New insights in the functional zonation of the canine adrenal cortex. J Vet Intern Med 2016;30:741–50.
7. Connell JM, MacKenzie SM, Freel EM, et al. A lifetime of aldosterone excess: long-term consequences of altered regulation of aldosterone production for cardiovascular function. Endocr Rev 2008;29:133–54.
8. Graham LH, Brown JL. Cortisol metabolism in the domestic cat and implications for non-invasive monitoring of adrenocortical function in endangered felids. Zoo Biol 1996;15:71–82.

9. Syme HM, Fletcher MG, Bailey SR, et al. Measurement of aldosterone in feline, canine and human urine. J Small Anim Pract 2007;48:202–8.
10. Williams GH. Aldosterone biosynthesis, regulation, and classical mechanism of action. Heart Fail Rev 2005;10:7–13.
11. Djajadiningrat-Laanen SC, Galac S, Kooistra HS. Primary hyperaldosteronism, expanding the diagnostic net. J Feline Med Surg 2011;13:641–50.
12. Young WF. Primary aldosteronism: renaissance of a syndrome. Clin Endocrinol (Oxf) 2007;66:607–18.
13. DeClue AE, Breshears LA, Pardo ID, et al. Hyperaldosteronism and hyperprogesteronism in a cat with an adrenal cortical carcinoma. J Vet Intern Med 2005;19: 355–8.
14. Djajadiningrat-Laanen SC, Galac S, Cammelbeeck SE, et al. Urinary aldosterone to creatinine ratio in cats before and after suppression with salt or fludrocortisone acetate. J Vet Intern Med 2008;22:1283–8.
15. Matsuda M, Behrend EN, Kemppainen R, et al. Serum aldosterone and cortisol concentrations before and after suppression with fludrocortisone in cats: a pilot study. J Vet Diagn Invest 2015;27:361–8.
16. Djajadiningrat-Laanen SC, Galac S, Boevé M, et al. Evaluation of the oral fludrocortisone suppression test for diagnosing primary hyperaldosteronism in cats. J Vet Intern Med 2013;27:1493–9.
17. MacKay AD, Holt PE, Sparkes AH. Successful surgical treatment of a cat with primary aldosteronism. J Feline Med Surg 1999;1:117–22.
18. Ash RA, Harvey AM, Tasker S. Primary hyperaldosteronism in the cat: a series of 13 cases. J Feline Med Surg 2005;7:173–82.
19. Rose SA, Kyles AE, Labelle P, et al. Adrenalectomy and caval thrombectomy in a cat with primary hyperaldosteronism. J Am Anim Hosp Assoc 2007;43:209–14.

Hyperthyroidism in Cats
Considering the Impact of Treatment Modality on Quality of Life for Cats and Their Owners

Mark E. Peterson, DVM*

KEYWORDS

- Feline • Thyroid • Antithyroid drug • Methimazole • Thyroidectomy • Radioiodine
- Radioactive iodine • Low-iodine diet

KEY POINTS

- Hyperthyroidism develops over time, transitioning from normal thyroid tissue to hyperplasia to adenoma (and, rarely, carcinoma). By the time cats are diagnosed with hyperthyroidism, almost all will have adenomatous disease (tumors), not hyperplasia.
- Hyperthyroidism is a progressive disease, and the underlying thyroid tumors will continue to grow over time, especially if left untreated or if hyperthyroidism is only controlled with antithyroid drugs or diet, and not removed or ablated with surgery or radioiodine.
- In cats, hyperthyroidism can be treated in 4 ways: medical management with methimazole or carbimazole, nutritional management (low-iodine diet), surgical thyroidectomy, and radioactive iodine (^{131}I). Medical and nutritional managements are "reversible" or palliative treatments, whereas surgical thyroidectomy and ^{131}I are "permanent" or curative treatments.
- Each form of treatment has advantages and disadvantages that should be considered when formulating a treatment plan for the individual hyperthyroid cat, with the goal of achieving the best long-term "quality of life," for both the cats and their owners. Treatment choices should be informed by factors such as age, thyroid disease severity, and clinically significant, nonthyroidal comorbidities.

INTRODUCTION

Hyperthyroidism is the most common feline endocrine disorder and an important cause of morbidity in middle-aged to older cats all around the world, affecting about 10% of senior to geriatric cats.[1–3] In cats, hyperthyroidism is typically a chronic progressive condition that, left untreated, can become life-threatening.[3–5] Therefore, almost all hyperthyroid cats will need to be treated, with veterinarians playing a primary role in advising and educating owners about treatment options.

Animal Endocrine Clinic, New York, NY, USA
* 220 Manhattan Avenue, New York, NY 11025.
E-mail address: drpeterson@animalendocrine.com

Vet Clin Small Anim 50 (2020) 1065–1084
https://doi.org/10.1016/j.cvsm.2020.06.004
0195-5616/20/© 2020 Elsevier Inc. All rights reserved.

Hyperthyroidism in cats can be treated in 4 ways, which include oral or transdermal antithyroid drugs, nutritional management with a low-iodine diet, surgical thyroidectomy, and radioiodine (^{131}I). All of these treatment options have the potential of resolving hyperthyroidism, but each treatment has its own advantages and disadvantages (**Table 1**).

When veterinarians recommend one of these options for a hyperthyroid cat, an important issue is frequently neglected—the impact that the selected treatment has on "quality of life" (QoL), for both the cat and their owners. This QoL issue is true, not only for the time when treatment is instituted but also during the weeks, months, and years during or following treatment, when the consequences of the chosen treatment option may still emerge.

This article illustrates how each treatment modality could actually be the optimal choice for a specific cat-owner combination, especially when the issue of long-term QoL for the hyperthyroid cat and its owner is considered. To that end, the article starts by reviewing the evolution of this feline disease and then discusses workup for concomitant diseases common in the senior to geriatric hyperthyroid cat. Finally, an in-depth review the of advantages and disadvantages of each treatment option is presented, because the clinician must have a comprehensive knowledge of this information in order to present the best, unbiased recommendation for each individual owner and their cat.

ETIOPATHOGENESIS OF FELINE HYPERTHYROIDISM

The veterinary clinician must have a firm grasp of the pathologic features of hyperthyroidism and how this thyroid tumor disease progresses in cats. Without this knowledge, the veterinarian cannot adequately advise the owner on the best treatment option for their cat.

Affected thyroid lobes of cats with hyperthyroidism contain single or multiple hyperplastic and adenomatous nodules,[3,6] which is most similar to the human disease of toxic nodular goiter (also known as Plummer disease), which occurs in elderly individuals.

Hyperthyroid disease develops and progresses over time, transitioning from normal thyroid tissue to thyroid hyperplasia to thyroid adenoma (and, rarely, carcinoma) (**Fig. 1**). By the time cats are diagnosed with hyperthyroidism, almost all cats will have nodular thyroid adenomas.[3]

The pathologic changes in the thyroid lobes of hyperthyroid cats are almost always benign.[6–8] Approximately 2% of hyperthyroid cats develop thyroid carcinoma, which can be classified as either follicular, papillary, or mixed.[9,10] However, the prevalence of malignancy in these cats appears to increase over time (see **Fig. 1**), especially if the thyroid tumor is not definitively treated with thyroidectomy or radioiodine.[4]

From a pathologic, morphologic, and functional perspective, thyroid tumors are not static. Once the adenomatous thyroid gland develops its autonomous state, both the size of the thyroid nodule (goiter) and the severity of the hyperthyroid state progress over time. Exposure to the environmental or nutritional disruptors that helped induce the cat's thyroid disease will likely be ongoing, and these factors may contribute to the continued progression of the disease.[1,3] Regardless of the specific molecular mechanisms responsible for the thyroid pathologic condition in hyperthyroid cats, the goiter grows and continues to secrete thyroid hormone autonomously. As the severity of the functional thyroid tumor disease worsens, these cats can develop more severe, and ultimately poorly responsive, hyperthyroidism.[5]

Table 1
Considerations regarding treatment options for feline hyperthyroidism

	Antithyroid Drugs	Low-Iodine Diet	Thyroidectomy	Radioiodine (^{131}I)
Control vs cure	Reversible, control Thyroid tumor continues to grow	Reversible, control Thyroid tumor continues to grow	Permanent, cure Removes thyroid tumors	Permanent, cure Irradiates and ablates thyroid tumors
Initial cost	Low	Low	High	High
Long-term cost	Moderate	Moderate	Low	Low
Success rate in controlling hyperthyroidism	Fairly high (75%)	About 50%	High (>90%)	Very high (>95%)
Prerequisites	None No special training required	Indoor cat Must be able to feed only the low-iodine diet	Preoperative preparation Skilled surgeon	Facility licensed to treat with ^{131}I
Ease for owner (easy, moderate, difficult)	Moderate to difficult for tablets Easier for liquid and transdermal routes	Easy (but low palatability issue in many cats)	Preoperative preparation moderately difficult Postoperative management easy unless hypocalcemia or hypothyroidism develop	Postdischarge radiation safety precautions moderately difficult Postoperative management easy unless hypothyroidism develops
Sedation or anesthesia	No	No	Anesthesia	Sedation (sometimes needed for thyroid imaging or treatment)
Hospitalization	No	No	1–3 d	3 d to 4 wk depending on regional legislation
Time to euthyroid	2–4 wk	6–8 wk	Within 24–48 h	Days to weeks
Clinical side effects	Mild side effects common Serious side effect rare	No, but many cats remain hyperthyroid	No	No

(continued on next page)

Table 1
(continued)

	Antithyroid Drugs	Low-Iodine Diet	Thyroidectomy	Radioiodine (^{131}I)
Hematologic side effects	Leukopenia, anemia possible	No	No	No
Hepatopathy	Possible	No	No	No
Hypothyroidism	Possible	No	Possible More likely after bilateral thyroidectomy	Possible More likely with bilateral tumors and higher ^{131}I doses
Hypoparathyroidism (hypocalcemia)	No	No	Not uncommon after bilateral thyroidectomy	No
Azotemic CKD	Possible More common if overdosed (iatrogenic hypothyroidism)	Possible, but unlikely	Possible More common with postoperative hypothyroidism	Possible More common with post-^{131}I hypothyroidism
Recurrence or relapse of hyperthyroidism	High T4 values common during long-term treatment Resistance to antithyroid drug can develop as thyroid tumor grows over time	Persistent hyperthyroidism relatively common Many cats do not regain lost weight	Recurrence after unilateral thyroidectomy common Relapse possible if bilateral thyroidectomy not complete	Relapse possible (<5%)
QoL for cat	Overall fair to good Poor in cats that develop side effects Many cats appear to dislike being medicated daily Bitter taste of medicine	Overall fair to good Poor in cats that refuse diet or are reluctant to eat it Poor in outdoor cats that must be kept indoor	Overall very good to excellent Poor in cats that develop hypocalcemia Fair in cats that develop hypothyroidism and must be treated with L-T4	Overall very good to excellent Fair in cats that develop hypothyroidism and must be treated with L-T4
QoL for owner	Fair to good Can become poor if cat develops "resistance" to medication Only fair if azotemia develops	Good if cat eats diet and hyperthyroidism is controlled Poor if diet fails to adequately lower serum T4 or if clinical signs persist	Overall good to excellent Poor if hypocalcemia develops (daily oral calcium and vitamin D) Only fair if hypothyroidism or azotemia develop	Overall good to excellent Only fair if hypothyroidism or azotemia develop

Normal thyroid
(with a few thyrocytes
predestined for growth)

Thyroid hyperplasia
(susceptible thyrocytes
proliferating)

Thyroid adenoma
(hyperplastic nodules
coalescing into
adenomas)

Thyroid carcinoma
(adenomas transforming
into multinodular
carcinoma)

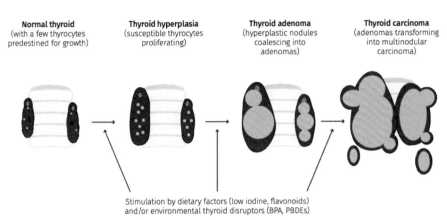

Stimulation by dietary factors (low iodine, flavonoids)
and/or environmental thyroid disruptors (BPA, PBDEs)

Fig. 1. Etiopathogenesis of adenomatous nodular goiter (thyroid adenoma and carcinoma) in cats with hyperthyroidism. In all likelihood, the normal feline thyroid gland contains a subset of thyrocytes (possibly stem cells) that are genetically predisposed to grow and form adenomatous nodules. These predisposed thyrocytes appear to have an exceedingly high natural, autonomous growth potential, reminiscent of, and possibly related to, that characterizing fetal thyroid cells (thyroid stem cells).[7,59,60] Therefore, adenomatous thyroid nodules of hyperthyroid cats are likely a late manifestation of this natural phenomenon of an inborn growth advantage in some thyrocytes resulting from the persistence of the enhanced growth behavior seen in embryonic stem cells into the adult life of some cells. Dietary factors (eg, mild iodine deficiency), or environmental thyroid disruptors (bisphenol A [BPA] or polybrominated diphenyl ethers [PBDEs]), or both can then act as multipliers to further stimulate these susceptible thyroid cells to grow and proliferate into adenomatous hyperplasia and then thyroid neoplasia (adenomas, and in some cases, carcinomas). (*From* Peterson ME. Hyperthyroidism: background, etiopathogenesis and changing prevalence of feline thyroid disease. In: Feldman EC, Fracassi F, Peterson ME, eds. Feline Endocrinology. Milan: EDRA; 2019:114-129; with permission.)

Although antithyroid drugs, such as methimazole or carbimazole, inhibit production of thyroid hormones, they do not slow or stop the progression of thyroid pathologic condition. The longer medical management is used, the larger the thyroid tumor becomes.[4] This progressive and relentless increase in the number of functional thyroid tumor cells explains the need to monitor and periodically increase the dose of antithyroid medication in order to maintain euthyroidism in hyperthyroid cats chronically managed with these drugs.[5,11]

The fact that feline hyperthyroidism is a progressive, benign thyroid neoplasia, with continued growth and an ability to transform into thyroid carcinoma (at least in some cats)[3,4] should influence the decision about treatment options for individual cats (see **Table 1**). Younger cats without concurrent disease that have a potential to live a long time might be better treated with a definitive treatment (ie, surgical thyroidectomy or ^{131}I), whereas geriatric cats with clinically significant concurrent disease (eg, chronic kidney disease [CKD] or neoplasia) might be better treated with antithyroid drugs or a low-iodine diet. Most hyperthyroid cats, however, fall somewhere in between these 2 extremes. Only the educated owner, with input from their veterinarian, can really decide what the best option is for both themselves and their cat.

RULE OUT CONCURRENT DISEASE

Almost all hyperthyroid cats are senior to geriatric, with more than 95% of cats being ≥10 years of age. Therefore, it should not be unexpected that such older hyperthyroid cats frequently suffer from comorbidities, which can further complicate the diagnosis and management of hyperthyroidism.

Concomitant diseases are common in hyperthyroid cats, with 20% to 35% of cats examined before ^{131}I therapy having at least 1 comorbidity.[12–14] The most common concurrent diseases detected in these hyperthyroid cats include cardiac, renal, and gastrointestinal (GI) disease.[12–15] Such comorbidities can either be a direct consequence of the hyperthyroid state or incidental findings, reflecting the older age of these cats.

All cats diagnosed with hyperthyroidism should have a thorough physical examination, hematologic and biochemical profile, and complete urinalysis. Particular attention should be paid to examination or laboratory findings not readily explained by a diagnosis of hyperthyroidism.[16] For example, small or irregularly shaped kidneys should increase suspicion of "masked" CKD. Thickened intestinal loops or jejunal lymphadenopathy detected on abdominal palpation should raise concern for enteropathy. Signs of dyspnea, cardiac murmur, or arrhythmia all suggest clinically significant heart disease. In these hyperthyroid cats, further workup with diagnostic imaging (eg, chest radiographs, echocardiography, abdominal ultrasound) is strongly recommended.

If coexisting disease is suspected or confirmed, it is important to discuss these issues with owners so that they do not falsely assume that all of their cat's clinical signs will resolve with treatment of hyperthyroidism alone.

Thyrotoxic Heart Disease

Clinical evidence of heart disease, such as tachycardia, murmur, arrhythmia, and ventricular hypertrophy, is a well-recognized consequence of hyperthyroidism.[17,18] Thyrotoxic heart disease becomes more common with increased severity of hyperthyroidism. In 1 study, concurrent cardiac disease was diagnosed in 37% of cats with mild hyperthyroidism versus 71% of cats with severe hyperthyroidism.[15] Clinical signs of heart failure (eg, dyspnea) were also more common in cats with severe disease (16%) compared with cats with mild disease (0%).[15]

Although rare in today's population of hyperthyroid cats, overt heart failure may result in pleural effusion or pulmonary edema, leading to respiratory distress.[13,15,16,18] Almost all cats that develop overt heart failure have severe and long-standing hyperthyroidism, many of which can no longer be controlled with antithyroid drugs.[5,15]

When assessing cardiac disease in hyperthyroid cats, one should focus on those with cardiac failure that need to be treated with diuretics. In hyperthyroid cats with stable cardiac disease, differentiating between underlying hypertrophic cardiomyopathy and thyrotoxic heart disease is difficult and is best done once the cat has been euthyroid for 6 months or longer.[18] Cats with subclinical thyrotoxic cardiac disease (without overt failure) rarely require additional therapy beyond treatment of hyperthyroidism itself.

Chronic Kidney Disease

Hyperthyroidism and CKD are both common disorders in older cats. Therefore, it should not be surprising that both disorders frequently occur in the same cat. Hyperthyroidism increases the renal blood flow as well as the glomerular filtration rate (GFR).[17,19,20] This increased GFR can "mask" underlying renal insufficiency by lowering serum concentrations of urea nitrogen and creatinine despite mild to moderate kidney disease. Decreased muscle mass, a common feature of hyperthyroidism, also contributes to the lowered serum creatinine concentration in these cats (because creatinine is derived from muscle metabolism).

Successful treatment of hyperthyroidism reduces serum thyroid hormone concentration to normal and, in cats without CKD, also normalizes the GFR.[17,19–21] In cats with CKD, however, the GFR will fall to the low-normal or subnormal levels expected with moderate renal dysfunction.[20] This decrease in GFR results in worsening of serum kidney function tests or the apparent development of renal disease.[17,19,20,22] Renal disease was already present before treatment but was masked by the hyperdynamic state.

Predicting which untreated hyperthyroid cats have underlying CKD can be difficult.[17,19,20] In the absence of methods for accurately measuring GFR, the serum urea and creatinine concentrations and urine specific gravity should be carefully evaluated. Serum symmetric dimethylarginine (SDMA) concentrations can also be helpful as an adjunctive test for masked CKD in these cats.[22] If the serum urea, creatinine, or SDMA concentrations are at the upper end of the reference interval (or borderline high), or if the urine specific gravity is dilute (<1.035, but certainly <1.020), then masked kidney disease should be suspected.

Because of the difficulties in predicting which hyperthyroid cats have masked CKD, a "methimazole trial" is commonly recommended as a test of renal function in these cats. If hyperthyroid cats do not develop worsening azotemia after the serum T_4 decreases to normal on antithyroid medication, then concurrent CKD can be excluded and a more definitive treatment option for hyperthyroidism is selected. However, this test frequently does not accurately predict or exclude CKD.[23] At least 3 to 6 months of euthyroidism are necessary to accurately assess renal function,[20,23] so a "normal" methimazole trial (lasting only 1 to 2 months) can never guarantee that the kidney function will not deteriorate after definitive therapy.

Approximately 25% of hyperthyroid cats can be expected to develop some degree of azotemia (serum creatinine $\geq$2.0 mg/dL; $\geq$175 µmol/L) within 3 to 6 months of successful treatment of hyperthyroidism. In most cats, this azotemia is only mild to moderate (International Renal Interest Society [IRIS] stage 2), tends to remain stable for prolong periods, and does not significantly affect survival, as long as euthyroidism is maintained.[23,24] Kidney parameters are unlikely to increase more than 1 IRIS stage. A few cats will develop more severe azotemic CKD (IRIS stage 3–4) after treatment, giving these cats a much poorer long-term prognosis.

On the other hand, cats that become hypothyroid after treatment have a higher prevalence of azotemia, with a subsequent decrease in QoL for both cats and owners. In addition, development of azotemia in cats with iatrogenic hypothyroidism has a negative impact on survival. In 1 study, survival of hypothyroid, azotemic cats was half of that of hypothyroid, nonazotemic cats (median 405 vs 905 days).[24] Thus, no matter what treatment is selected, the aim is to maintain total T_4 concentrations within the middle half of the reference interval to ensure euthyroidism, but to avoid overt or subclinical hypothyroidism (low to low-normal T_4 with high serum TSH concentrations).[25,26] If iatrogenic hypothyroidism develops after definitive therapy (^{131}I or thyroidectomy), supplementation with levothyroxine (L-T_4) will lower serum creatinine concentrations in many of these cats and improve survival.[27]

Gastrointestinal Disease

In 1 study of untreated hyperthyroid cats, the most commonly identified concurrent diseases were chronic enteropathy and alimentary lymphoma. Therefore, although GI signs can be due to hyperthyroidism itself, one must always consider that these signs may be due to concurrent GI disease. For example, vomiting is reported in just under half of cats diagnosed with hyperthyroidism. Owners often indicate that this occurs shortly after eating, leading to the suspicion that it is secondary to rapid overeating. Vomiting should resolve once euthyroidism has been restored. A cat that continues to vomit after effective treatment for hyperthyroidism should raise suspicion for undiagnosed GI comorbidity.

Changes in defecation, mainly diarrhea and increased fecal volume, are less commonly seen in hyperthyroid cats. These findings can result from intestinal hypermotility and malabsorption associated with the hyperthyroid state. Some hyperthyroid cats will also develop steatorrhea.[16,28] However, most hyperthyroid cats that present with moderate to severe diarrhea as one of their primary clinical signs have concurrent GI disease (eg, inflammatory bowel disease, alimentary lymphoma).[13] In these cats, further diagnostic workup, including an abdominal ultrasound, endoscopy, or intestinal biopsy, should be considered, especially before definitive treatment. Short-term use of an antithyroid drug trial can also help determine if the diarrhea is due to hyperthyroidism or primary GI disease. If signs of diarrhea persist despite adequate control of the hyperthyroidism, then concurrent GI disease is likely.

SELECTING THE BEST TREATMENT FOR THE INDIVIDUAL HYPERTHYROID CAT (AND THEIR OWNER)
Owner Needs and Circumstances

Education about details of treatment options
The 4 treatment options include oral or transdermal antithyroid drugs, nutritional management with a low-iodine diet, surgical thyroidectomy, and ^{131}I (radioiodine) thyroid tumor ablation. All of these treatment options have the potential of resolving clinical signs of hyperthyroidism, but each has advantages and disadvantages (see **Table 1**).

The options differ in their potential efficacy, side effects, costs, ease of administration, and availability (see **Table 1**), and some cats will receive or require multiple modes of treatment over time. Veterinarians need to clearly communicate and discuss details of all 4 treatment options with the owner, including potential costs, adverse effects, risks, and expected outcome for each option (see **Table 1**). Only after informing the owner about the pros and cons of each option can they decide the best way to treat their hyperthyroid cat—one that will result in the best QoL for both cat and the owner.

However, in many veterinary practices, communication appears inadequate. One survey of owners of hyperthyroid cats found that almost 20% would have liked a more detailed explanation of treatment options by their veterinarian, and more than 30% would have liked more information on long-term management of their hyperthyroid cats.[29]

Cat owner issues or circumstances
Cat owner issues or circumstances, such as cost of therapy, is a major consideration in many instances (see **Table 1**). Definitive treatments, such as surgical thyroidectomy or ^{131}I, have a higher initial expense. Medical or nutritional therapy costs far less initially. However, the cost of ongoing monitoring can exceed that of thyroidectomy or ^{131}I therapy over a period of many months to years.

Other factors may be important. For example, nutritional therapy may not be a practical option for owners with multiple cats, especially when the other cats are on prescription diets for other disorders, such as CKD. Some owners find medicating difficult, whereas others are wary of radiation therapy. All of these owner factors must be considered when deciding on the "best" treatment of an individual hyperthyroid cat.

Potential Long-Term Risks of Not Addressing the Underlying Cause of Hyperthyroidism

Surgery and ^{131}I are considered "definitive" treatment options in that all abnormal thyroid tumor tissue is either removed or destroyed, and hyperthyroidism is permanently resolved (see **Table 1**). By contrast, antithyroid drugs and low-iodine diets are only effective in keeping the circulating T_4 within the reference interval when administered on a continued basis, making these 2 treatment choices "palliative."

Using either of these "palliative choices" initially can counteract cardiac and metabolic consequences of hyperthyroidism while an owner is deciding on other possible options, to prepare the cat for surgery, or to stabilize the cat before [131]I. It is important that owners understand that neither pharmacologic nor dietary treatment options directly address the cause of the disease (ie, the thyroid adenomatous hyperplasia/neoplasia), and the thyroid tumor remains.

Hyperthyroidism is a progressive disease and does not stop or slow with antithyroid medication. In cats treated with antithyroid drugs, a gradual increase in thyroid tumor size over time is expected. The prevalence of severe signs, large thyroid masses, multifocal disease, intrathoracic thyroid masses, and suspected thyroid malignancy all increase with duration of hyperthyroidism.[4,5] The rate of progression varies from cat to cat and is unpredictable, and owners should be aware of the potential for benign tumor to transform and become malignant.

Antithyroid Drug Management

Prevalence of antithyroid drug use in cats

One online survey reported that antithyroid medication was offered as initial treatment to 92% of hyperthyroid cat owners.[29] Indeed, it is likely that worldwide, most hyperthyroid cats receive antithyroid drugs at least at some point during their treatment. Many are treated lifelong, whereas others are treated for a short period (ie, trial to help exclude masked CKD; to prepare for thyroidectomy, or awaiting appointment for ^{131}I). Hence, antithyroid medications seem to be the most commonly used treatment option for feline hyperthyroidism worldwide.

However, in Caney's[29] survey of hyperthyroid cat owners, 30% had *only* been offered oral antithyroid medication as a treatment, with no discussion of other options. Reasons for this are unclear, but it appears that many primary veterinarians decide on their own that surgery or ^{131}I is not appropriate treatment for cats, without informing the owner about other treatment options. In support of that, another survey of veterinarians reported that almost 60% agreed with the statement "radioiodine is the gold-standard treatment for hyperthyroidism," but more than half of these veterinarians did not refer cats for ^{131}I treatment.[30]

Which cats should be treated with antithyroid drugs?

Box 1 outlines the pros and cons of short- and long-term antithyroid medication. Because of the progressive nature of hyperthyroid disease, most younger and healthy cats are best treated with definitive treatments, such as surgical thyroidectomy or [131]I. Long-term medical management is best reserved for cats of advanced age (that would not be expected to live long enough for the thyroid tumor size to dramatically increase in size or undergo malignant transformation[4,5]) or for those cats with moderate to severe concurrent disease (expected to shorten their lifespan). Finally, antithyroid drugs are the treatment of choice when owners refuse definitive treatment.

Nutritional Management with Low-Iodine Diet

Nutritional management with a low-iodine diet (Hill's Prescription Diet y/d) has the lowest rate of treatment success (see **Table 1**). Therefore, this option is generally best for management of cats that are not good candidates for the other more efficacious treatments. The basis for using a low-iodine diet to manage cats with

---

Box 1
Pros and cons of antithyroid medication

Pros of antithyroid medication

- Medical management requires no special facilities.
- Cost of these drugs is relatively cheap.
- Anesthesia is avoided, as are the surgical complications associated with thyroidectomy.
- Long-term control of hyperthyroidism can be achieved in about 75% of treated cats.[11,31,32]
- In addition to long-term treatment, medication is also recommended before surgical thyroidectomy to decrease the metabolic and cardiac complications associated with hyperthyroidism.[33]
- Short-term medical management is often recommended as trial therapy before ^{131}I therapy to determine the effect of restoring euthyroidism on renal function.

Cons of antithyroid medication

- Medical treatment is not curative, is highly dependent on owner and cat compliance, and requires regular biochemical monitoring to ensure efficacy of treatment.
- Adverse signs effects, mostly mild but some serious (life-threatening), are relatively common **(Tables 2 and 3).**[31,32] Because of the multitude of clinical and laboratory-related side effects, one should closely monitor the cat's hematology, renal function, and thyroid function, especially over the first 3 months.[11,31,32]
- Iatrogenic hypothyroidism may occur from excessive doses.[11,26,34] Monitoring thyroid and renal function is critical because hypothyroidism can contribute to development or worsening azotemia and shorten survival.[24]
- Euthyroidism can be difficult to maintain in cats treated chronically with these drugs.[31,32]
- Antithyroid drugs have no effect on the underlying thyroid tumor, and the thyroid mass continues to grow during treatment.[4,5] This necessitates a progressive increase in the drug dose over time, with some cats becoming "resistant" to the thyroid-lowering effects of the medication, as the thyroid nodules grow in size.
- Cats with long-standing thyroid tumor disease are much more difficult to treat with definitive methods. After many months to years, large benign thyroid tumors may transform to thyroid carcinoma in some cats.[4,5]
- Owners must be informed of the risk to themselves and their thyroid function. Methimazole or carbimazole tablets should never be crushed or divided, because this increases human exposure. Owners who administer transdermal antithyroid drugs must use appropriate gloves or finger protection to avoid self-medicating.
- Furthermore, these drugs are potentially teratogenic.[11,32] Pregnant women should not administer these drugs (oral or transdermal) and should avoid contact with the litter box.

Data from Refs.[4,5,11,24,26,31–34]

---

hyperthyroidism is that iodine is an essential component of the thyroid hormones; T_4 contains 4 iodine atoms per molecule, whereas T_3 contains 3 atoms per molecule.[35] Without sufficient amounts of dietary iodine, the thyroid cannot produce excess thyroid hormones.

Hill's Prescription Diet y/d is an iodine-deficient diet, containing levels below the minimum daily requirement for adult cats.[36] Although limiting the intake of dietary iodine blunts the synthesis and secretion of thyroid hormone, the autonomous thyroid adenoma remains and the disease is not cured. It will not effectively suppress high thyroid hormone concentrations in all hyperthyroid cats (**Box 2**; see **Table 1**).

Table 2
Frequency of non-life-threatening suspected adverse reactions to methimazole and carbimazole

	Oral Methimazole	Transdermal Methimazole	Oral Carbimazole
Lethargy, GI signs (anorexia, vomiting)	23%	4%	33%
Mild hematologic abnormalities (leukopenia, eosinophilia, lymphocytosis)	16%	Not reported	35%
Facial/cervical self-induced excoriations (pruritis)	4%	8%	12%
Generalized peripheral lymphadenopathy	Few case reports	Not reported	Not reported

Data from Daminet S, Kooistra HS, Fracassi F, et al. Best practice for the pharmacological management of hyperthyroid cats with antithyroid drugs. J Small Anim Pract 2014;55:4-13; and Daminet S. Treatment of hyperthyroidism: antithyroid drugs. In: Feldman EC, Fracassi F, Peterson ME, eds. Feline Endocrinology. Milan: EDRA; 2019:198-210.

Which cats should be managed with a low-iodine diet?

Box 2 outlines the pros and cons of nutritional management with a low-iodine diet. In general, dietary management with a low-iodine diet should be considered as the last option for most hyperthyroid cats and be reserved for situations in which definitive therapy is not possible, the cat cannot tolerate, or the owner is unable to administer, long-term medical therapy.

Surgical Thyroidectomy

Surgical thyroidectomy is an extremely effective definitive treatment for cats with hyperthyroidism. With experience, a surgeon can become highly proficient at complete removal of all adenomatous thyroid tissue while preserving at least 1 functional parathyroid gland. Because 65% of cats have thyroid tumors of both thyroid lobes,[46,47] most will require bilateral thyroidectomy. To help mitigate the prevalence of iatrogenic hypoparathyroidism (**Box 3**; see **Table 1**), bilateral thyroidectomy can be staged, with a waiting period of 4 weeks between surgeries. This protocol allows time for parathyroid tissue to revascularize and recover from surgical trauma but also requires a second anesthetic procedure.[33,48]

Table 3
Frequency of life-threatening suspected adverse reactions to methimazole

	Oral Methimazole	Transdermal Methimazole
Hepatopathy (icterus/anorexia)	3%	4%
Bleeding diathesis (epistaxis, oral bleeding, prolonged clotting time)	3%	Not reported
Severe thrombocytopenia (platelet count <75,000/μL)	3%	8%
Agranulocytosis (severe leukopenia; total granulocyte count <500/μL) and neutropenia	3%	6%
Myasthenia gravis	Few case reports	One case report
Anemia (including aplastic anemia)	Few case reports	Not reported

Data from Daminet S, Kooistra HS, Fracassi F, et al. Best practice for the pharmacological management of hyperthyroid cats with antithyroid drugs. J Small Anim Pract 2014; 55:4-13; and Daminet S. Treatment of hyperthyroidism: antithyroid drugs. In: Feldman EC, Fracassi F, Peterson ME, eds. Feline Endocrinology. Milan: EDRA; 2019:198-210.

Box 2
Pros and cons of nutritional management with low-iodine diet

Pros of nutritional management

- Dietary management can be a feasible alternative in cats that are not candidates for definitive treatment of the underlying thyroid tumor(s), or when finances are limited.

- A low-iodine diet can be considered in cats whose owners are not able to give oral medication, in cats that develop side effects from methimazole or carbimazole, or in cats with concurrent nonthyroidal illness (eg, CKD)

Cons of nutritional management

- One major drawback is poor palatability; over a third of cats will not eat the diet.[37] If a cat refuses to eat the low-iodine diet, the T_4 concentrations do not fall.

- This diet must be fed exclusively. No treats, table food, flavored medications, or other cat food can be given, or relapse will occur. Some owners find this level of dietary restriction to be unacceptable. Owners with multiple cats that are fed multiple diets will often find it difficult to restrict access of the hyperthyroid cat to other food. Likewise, nutritional management is not a good option for cats that go outside and can access other sources of dietary iodine (rodents, birds), or for cats that need to be on a therapeutic diet to manage concurrent illnesses.

- The macronutrient composition is suboptimal for an obligate carnivore, especially in an older hypermetabolic cat with severe muscle wasting or sarcopenia.[37] Protein levels are lower, and carbohydrates levels are higher than ideal.[37] Nutritional recommendations for hyperthyroid cats are to feed a diet containing 40% or more of daily calories from protein, or greater than or equal to 12 g/100 kcal metabolizable energy, which is similar to that recommended for senior to geriatric cats.[37,38] This amount of dietary protein ingested is similar to the dietary intake of cats reported in the wild.[39]

- Use of a low-iodine diet takes a few weeks to lower high serum T_4 concentrations, and the diet will fail to normalize thyroid hormone concentrations in 30% of cats.[37,40–45] Even when the serum T_4 concentrations normalize, published studies show that dietary management can fail to completely reverse all clinical signs of hyperthyroidism, with weight loss, muscle wasting, and tachycardia persisting.[37,40–45]

- One reason for this lack of improvement may be because the serum T_4 concentrations in many cats fed this diet only fall into the upper third of the reference interval. Those cats that achieve a reduction of T_4 concentrations into the mid to lower end range of reference interval tend to better resolution of clinical signs. The iodine-restricted food did not restore complete euthyroidism in all cats in 1 study even when the serum T_4 normalized.[40] Dietary management is unlikely to resolve the clinical signs of hyperthyroidism as well as treatment with methimazole, thyroidectomy, or radioiodine.

Data from Refs.[37–45]

Which cats should be treated with surgery?

Box 3 outlines the pros and cons of surgical thyroidectomy. Because of the progressive nature of hyperthyroid disease, younger and healthy cats are best treated with a definitive treatment to cure the disease, such as surgical thyroidectomy. The success rate for a cure of hyperthyroidism with this option is very high (>90%); surgery requires only a short hospital stay, and thyroidectomy will lower the serum thyroid hormone concentrations to normal within 24 to 48 hours, making it the fastest way to control hyperthyroidism. It is the definitive treatment of choice if ^{131}I is unavailable or the owners decline ^{131}I treatment.

Many owners worry about risks of anesthesia and surgery, especially if their cat is geriatric or has concomitant nonthyroidal illness. Thyroidectomy comes with an

Box 3
Pros and cons of surgical thyroidectomy

Pros of thyroidectomy

- Thyroidectomy offers a permanent cure for cats with hyperthyroidism, with a success rate of more than 90%.[46]
- It is relatively simple and does not require specialized equipment.
- Serum T_4 and T_3 concentrations will decrease to normal within 24 to 48 hours, making it the fastest way to control hyperthyroidism in cats.
- It is the definitive treatment of choice if ^{131}I is unavailable or the owners decline ^{131}I treatment.

Cons of thyroidectomy

- Most hyperthyroid cats are aged and have comorbidities (eg, renal or cardiac disease) adding to the risks of general anesthesia. Careful perioperative support is essential.
- Common complications include iatrogenic hypoparathyroidism, hypothyroidism, and persistent hyperthyroidism. Rare complications include laryngeal nerve damage and Horner syndrome.[33]
- Failure to preserve at least 1 parathyroid gland during bilateral thyroidectomy causes hypoparathyroidism and signs of life-threatening hypocalcemia (eg, muscle twitching, tetany, or seizures).[48,49] Iatrogenic hypoparathyroidism greatly increases the cost because it lengthens hospital stay and requires treatment with oral calcium and vitamin D for at least a few weeks.
- Most hyperthyroid cats undergoing unilateral thyroidectomy will develop temporary hypothyroidism, with serum T_4 and T_3 concentrations falling to subnormal levels for 3 to 6 months. Short-term thyroid hormone replacement (L-T_4) is recommended, especially if they become lethargic or develop new or worsening azotemia.[26]
- Following bilateral thyroidectomy, cats are expected to develop hypothyroidism within 24 to 48 hours. L-T_4 should be started on the day of discharge, and life-long replacement therapy might be necessary.[26]
- Although surgical thyroidectomy has a success rate of greater than 90%, hyperthyroidism persists in a few cats. Causes for treatment failure include:
  - Presence of unidentified ectopic thyroid tumors[33,46] at the base of the tongue or in the anterior mediastinum,[46,47] sites not accessible during cervical exploration. These are present in 4% of hyperthyroid cats.[5,47]
  - Gravitation of a large thyroid tumor through the thoracic inlet into the thoracic cavity.[4,5,47] These large thyroid tumors can generally be pulled back out of the chest through the thoracic inlet for removal.
  - Invasion of large and vascular thyroid carcinomas into adjacent soft tissues and through the thoracic inlet into the thoracic cavity or metastasis to regional lymph nodes or distant sites.[9,47]
- Rarely hyperthyroidism can recur months to years after surgery:
  - Following unilateral thyroidectomy, when the smaller, contralateral thyroid lobe becomes adenomatous and enlarges to cause hyperthyroidism.[50]
  - Following bilateral surgery, with growth of a residual piece of adenomatous thyroid tissue left in situ at time of surgery.[33,49]
  - Cats with persistent or recurrent hyperthyroidism after thyroidectomy are best reevaluated with thyroid scintigraphy to determine the cause of relapse.[5,47]

Data from Refs.[4,5,9,26,33,46–50]

extensive list of potential, albeit rare, complications. These issues should be discussed in detail with owners when contemplating the best treatment option for their cat.

Radioiodine Therapy

Radioiodine is considered by most to be the gold-standard treatment of choice for hyperthyroid cats. Treatment with ^{131}I has many advantages over other treatment methods. Most consider ^{131}I the treatment of choice owing to its curative outcome, high success rate (>95%), noninvasiveness, low prevalence of complications, and longer survival time.[51–53] In addition, it is simple and relatively stress free for most cats. In 1 survey of owners of cats treated with ^{131}I, 91% were happy with their decision to choose this treatment option for their cat.[54] When the same owners rated their cat's QoL, on a scale of 1 (very poor) to 10 (excellent]), results showed a QoL rating of 4/10 before ^{131}I treatment rising to 9/10 after ^{131}I treatment.[54]

Which cats should be treated with radioiodine?

Box 4 outlines the pros and cons for the use of ^{131}I therapy. Most endocrinologists consider ^{131}I the treatment of choice for most hyperthyroid cats because of its lack of serious complications and high cure rate. Radioiodine treatment should be strongly considered in all newly diagnosed hyperthyroid cats that are expected to live for longer than 2 to 3 years (eg, younger cats ≤12 years and even very healthy geriatric cats ≤16 years). The ^{131}I treatment irradiates and destroys the functional thyroid tumor nodule or nodules and prevents the progression of hyperthyroid disease over many months to years. Cats with ectopic thyroid tumors or thyroid carcinomas are best treated with [131]I.

Cats must be relatively stable before ^{131}I therapy is considered. Those with clinically significant or unstable cardiovascular, renal, GI, endocrine (eg, diabetes), or neurologic disease may not be very good candidates, especially because of the length of boarding required after the ^{131}I treatment is administered. For owners of cats that cannot pill their cats, ^{131}I may not be the best option because of the potential for iatrogenic hypothyroidism, which would require daily (and generally life-long) replacement with L-T$_4$. In these cats, use of a lower dose of ^{131}I will help minimize the chance of hypothyroidism, but with a slightly lowered cure rate.

The prognosis for most cats treated with ^{131}I is good to excellent, with almost all treated cats improving clinically and achieving a better QoL,[54] with increased survival.[52]

BOTTOM LINE—WHAT'S THE BEST TREATMENT?

With hyperthyroid cats, treatment is aimed at either removing or destroying the hyperfunctioning thyroid tumor or inhibiting thyroid hormone synthesis and release. Surgical thyroidectomy and radioactive iodine remain the only curative options available. Management of hyperthyroidism with antithyroid medication and a low-iodine diet are noncurative, life-long treatments because the thyroid tumor is not removed or destroyed and will continue to grow.

One must tailor the treatment to each individual cat, with the following factors all considered when selecting the "best" treatment. The long-term effect of the selected treatment on QoL for the cat and its owner should play a major role in the decision process:

- Age of cat
- Presence/absence of significant concurrent disease

Box 4
Pros and cons of radioiodine therapy

Pros of radioiodine treatment

- Radioiodine avoids inconvenience of daily oral (or transdermal) administration and side effects associated with antithyroid drugs, the restrictions associated with the lifelong feeding of an iodine-deficient diet, and the risks and postoperative complications associated with surgical thyroidectomy.

- This treatment does not require general anesthesia, which may be contraindicated in elderly cats.[53]

- Treatment with ^{131}I irradiates and destroys all tumor nodules, resulting in definitive cure of the hyperthyroidism.

- Indicated for cats with ectopic or intrathoracic thyroid tumor tissue that cannot be easily removed surgically, as well as for cats with invasive or metastatic thyroid carcinoma.[9,10,53,55]

- Best treatment for cats that develop serious adverse reactions to antithyroid medication (eg, facial excoriation, hepatopathy, or blood dyscrasias)[31,32] or in cats that become resistant to the effects of antithyroid medication.[4,5]

Cons of radioiodine treatment

- Use of ^{131}I requires special licensing and hospitalization facilities, nuclear medicine equipment, and compliance with local radiation safety regulations.

- Because a ^{131}I-treated cat will be radioactive for 3 to 4 weeks, cats must be kept for a few days in a special radioactive facility isolated from other animals, as well as from the general public and veterinary personnel not trained and authorized to care for radioactive cats.[56] Owners cannot visit their treated cat during this period. Attending personnel must wear protective clothing and gloves, as well as dosimetry badges to monitor their radiation exposure. The length of hospitalization varies according to the ^{131}I dose administered and local regulations.

- The one-time expense of radioiodine treatment is a downside of this treatment for many veterinarians and owners.[30]

- Some owners are reluctant to isolate their cat for this hospitalization period. One study assessing owners' feelings about ^{131}I treatment reported a moderate level of concern about the boarding period, including the possibility of the cat being unhappy (82% of owners), owner missing the cat (65% of owners), and worry about the cat not eating well while away from home (32%).[54] This emphasizes the importance of the human-animal bond, and the need for proper information and reassurance from specialists providing radioiodine services, as well as the primary veterinarian.

- Once treated, ^{131}I-treated cats will continue to excrete small amounts of ^{131}I in urine, with a smaller amount in feces and saliva, for up to 4 weeks. Therefore, owners must follow radiation safety guidelines to reduce human exposure to radiation emitted from the ^{131}I-treated cat and its waste during this period, as mandated by local regulations (which vary regionally).[53,56] These include minimizing close contact with the ^{131}I-treated cat and not sleeping with the cat at night. Children or pregnant women must avoid contact with the ^{131}I-treated cat. For owners afraid of the potential human health risks, education and counseling are needed to relieve these fears or help them choose another treatment option.

- About 5% of cats fail to achieve euthyroidism 3 to 6 months after initial ^{131}I treatment. Almost all cats with persistent hyperthyroidism can be cured by a second ^{131}I treatment, especially if thyroid scintigraphy is used to restage the disease and individualize the ^{131}I dose.[53,57]

- Overt iatrogenic hypothyroidism is relatively common after ^{131}I treatment, with a prevalence of less than 5% to more than 30% depending on the ^{131}I dose regimen.[58] These cats may show few, if any, clinical signs for months, and therefore, can be difficult to diagnose on clinical grounds alone.
  - Because hypothyroidism leads to a decrease in renal blood flow and GFR, one should exclude hypothyroidism in all cats that develop new or worsening kidney disease.

> ○ Diagnosing hypothyroidism requires measurement of both serum T_4 and TSH.[26,27] Serum TSH concentration is a very sensitive and specific diagnostic test for iatrogenic (^{131}I-induced) hypothyroidism in cats, especially in those cats that develop azotemic CKD after treatment.[27] If the serum T_4 becomes low-normal or subnormal and serum TSH increases significantly (eg, >0.9 ng/mL, 2 to 3 times the upper limit of the TSH reference interval), a diagnosis of iatrogenic hypothyroidism is made.[26,27]
> ○ Treatment with L-T_4 is recommended, especially if a new or worsening moderate azotemia is detected.[26,27]
>
> *Data from* Refs.[4,5,9,10,26,27,30–32,53–58]

- Severity of clinical hyperthyroidism
- Size of goiter (thyroid tumor)
- Availability of skilled surgeon
- Access to ^{131}I treatment facility
- Owner ability to administer tablets/transdermal medication
- Cat compliance for oral or transdermal medication
- Willingness of cat to eat low-iodine diet
- Multicat household or outdoor cat that hunts
- Immediate and long-term costs of each treatment
- Potential complications of treatments

In younger cats without concurrent disease, definitive treatment with either surgery or radioiodine is recommended whenever possible. In contrast, long-term medical or nutritional management is best reserved for cats of advanced age or for those with concurrent diseases, and when owners refuse either surgery or [131]I. Cats with more severe hyperthyroidism and larger thyroid tumors are more likely to become resistant to the effects of antithyroid drugs or dietary therapy; in these cats, a definitive treatment is best selected sooner rather than later (when the cat may no longer be a candidate because of overall body condition or cardiac failure).

Most cats that the veterinary clinician diagnoses and treats, however, fall into the intermediate age range (13–16 years). In these cats, clinicians must recommend the best treatment for that individual cat, based on the cat's age and condition at the time of diagnosis, severity and duration of the hyperthyroid disease, and the presence of severe or life-threatening concurrent diseases (eg, CKD or heart disease).

Veterinarians play a key role in educating the cat owner to help direct the best treatment option of choice for each cat-owner combination according to the individual circumstances. Discussing the intricacies of each modality with regards to reversibility/cure, initial and long-term (ongoing) costs, treatment options, risks, costs, and outcomes is essential to end up with the best QoL for both the owner and their cat.

DISCLOSURE

The author has nothing to disclose.

REFERENCES

1. Peterson M. Hyperthyroidism in cats: what's causing this epidemic of thyroid disease and can we prevent it? J Feline Med Surg 2012;14:804–18.
2. McLean JL, Lobetti RG, Schoeman JP. Worldwide prevalence and risk factors for feline hyperthyroidism: a review. J S Afr Vet Assoc 2014;85:1097.

3. Peterson ME. Hyperthyroidism: background, etiopathogenesis and changing prevalence of feline thyroid disease. In: Feldman EC, Fracassi F, Peterson ME, editors. Feline endocrinology. Milan (Italy): EDRA; 2019. p. 114–29.

4. Peterson ME, Broome MR, Rishniw M. Prevalence and degree of thyroid pathology in hyperthyroid cats increases with disease duration: a cross-sectional analysis of 2096 cats referred for radioiodine therapy. J Feline Med Surg 2016;18: 92–103.

5. Broome MR, Peterson ME. Treatment of hyperthyroidism: severe, unresponsive, or recurrent hyperthyroidism. In: Feldman EC, Fracassi F, Peterson ME, editors. Feline endocrinology. Milan (Italy): EDRA; 2019. p. 267–80.

6. Gerber H, Peter H, Ferguson DC, et al. Etiopathology of feline toxic nodular goiter. Vet Clin North Am Small Anim Pract 1994;24:541–65.

7. Peter HJ, Gerber H, Studer H, et al. Autonomy of growth and of iodine metabolism in hyperthyroid feline goiters transplanted onto nude mice. J Clin Invest 1987;80: 491–8.

8. Wakeling J, Smith K, Scase T, et al. Subclinical hyperthyroidism in cats: a spontaneous model of subclinical toxic nodular goiter in humans? Thyroid 2007;17: 1201–9.

9. Turrel JM, Feldman EC, Nelson RW, et al. Thyroid carcinoma causing hyperthyroidism in cats: 14 cases (1981-1986). J Am Vet Med Assoc 1988;193: 359–64.

10. Hibbert A, Gruffydd-Jones T, Barrett EL, et al. Feline thyroid carcinoma: diagnosis and response to high-dose radioactive iodine treatment. J Feline Med Surg 2009; 11:116–24.

11. Daminet S. Treatment of hyperthyroidism: antithyroid drugs. In: Feldman EC, Fracassi F, Peterson ME, editors. Feline endocrinology. Milan (Italy): EDRA; 2019. p. 198–210.

12. Boland LA, Hibbert A, Harvey AM. Incidence of comorbid disease in cats referred for radioiodine treatment (abstract). J Vet Intern Med 2009;23:1347.

13. Puig J, Cattin I, Seth M. Concurrent diseases in hyperthyroid cats undergoing assessment prior to radioiodine treatment. J Feline Med Surg 2015;17: 537–42.

14. Nussbaum LK, Scavelli TD, Scavelli DM, et al. Abdominal ultrasound examination findings in 534 hyperthyroid cats referred for radioiodine treatment between 2007-2010. J Vet Intern Med 2015;29:1069–73.

15. Watson N, Murray JK, Fonfara S, et al. Clinicopathological features and comorbidities of cats with mild, moderate or severe hyperthyroidism: a radioiodine referral population. J Feline Med Surg 2018;20:1130–7.

16. Miller ML, Randolph JF, Peterson ME. Hyperthyroidism: clinical signs and physical examination findings. In: Feldman EC, Fracassi F, Peterson ME, editors. Feline endocrinology. Milan (Italy): EDRA; 2019. p. 130–40.

17. Syme HM. Cardiovascular and renal manifestations of hyperthyroidism. Vet Clin North Am Small Anim Pract 2007;37:723–43.

18. Sangster JK, Panciera DL, Abbott JA. Cardiovascular effects of thyroid disease. Compendium 2013;35:E1–10.

19. Vaske HH, Schermerhorn T, Grauer GF. Effects of feline hyperthyroidism on kidney function: a review. J Feline Med Surg 2016;18:55–9.

20. van Hoek I, Lefebvre HP, Peremans K, et al. Short- and long-term follow-up of glomerular and tubular renal markers of kidney function in hyperthyroid cats after treatment with radioiodine. Domest Anim Endocrinol 2009;36:45–56.

21. Williams T. Thyroid and kidney disease in cats. In: Feldman EC, Fracassi F, Peterson ME, editors. Feline endocrinology. Milan (Italy): EDRA; 2019. p. 156–68.
22. Peterson ME, Varela FV, Rishniw M, et al. Evaluation of serum symmetric dimethylarginine concentration as a marker for masked chronic kidney disease in cats with hyperthyroidism. J Vet Intern Med 2018;32:295–304.
23. Syme H. Are methimazole trials really necessary?. In: Little SE, editor. August's consultations in feline internal medicine. Philadephia: Elsevier; 2016. p. 276–81.
24. Williams TL, Elliott J, Syme HM. Association of iatrogenic hypothyroidism with azotemia and reduced survival time in cats treated for hyperthyroidism. J Vet Intern Med 2010;24:1086–92.
25. Peterson ME. Diagnosis and management of iatrogenic hypothyroidism. In: Little SE, editor. August's consultations in feline internal medicine. Philadephia: Elsevier; 2016. p. 260–9.
26. Peterson ME. Hypothyroidism. In: Feldman EC, Fracassi F, Peterson ME, editors. Feline endocrinology. Milan (Italy): EDRA; 2019. p. 281–316.
27. Peterson ME, Nichols R, Rishniw M. Serum thyroxine and thyroid-stimulating hormone concentration in hyperthyroid cats that develop azotaemia after radioiodine therapy. J Small Anim Pract 2017;58:519–30.
28. Peterson ME, Kintzer PP, Cavanagh PG, et al. Feline hyperthyroidism: pretreatment clinical and laboratory evaluation of 131 cases. J Am Vet Med Assoc 1983;183:103–10.
29. Caney SM. An online survey to determine owner experiences and opinions on the management of their hyperthyroid cats using oral anti-thyroid medications. J Feline Med Surg 2013;15:494–502.
30. Higgs P, Murray JK, Hibbert A. Medical management and monitoring of the hyperthyroid cat: a survey of UK general practitioners. J Feline Med Surg 2014; 16:788–95.
31. Peterson ME, Kintzer PP, Hurvitz AI. Methimazole treatment of 262 cats with hyperthyroidism. J Vet Intern Med 1988;2:150–7.
32. Daminet S, Kooistra HS, Fracassi F, et al. Best practice for the pharmacological management of hyperthyroid cats with antithyroid drugs. J Small Anim Pract 2014;55:4–13.
33. Flanders JA. Treatment of hyperthyroidism: surgical thyroidectomy. In: Feldman EC, Fracassi F, Peterson ME, editors. Feline endocrinology. Milan (Italy): EDRA; 2019. p. 211–26.
34. Aldridge C, Behrend EN, Martin LG, et al. Evaluation of thyroid-stimulating hormone, total thyroxine, and free thyroxine concentrations in hyperthyroid cats receiving methimazole treatment. J Vet Intern Med 2015;29:862–8.
35. Zbigniew S. Role of iodine in metabolism. Recent Pat Endocr Metab Immune Drug Discov 2017;10:123–6.
36. Wedekind KJ, Blumer ME, Huntington CE, et al. The feline iodine requirement is lower than the 2006 NRC recommended allowance. J Anim Physiol Anim Nutr (Berl) 2010;94:527–39.
37. Loftus JP, Peterson ME. Treatment of hyperthyroidism: diet. In: Feldman EC, Fracassi F, Peterson ME, editors. Feline endocrinology. Milan (Italy): EDRA; 2019. p. 255–66.
38. Peterson ME, Eirmann L. Dietary management of feline endocrine disease. Vet Clin North Am Small Anim Pract 2014;44:775–88.

39. Plantinga EA, Bosch G, Hendriks WH. Estimation of the dietary nutrient profile of free-roaming feral cats: possible implications for nutrition of domestic cats. Br J Nutr 2011;106(Suppl 1):S35–48.
40. van der Kooij M, Becvarova I, Meyer HP, et al. Effects of an iodine-restricted food on client-owned cats with hyperthyroidism. J Feline Med Surg 2013;14:491–8.
41. Hui TY, Bruyette DS, Moore GE, et al. Effect of feeding an iodine-restricted diet in cats with spontaneous hyperthyroidism. J Vet Intern Med 2015;29:1063–8.
42. Scott-Moncrieff JC, Heng HG, Weng HY, et al. Effect of a limited iodine diet on iodine uptake by thyroid glands in hyperthyroid cats. J Vet Intern Med 2015;29:1322–6.
43. Vaske HH, Armbrust L, Zicker SC, et al. Assessment of renal function in hyperthyroid cats managed with a controlled iodine diet. Intern J Appl Res Vet Med 2016;14:38–48.
44. Grossi G, Zoia A, Palagiano P, et al. Iodine-restricted food versus pharmacological therapy in the management of feline hyperthyroidism: a controlled trial in 34 cats. Open Vet J 2019;9:196–204.
45. Loftus JP, DeRosa S, Struble AM, et al. One-year study evaluating efficacy of an iodine-restricted diet for the treatment of moderate-to-severe hyperthyroidism in cats. Vet Med (Auckl) 2019;10:9–16.
46. Naan EC, Kirpensteijn J, Kooistra HS, et al. Results of thyroidectomy in 101 cats with hyperthyroidism. Vet Surg 2006;35:287–93.
47. Peterson ME, Broome MR. Thyroid scintigraphy findings in 2,096 cats with hyperthyroidism. Vet Radiol Ultrasound 2015;56:84–95.
48. Flanders JA, Harvey HJ, Erb HN. Feline thyroidectomy. A comparison of postoperative hypocalcemia associated with three different surgical techniques. Vet Surg 1987;16:362–6.
49. Welches CD, Scavelli TD, Matthiesen DT, et al. Occurrence of problems after three techniques of bilateral thyroidectomy in cats. Vet Surg 1989;18:392–6.
50. Swalec KM, Birchard SJ. Recurrence of hyperthyroidism after thyroidectomy in cats. J Am Anim Hosp Assoc 1990;26:433–7.
51. Peterson ME, Becker DV. Radioiodine treatment of 524 cats with hyperthyroidism. J Am Vet Med Assoc 1995;207:1422–8.
52. Milner RJ, Channell CD, Levy JK, et al. Survival times for cats with hyperthyroidism treated with iodine 131, methimazole, or both: 167 cases (1996-2003). J Am Vet Med Assoc 2006;228:559–63.
53. Peterson ME, Xifra MP, Broome MR. Treatment of hyperthyroidism: radioiodine. In: Feldman EC, Fracassi F, Peterson ME, editors. Feline endocrinology. Milan (Italy): EDRA; 2019. p. 227–54.
54. Boland LA, Murray JK, Bovens CP, et al. A survey of owners' perceptions and experiences of radioiodine treatment of feline hyperthyroidism in the UK. J Feline Med Surg 2014;16:663–70.
55. Guptill L, Scott-Moncrieff CR, Janovitz EB, et al. Response to high-dose radioactive iodine administration in cats with thyroid carcinoma that had previously undergone surgery. J Am Vet Med Assoc 1995;207:1055–8.
56. Puille M, Puille N, Neiger R, et al. Radioiodine treatment of feline hyperthyroidism: radiation safety of contact persons. Tierarztl Prax Ausg K Kleintiere Heimtiere 2005;22:291–5.
57. Peterson ME, Varela FV, Rishniw M. Radioiodine treatment of cats with hyperthyroidism: evaluation of a novel algorithm for individual dose calculation based on thyroid scintigraphy, serum thyroid hormone concentrations, and thyroid uptake of radioiodine (abstract). J Vet Intern Med 2018;32:2139–40.

58. Lucy JM, Peterson ME, Randolph JF, et al. Efficacy of low-dose (2 millicurie) versus standard-dose (4 millicurie) radioiodine treatment for cats with mild-to-moderate hyperthyroidism. J Vet Intern Med 2017;31:326–34.

59. Studer H, Peter HJ, Gerber H. Natural heterogeneity of thyroid cells: the basis for understanding thyroid function and nodular goiter growth. Endocr Rev 1989;10: 125–35.

60. Derwahl M. Linking stem cells to thyroid cancer. J Clin Endocrinol Metab 2011;96: 610–3.

Updates in Feline Diabetes Mellitus and Hypersomatotropism

Linda Fleeman, BVSc (Hons), PhD, MANZCVS[a],
Ruth Gostelow, BVetMed (Hons), PhD, FHEA, MRCVS[b],*

KEYWORDS

- Ketoacidosis • Remission • Acromegaly • Glycemic variability

KEY POINTS

- Flash glucose monitoring is a useful addition to standard blood glucose monitoring and can provide frequent, noninvasive glucose measurements in a variety of settings.
- Hypophysectomy is the gold standard treatment of hypersomatotropism-associated diabetes in cats and offers a good chance of cure of hypersomatotropism and diabetes mellitus.
- Toujeo insulin glargine seems to provide a more flat, constant activity profile than other long-acting insulins and could be particularly effective in cats with glycemic variability.

This article uses a case-based approach to explore the current evidence on feline diabetes mellitus (DM) treatment and how to best apply this evidence in clinical situations. These cases also discuss novel concepts in feline DM management, including flash glucose monitoring, novel insulin preparations, and hypophysectomy for the treatment of hypersomatotropism (HS).

CASE 1: SICK DIABETIC CAT, MONKEY, A 12-YEAR-OLD NEUTERED MALE DOMESTIC SHORTHAIR

Presentation

- Inappetence for 3 days
- Vomited once yesterday
- Increased thirst for 1 week
- Depressed mentation for 1 day
- Plantigrade gait for 1 day

[a] Animal Diabetes Australia, 9-11 Miles Street, Mulgrave, Victoria 3170, Australia;
[b] Department of Clinical Science and Services, The Royal Veterinary College, Hawkshead Lane, North Mymms, Hertfordshire AL9 7TA, UK
* Corresponding author.
E-mail address: rgostelow@rvc.ac.uk

Vet Clin Small Anim 50 (2020) 1085–1105
https://doi.org/10.1016/j.cvsm.2020.06.005   vetsmall.theclinics.com

- No other recent health concerns

Initial Examination

- Weight: 7.8 kg
- Body condition score (BCS): 7.5/9
- Muscle score: 2/3 (mild muscle loss)
- Mentation: quiet, responsive
- Hydration: slightly tacky oral mucosa
- Vital signs: heart rate 170/min, respiratory rate 24/min, temperature 38.3°C (**Box 1**)

Assessment

Does this cat have diabetes mellitus or stress hyperglycemia?

Presence of ketosis is useful to distinguish diabetic from nondiabetic sick cats and is more reliable than fructosamine.[1] Although there is no information yet about blood ketones in this case, the presence of ketonuria indicates that ketosis and therefore DM is likely. Semiquantitative blood/serum ketone measurement is easily performed by applying a drop of serum or plasma to the ketone test patch of a urine dipstick, which provides a colorimetric indication of acetoacetate ± acetone concentration.[2] Point-of-care handheld ketone meters, which measure β-hydroxybutyrate, are also reliable in cats. These are likely to be more sensitive for the detection of ketosis due to β-hydroxybutyrate being the predominant ketone body in ketosis secondary to DM. They also provide a rapid, quantitative measurement, which can be used to monitor patient progress.[3,4]

Is there ketoacidosis (diabetic ketoacidosis) and/or hyperosmolality?

Although ketosis is likely, identification of decreased blood pH and/or decreased plasma bicarbonate concentration is required to diagnose acidosis. However, when this is unavailable, the European Society of Veterinary Endocrinology ALIVE guidelines recommends that diabetic patients who are unwell "should be suspected of suffering

---

Box 1
Initial in-house clinical pathology results for monkey

Blood glucose (BG): 513 mg/dL (reference interval [RI] 70 to 150 mg/dL) (28.5 mmol/L [RI 3.9–8.3 mmol/L])

Plasma albumin: 4.5 g/dL (RI 2.2–4.4 g/dL) (45 g/L [RI 22–44 g/L])

Plasma urea: 38.8 mg/dL (RI 10.0–30.0 mg/dL) (13.6 mmol/L [RI 3.6–10.7 mmol/L])

Plasma creatinine: 2.32 mg/dL (RI 0.30–2.00 mg/dL) (211 μmol/L [RI 27–186 μmol/L])

Plasma alanine aminotransferase: 107 U/L (RI 20–100 U/L)

Plasma alkaline phosphatase: 48 U/L (RI 10–90 U/L)

Plasma sodium: 147 mEq/L (RI 142–164 mEq/L) (147 mmol/L [RI 142–164 mmol/L])

Plasma potassium: 3.9 mEq/L (RI 3.7–5.8 mEq/L) (3.9 mmol/L [RI 3.7–5.8 mmol/L])

Plasma chloride: 110 mEq/L (RI 110–126 mEq/L) (110 mmol/L [RI 110–126 mmol/L])

Urine specific gravity: 1.023

Urine glucose: 4+

Urine ketones: 2+

from diabetic ketoacidosis (DKA)."[5] Diabetic cats that are inappetent or anorexic should be assumed to be unwell because DM generally causes polyphagia, unless complicated by another condition.

Estimated osmolality is 344 mOsm/kg (**Box 2**). Patients are considered hyperosmolar at an osmolality greater than 320 mOsm/kg, whereas the more complicated hyperosmolar hyperglycemic state is usually associated with osmolality greater than 340 mOsm/kg and BG greater than 600 mg/dL (>33 mmol/L).[6]

Therefore, Monkey should commence treatment of DKA and possible hyperosmolar hyperglycemic state. Treatment of these two conditions is similar and, although it will be useful to have additional diagnostic information in due course, there is already sufficient information to begin treatment without delay. Importantly, DKA in cats with newly diagnosed DM does not affect survival time,[7] and these cases can often go on to achieve diabetic remission.[8] One important negative prognostic indicator in cats with newly diagnosed DM is higher plasma creatinine concentration.[7] It is therefore noteworthy that Monkey's creatinine is only mildly increased, despite dehydration and hyperosmolality. Although it is difficult to assess renal function in diabetic cats with dehydration and osmotic diuresis, chronic kidney disease is not more frequent than in nondiabetic cats.[9]

Goals of Treatment in Sick Diabetic Cats

- Gradually replace body fluid deficit
- Slowly decrease plasma osmolality and BG concentration
- Halt and prevent ketogenesis
- Restore electrolyte and acid-base balance
- Identify and manage any underlying or precipitating factors

Fluid and Electrolyte Therapy

- No published studies have compared the efficacy of different fluid types in sick diabetic cats, but 0.9% saline or lactated Ringer solutions are commonly recommended.[6,10,11]
- A conservative fluid rate is recommended to avoid overhydration and major osmotic shifts. Flow rates 1.5 to 2 times normal maintenance requirements (4–6 mL/kg/h) are therefore appropriate. This aligns with the current perspective for human pediatric patients with DKA that advocates a "one size fits all" strategy with slow and even correction of fluid deficit.[12]
- It is important to calculate rates based on estimated ideal body weight in underweight or overweight cats. Because Monkey has an overweight body condition, it

---

Box 2
Estimation of plasma osmolality

Estimated osmolality (mOsm/kg) = 2*(Na$^+$ + K$^+$) + glucose (mg/dL)/18 + blood urea nitrogen (mg/dL)/2.8

[or 2*(Na$^+$ + K$^+$) + glucose (mmol/L) + blood urea nitrogen (mmol/L)]

The main determinant of osmolality is sodium; glucose has less impact unless there is severe hyperglycemia. Therefore, effective osmolality can alternatively be calculated using the simplified formula:

Effective osmolality = 2*Na$^+$ + glucose (mg/dL)/18 [or 2*Na$^+$ + glucose (mmol/L)]

is prudent to use an estimation of ideal body weight (eg, 5.5 kg) for all dose calculations.

- Maintenance fluids should be supplemented with 30 to 40 mEq/L (30–40 mmol/L) of potassium (KCl or a 50:50 combination of KCl and KPO_4) from the outset. Sick diabetic cats have a high risk of hypokalemia even if plasma potassium concentration is not decreased at presentation. Potassium depletion results from reduced intake caused by anorexia, and increased loss caused by vomiting and diuresis. Fluid therapy causes dilution of circulating potassium concentrations and promotes further renal loss, whereas insulin therapy and correction of acidosis results in movement of potassium out of the extracellular space into cells. In critically ill patients, adjustment of fluid potassium supplementation should ideally be based on results of plasma potassium concentration monitoring.[6,11] Such intensive monitoring is usually not required for cats that rapidly recover a normal or polyphagic appetite while treated with fluids supplemented with potassium as recommended previously.

Insulin Therapy

- Insulin treatment should commence when practical. Cats with DKA recover more rapidly if insulin treatment commences within 6 hours after admission[13] and higher concentrations of intravenous (IV) insulin result in better clinical outcomes.[14] Although fluid therapy corrects many metabolic derangements and causes BG to decrease, it does not switch off ketogenesis, which is the catalyst for DKA. In fact, before insulin was commercially available, DKA was almost uniformly fatal.
- Rapid-acting insulin, such as regular (soluble) insulin, is administered as an IV constant rate infusion (CRI) or as repeated intramuscular (IM) and subcutaneous (SC) injections.[6,10,11] Other rapid-acting options are insulin lispro[15] and aspart.[16] If rapid-acting insulin is unavailable, Lantus glargine is substituted in CRI protocols because it has a similar action to regular insulin when delivered by IV.[17]
- CRI protocols are often simpler and less labor intensive for prolonged management of sick diabetic cats. The main constraint is that a separate fluid infusion pump is required in addition to that used for supportive fluid therapy. **Box 3** and **Fig. 1** provide a simple, "one size fits all" insulin CRI protocol that is appropriate for Monkey.
- Protocols of repeated IM and SC injections are also effective. The most common protocol comprises an initial 0.2 U/kg dose of regular insulin administered IM and followed with SC doses at 0.1 U/kg every hour. Ongoing insulin doses are then adjusted based on BG monitoring at least once hourly.[18]
- Glargine can also be used IM and SC for the management of sick diabetic cats.[19,20] A protocol using intermittent IM/SC injections of glargine and regular insulin was established as an alternative to insulin CRI for treatment of DKA in cats.[20] Glargine was administered at a dose of 0.25 U/kg every 12 hours. BG was checked every 2 to 4 hours and the following actions taken:
  - 1 U regular insulin was administered every 6 hours when BG was greater than 250 mg/dL (>14 mmol/L)
  - 2.5% glucose CRI was given when BG was 80 to 250 mg/dL (4.4–13.8 mmol/L)
  - An IV bolus of glucose plus ongoing CRI with 5% glucose was given if BG was less than 80 mg/dL (<4.4 mmol/L).[20]

Box 3
"One size fits all" insulin CRI protocol for sick diabetic cats

- Add 25 U (0.25 mL) regular insulin to 500 mL saline or lactated Ringer solution (or 50 U [0.5 mL] to 1000 mL solution), resulting in a 50 mU/mL solution. Cover the fluid bag to protect insulin from light.

- Priming the line is unnecessary. Some insulin adsorbs to the lining of the infusion bag and giving set, but this soon reaches steady state and all remaining insulin is delivered to the animal. It is also not necessary to run the insulin CRI through a separate IV catheter. In fact, it is prudent to run concurrent insulin and glucose infusions through the same catheter to ensure that both infusions cease at the same time if the catheter fails.

- An initial insulin infusion rate of 50 mU/kg/h is recommended, achieved by administering the previously mentioned solution at 1 mL/kg/h (calculated using estimated ideal body weight).

- This rate is halved to 25 mU/kg/h (0.5 mL/kg/h of this solution) when BG reaches 180 to 270 mg/dL (10–15 mmol/L). At the same time, maintenance fluids should be changed to contain 2.5% dextrose in 0.45% saline supplemented with 30 to 40 mEq/L (30–40 mmol/L) potassium.

- A reliable means of achieving a fairly stable BG concentration in an anorexic diabetic cat is to balance IV infusion of insulin at 25 mU/kg/h (0.5 mL/kg/h) with 2.5% dextrose in 0.45% saline supplemented with potassium at 6 mL/kg/h. This is the safest option whenever close monitoring is not possible.

- Insulin infusion rate is adjusted up or down to maintain BG at 145 to 270 mg/dL (8–15 mmol/L). If the cat's illness is associated with substantial insulin resistance (IR), an insulin infusion rate of up to 150 mU/kg/h (3 mL/kg/h of the solution described previously) may be required to maintain BG at 145 to 270 mg/dL (8–15 mmol/L).

- When a previously anorexic diabetic cat begins to eat, the IV insulin rate might need to be increased to manage increased glycemia.

- See **Fig. 1** for an example flow chart for hospital use.

Glucose Monitoring

- The standard method for monitoring glucose response to treatment is serial measurement of BG concentration. Blood samples can be obtained by direct venipuncture, although use of a central venous catheter or the marginal ear vein are typically more comfortable and less stressful for the cat.[10]

- Veterinary glucose meters that have been validated using feline samples are recommended for monitoring sick diabetic cats, although meters intended for human use can also be reliable.[21–23]

- Continuous glucose monitors (CGMs) measure interstitial glucose and can supplement traditional BG measurement in hospitalized cats.[24] CGMs may be less accurate in cats when there is hypoglycemia,[25] but importantly can detect low glucose values that would have been missed by intermittent BG testing.[26] The working range of these systems is not a practical limitation in the clinical setting. For treatment decisions, it is usually sufficient to know that an animal's glucose concentration is less than 40 mg/dL (<2.2 mmol/L) or greater than 400 mg/dL (>22.2 mmol/L). In this situation, BG measurement is performed if a more accurate result is required.

- The Abbott FreeStyle Libre glucose monitoring system (Abbott Park, Illinois) is an innovative and inexpensive means of monitoring interstitial glucose that is simple to use.[27] The FreeStyle Libre system consists of an adhesive sensor, which samples interstitial glucose concentration every minute and stores these readings for

Fluid therapy for diabetic dogs and cats

Diabetic dogs and cats that need to be on a drip for any reason should also receive their insulin intravenously. Intravenous insulin therapy should continue until the time when long-acting insulin injections are started/resumed.

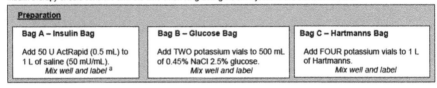

Preparation

Bag A – Insulin Bag	Bag B – Glucose Bag	Bag C – Hartmanns Bag
Add 50 U ActRapid (0.5 mL) to 1 L of saline (50 mU/mL). *Mix well and label* [a]	Add TWO potassium vials to 500 mL of 0.45% NaCl 2.5% glucose. *Mix well and label*	Add FOUR potassium vials to 1 L of Hartmanns. *Mix well and label*

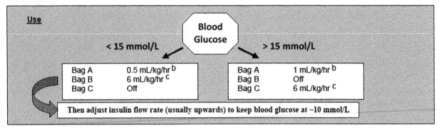

Use

Blood Glucose

< 15 mmol/L

Bag A	0.5 mL/kg/hr [b]
Bag B	6 mL/kg/hr [c]
Bag C	Off

> 15 mmol/L

Bag A	1 mL/kg/hr [b]
Bag B	Off
Bag C	6 mL/kg/hr [c]

Then adjust insulin flow rate (usually upwards) to keep blood glucose at ~10 mmol/L

Fig. 1. Example of a fluid therapy flow chart for use in hospitalized diabetic cats. [a] Cover bag to avoid exposure to light. [b] Flow rates are a guide only. Adjust to achieve desired blood glucose concentration. [c] This is approximately twice maintenance. Animals with increased fluid requirements can have the remaining additional fluid rates provided by Bag C. All doses should be based on estimated ideal body weight and not actual body weight.

up to 8 hours (**Fig. 2**). Whenever the sensor is scanned with the provided scanner, or smartphone App, a flash of the current and previous 8 hours of interstitial glucose data are obtained and a trend arrow is displayed to show whether glucose is increasing, decreasing, or changing slowly. The system requires no calibration and each sensor lasts up to 14 days, although sensor life is typically shorter in cats.

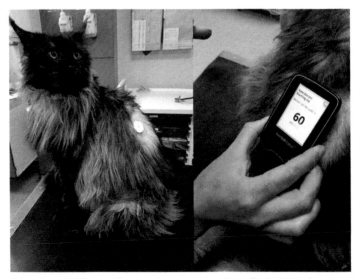

Fig. 2. A Maine Coon with an adhesive glucose sensor for a flash CGM placed on its epaxial area (*left*). The sensor can be scanned to download glucose data (*right*).

- Treatment decisions should not be based solely on interstitial glucose monitoring results. Instead, the FreeStyle Libre can identify changing glucose trends that are confirmed by standard BG testing and thereby facilitate timely treatment decisions. If used correctly, flash glucose monitoring can thus improve patient comfort by decreasing needle sticks while also reducing staff workload. **Box 4** provides tips for use of FreeStyle Libre flash glucose monitoring in sick diabetic cats.

Outcome

- Monkey improved rapidly with fluid and insulin therapy, along with SC maropitant to manage nausea. When hematology, biochemistry, and urinalysis results were returned from the external reference laboratory, they did not identify any significant concurrent problems. He regained a polyphagic appetite within 12 hours and was discharged home after 24 hours with long-acting insulin therapy every 12 hours for maintenance. The FreeStyle Libre sensor remained in place to provide glucose monitoring and helpful feedback to his owners as they became accustomed to the home treatment regimen.
- Monkey continued to have a weak hind leg gait at home, which progressed to generalized weakness unassociated with hypoglycemia. Oral potassium gluconate supplementation resulted in rapid resolution of severe weakness, although a mild plantigrade gait persisted. Potassium depletion myopathy is an important differential diagnosis in cats for diabetic neuropathy and hypoglycemia. Factors that promote potassium depletion in diabetic cats include polyuria and insulin treatment.[28] Improvement in response to oral potassium gluconate supplementation typically occurs within 1 to 2 days with full recovery within 2 to 3 weeks.[29]
- Monkey achieved diabetic remission that lasted for many years after 7 weeks of insulin treatment.
- The residual plantigrade gait presumably caused by diabetic neuropathy gradually resolved by 3 months.

Box 4
Tips for use of FreeStyle Libre glucose monitoring in hospitalized diabetic cats

- A FreeStyle Libre glucose sensor should be applied when practical after hospital admission. This allows glucose monitoring during hospitalization and also for several days after discharge.
- Interstitial and BG results must be clearly differentiated on hospital charts. Two separate columns/rows are therefore required.
- The system does not provide alarms for high or low glucose so must be actively monitored. For example, a veterinarian may write an order to "decrease the insulin CRI rate to 2 mL/h when the BG is <270 mg/dL (<15 mmol/L)." A technician can then periodically scan the sensor every 1 to 2 hours without disturbing the cat and record the times and glucose results on the patient's chart. Once interstitial glucose concentration decreases to less than 270 mg/dL (<15 mmol/L), this is confirmed by testing BG and the insulin treatment adjusted.
- It is helpful to pay attention to the trend arrows and review the graph displayed on the device's reader.
- Any unexpected interstitial glucose results should be checked against BG concentration.
- Once every 24 hours, it is helpful to use the FreeStyle Libre software or LibreView to generate a detailed PDF report and attach this to the patient's file so it is readily accessed by the veterinarian when reviewing overall progress.

- He steadily lost weight and achieved an ideal body weight of 5.5 kg after 5 months.

CASE 2: CAT WITH HYPERSOMATOTROPISM-ASSOCIATED DIABETES MELLITUS, BONNIE, AN 11-YEAR-OLD FEMALE NEUTERED DOMESTIC LONGHAIR

Presentation

- DM diagnosed 4 months previously and treated with Lantus insulin glargine every 12 hours since diagnosis.
- Persistently poor glycemic control, despite increasing insulin dosage.
- Obvious polyuria and polydipsia (PUPD), and extreme polyphagia. Overweight with minimal weight loss (200 g) since diagnosis.
- Currently receiving 10 U (1.8 U/kg) glargine every 12 hours and fed a carbohydrate-restricted, wet commercial diet.
- Recent serum fructosamine 680 μmol/L (RI 249–320 μmol/L).
- Home BG measurements persistently greater than 360 mg/dL (>20 mmol/L) throughout the day.
- Presented for assessment of IR.

Examination

- See **Fig. 3** for patient photograph and oral examination
- Weight: 5.5 kg
- BCS: 6/9
- Muscle condition score: 2/3 (mild muscle loss)
- Alert, appropriate mentation
- Moderate hepatomegaly, mild prognathism inferior (see **Fig. 3**B); examination otherwise unremarkable

Assessment

It is vital to first exclude problems of insulin administration and/or storage when assessing cats with apparent IR. These were excluded in Bonnie's case. Many concurrent conditions can contribute to IR in feline diabetics (**Box 5**), but several features make HS a likely cause in Bonnie's case. HS can cause particularly profound IR compared with other comorbidities, which is consistent with Bonnie's persistent, marked hyperglycemia, despite substantial insulin dosing. Extreme polyphagia, as

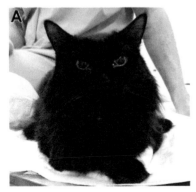 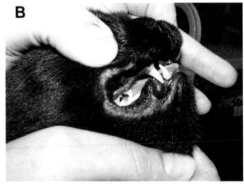

Fig. 3. Patient photographs demonstrating subjectively broad facial features (A) and prognathism inferior (B).

Box 5
Causes of insulin resistance in cats with DM (not exhaustive)

Obesity

Hypersomatotropism

Hyperadrenocorticism

Hyperthyroidism

Exogenous glucocorticoids or progestogens

Pancreatitis

Chronic kidney disease

Gastrointestinal disease

Any chronic inflammatory disease

---

seen in Bonnie, is a common finding in cats with HS.[30] Bonnie's subjective facial broadening and prognathism inferior (see **Fig. 3**) suggest she is affected by acromegaly, which results from the mitogenic effects of excess growth hormone. However, only a proportion of cats with HS-associated DM have noticeable acromegaly and its absence should not exclude the possibility of HS.[30,31] Index of suspicion for HS would be particularly great if practicing in a country with a high reported prevalence of HS among diabetic cats. HS has been estimated to cause approximately 25% of feline DM cases in the United Kingdom.[30] However, this could be an overestimation because of veterinarians' being more likely to submit samples for the study's free insulin-like growth factor-1 (IGF-1) measurement from cats with possible signs of HS. An alternative study from Switzerland and the Netherlands reported an estimated prevalence of 17.8% among diabetic cats.[32]

Serum IGF-1 measurement was submitted and was supportive of HS (239 nmol/L [1825 ng/mL]; RI <130 nmol/L [<1000 ng/mL]).

Are further diagnostic tests necessary to confirm hypersomatotropism?

A serum IGF-1 concentration of greater than 130 nmol/L (>1000 ng/mL) has a positive predictive value of 95%[30] for HS so, in combination with Bonnie's consistent clinical findings, is highly suggestive of HS. Pituitary imaging with computed tomography or, less often, MRI is often used to support the diagnosis by demonstrating pituitary enlargement. Despite this, 3% to 4% of cases have a normal pituitary size on diagnostic imaging[30] and this percentage is likely to increase with improved awareness and earlier detection of cats with HS. HS should therefore not be excluded based on a normal pituitary appearance on advanced imaging. Pituitary imaging also provides information that is relevant to several treatment modalities (**Table 1**).

What are the major treatment options for hypersomatotropism-associated diabetes mellitus?

Table 1 shows the main treatment options for HS-associated DM in cats.

Treatment Plan

Bonnie underwent hypophysectomy to provide the greatest chance of cure of HS and resolution of DM. Preoperative cranial computed tomography revealed moderate pituitary enlargement (ventrodorsal height 8 mm, normal ≤4 mm[33]) (**Fig. 4**). The extent of

Table 1
Main treatment options for cats with HS-associated DM

Treatment	Rationale	Advantages and Disadvantages

Standard DM management only	Attempts to manage the diabetogenic effects of GH excess only	Advantages
		  Widely accessible option
		  Might maintain an acceptable quality of life for a period of time
		Disadvantages
		  Does not treat the pituitary tumor or mitogenic effects of GH (eg, acromegalic changes)
		  DM control often poor with severe ongoing DM signs
		  Large insulin doses potentially required, which is costly
		  Large insulin dosage makes hypoglycemic episodes possible when pulsatile GH secretion is low

Radiotherapy	Targeted radiation energy preferentially damages pituitary tumor tissue
	Several protocols described including, recently, stereotactic[46–48]
		Advantages
		  Improved DM control common, with 30%–40% diabetic remission rate
		  Might shrink tumor, and thus improve any neurologic signs
		Disadvantages
		  Typically, weeks to months for improvement to become apparent
		  IGF-1 and mitogenic effects of GH do not normalize
		  Relapse common
		  Limited availability
		  Costly
		  Repeated anesthesia required (fewer with stereotactic)

Transsphenoidal Hypophysectomy	Surgical pituitary removal	Advantages[49]
		  Removes tumor
		  Normalization of IGF-1 and cure of HS in >90% of cats
		  Approximately 70% DM remission rate
		Disadvantages
		  Limited availability
		  Costly
		  Associated mortality (<10%)
		  Long-term hormonal replacement required

Cryohypophysectomy	Surgical cryoablation of the pituitary gland	Advantages
		  Destroys tumor tissue
		  Decreased IGF-1 in the only 2 cases reported[50,51]
		Disadvantages
		  Little clinical experience, limited availability
		  Costly

(continued on next page)

Table 1 (continued)		
Treatment	Rationale	Advantages and Disadvantages
Pasireotide	Injectable somatostatin analogue; inhibits GH secretion from pituitary tumor	Advantages Improved DM control common, with diabetic remission rates of approximately 20%–25%[52] Generally well-tolerated Disadvantages IGF-1 and mitogenic effects of GH do not normalize Does not treat tumor Limited availability Costly Self-limiting diarrhea common
Cabergoline	Dopamine agonism causing inhibition of pituitary GH release	Advantages Widely available Low-cost Generally well-tolerated Disadvantages Little clinical experience, might improve glycemic control in individual cats at dose of 5–10 μg/kg PO SID,[53] further research warranted

Abbreviation: GH, growth hormone.

acromegalic cardiomyopathy was assessed preoperatively using echocardiography to guide anesthesia and perioperative fluid therapy.

Preoperatively, an Abbott FreeStyle Libre flash glucose monitoring system was applied to provide frequent, noninvasive interstitial glucose measurement during the perioperative period (**Fig. 5**). Hypophysectomy was performed via a transsphenoidal approach through the oral cavity (**Fig. 6**).[34]

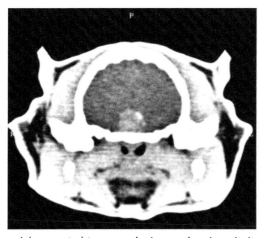

Fig. 4. Transverse cranial computed tomography image showing pituitary enlargement.

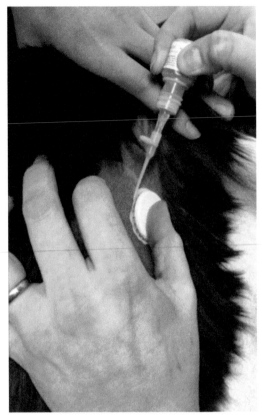

Fig. 5. A flash glucose sensor is applied to Bonnie's lateral thoracic wall. Small drops of tissue glue are applied to the adhesive layer for additional security.

What Are the Medical Considerations Following Hypophysectomy?

- To control hyperglycemia, cats receive a CRI of 0.9% NaCl with soluble insulin ± dextrose from anesthesia induction until willing to eat postoperatively, when long-acting maintenance insulin can be reintroduced. At the author's (RG) hospital, a maximum hourly rate of 4 mL/kg/h for all infusions is used to limit risk of volume overload. Cats often eat within 24 hours postsurgery. Insulin sensitivity can rapidly improve following successful surgery (**Fig. 7**) so glucose concentration must be frequently monitored and insulin dose adjusted. Maintenance insulin is typically restarted at a reduced dose compared with preoperatively because of improved insulin sensitivity.
- Treated cats require lifelong glucocorticoid and thyroxine supplementation because of absolute lack of adrenocorticotrophic hormone and thyroid-stimulating hormone, respectively, following hypophysectomy. A hydrocortisone sodium succinate CRI is started immediately before pituitary removal and is continued postoperatively until oral glucocorticoid therapy is introduced. Oral levothyroxine is started once cats can tolerate oral medication.
- Antidiuretic hormone supplementation is required at time of surgery and postoperatively to treat central diabetes insipidus because hypophysectomy causes cessation of antidiuretic hormone secretion by the neurohypophysis.

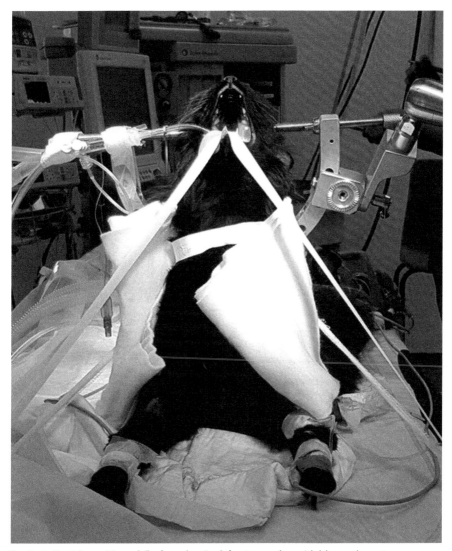

Fig. 6. Patient is positioned (before draping) for transsphenoidal hypophysectomy.

Supplementation can eventually be discontinued in some cats because antidiuretic hormone from the hypothalamus can still be secreted into the systemic circulation via the portal capillaries of the median eminence.[35]

- Prophylactic amoxicillin-clavulanate therapy is given for 2 weeks postoperatively.

Outcome

Bonnie's hypophysectomy proceeded without complication and she was alert and willing to eat within 18 hours of surgery. Conjunctival desmopressin (1 drop every 8 hours) was started during surgery. Hydrocortisone CRI was replaced with oral hydrocortisone (0.5 mg/kg every 12 hours) the day following surgery. Oral levothyroxine (0.1 mg total dose every 24 hours) and a reduced dose of Lantus glargine (3 U every

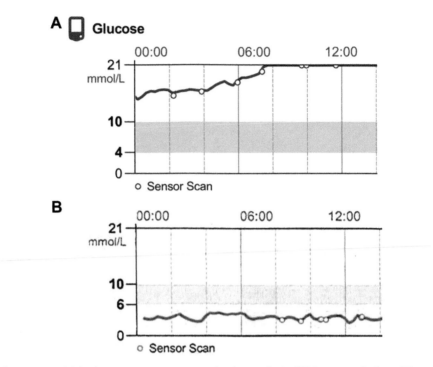

Fig. 7. Interstitial glucose curves, generated using a flash CGM system, before (*A*) and 5 days' after (*B*) hypophysectomy, showing greatly improved insulin sensitivity. (*Courtesy of* J. Cockerill, BVMS, Eaton, Australia.)

12 hours) was introduced 2 days after surgery. Insulin sensitivity noticeably improved during postoperative hospitalization (see **Fig. 7**) and Bonnie was discharged 1 week postsurgery on a Lantus glargine dose of 1 U SC every 12 hours. Hydrocortisone dose was reduced to 0.5 mg/kg every 24 hours at the time of discharge. One month postoperatively, IGF-1 measurement revealed resolution of HS (8.4 nmol/L [64 ng/mL]), and a serum total thyroxine measurement 5 hours postpill was 55 nmol/L (RI 19–65 nmol/L [4.3 μg/dL (RI 1.5–5.0 μg/dL)]), supporting adequate levothyroxine supplementation. Bonnie was able to discontinue insulin therapy 3 weeks after surgery and went on to achieve sustained diabetic remission. Conjunctival desmopressin frequency was reduced over 3 months following surgery, but discontinuing treatment resulted in PUPD. Therapy was therefore reinstated and continued at 1 drop every 24 hours indefinitely.

CASE 3: EXCESSIVE GLYCEMIC VARIABILITY IN A DIABETIC CAT, MU, A 16-YEAR-OLD NEUTERED FEMALE BURMESE
Presentation

- DM was first diagnosed 6 years ago; remission readily achieved within a few months.
- DM relapsed 2 years ago and Mu subsequently remained insulin-dependent.
- Stable glycemic control has been difficult to achieve over the last year, despite careful adjustment of insulin dose, and Mu has experienced several unexpected episodes of hypoglycemia with mild to severe clinical signs.

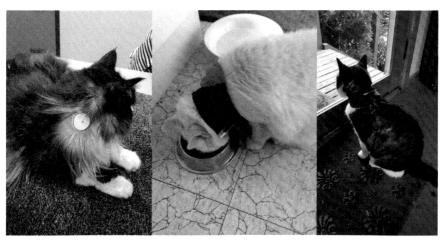

Fig. 8. A loose "scarf" (*middle* and *right*) can protect a flash CMS sensor applied to the side of the neck (*left*) and so extend the life of sensors worn in the home environment. This is simply fashioned by pinning together the top and toe of a sock around the neck.

- Insulin treatment was changed 9 months ago from veterinary porcine lente insulin (Vetsulin/Caninsulin) administered every 12 hours with U-40 syringes to Lantus glargine insulin administered every 12 hours with a SoloStar insulin dosing pen. Current dose is 1 U every 12 hours.

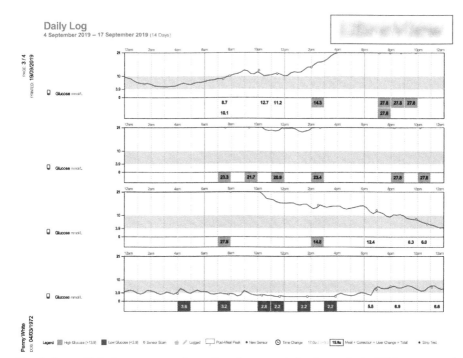

Fig. 9. Interstitial glucose curves from Case 3, generated using a flash CGM system and demonstrating excessive glycemic variability ranging less than 40 to greater than 400 mg/dL (<2.2 to >27.8 mmol/L).

- BG monitoring at home is limited because the owner works long hours. In addition to occasional hypoglycemia, results over several months also frequently identified moderate and severe hyperglycemia (range, 30–685 mg/dL [1.7–38 mmol/L]).
- Mu has a stable body weight, but is often PUPD, and has polyphagia. Urine dipstick testing at home is usually positive for glucose, but a negative result is obtained about once weekly.

Examination

- Weight: 4.7 kg
- BCS: 6/9
- Muscle score: 3/3
- Mentation: alert, appropriately responsive
- Unremarkable physical examination with a soft glossy coat

Assessment

- Several features of Mu's case are consistent with excessive "glycemic variability,"[36] a condition that anecdotally seems to be more common in cats with long duration of DM.
- "Somogyi effect" is also often used to explain periods when hypoglycemia and hyperglycemia occur. A more appropriate term that has been adopted in human

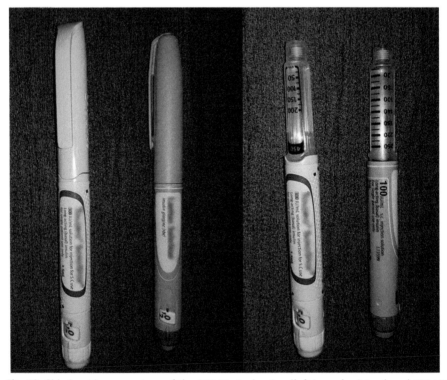

Fig. 10. Side-by-side comparison of the 300 U/mL glargine (*left* in each picture) and 100 U/mL glargine (*right* in each picture) insulin dosing pens. Note all staff and clients must be educated to never draw the 300 U/mL insulin from the dosing pen using a syringe. (*Courtesy of* Sanofi US, Bridgewater, NJ.)

medicine is "glycemic variability."[36–38] The term "brittle DM" has also been used, although this is now less preferred.

- A key observation is failure of increased insulin doses to resolve hyperglycemia. Instead, the cat continues to have poor diabetic control with higher insulin doses but might become prone to unexpected hypoglycemia. Decreasing insulin dose

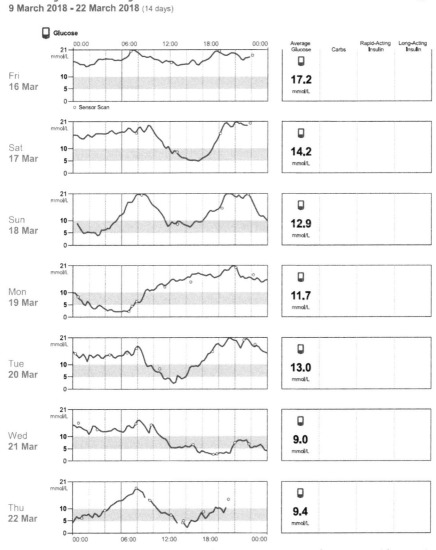

Fig. 11. Interstitial glucose curves generated using a CGM system from a cat with excessive glycemic variability and a history of unexpected episodes of neuroglycopenia. The change from 100 U/mL Lantus glargine to 300 U/mL Toujeo glargine insulin at the same dose occurred on Monday March 19th. Glycemic variability then subjectively reduced and the average daily interstitial glucose decreased to 170 mg/dL (9.4 mmol/L).

sometimes results in improvement of clinical signs, especially if the dose was high,[39] but often the outcome of insulin dose reduction is lower risk for hypoglycemia but persistence of poor diabetic control. Fluctuation between hyperglycemia and hypoglycemia often seems to follow a 3-day cycle.

- Availability of CGM has provided insight in humans with diabetes that was not possible from intermittent BG measurements. Individuals with increased glycemic variability present with poor diabetic control because of the occurrence of frequent hyperglycemia, whereas most of the hypoglycemic events are associated with no clinical signs and would be missed by standard intermittent BG monitoring. Nevertheless, the frequent hypoglycemia can induce physiologic unawareness of hypoglycemia and impaired glucose counterregulation, which in turn predisposes to increased risk of neuroglycopenia.[40] Whereas the periods of hypoglycemia are likely caused by excess exogenous insulin, the mechanisms for the periods of hyperglycemia are poorly understood and probably relate to the multiple causes of hyperglycemia and IR in DM.

- Longer-acting insulin preparations are generally recommended for treatment of DM in cats.[41–43] because they typically result in less potent and more prolonged duration of action than intermediate-acting products. Recently, a new 300 U/mL glargine insulin product (Toujeo) was shown to have a significantly longer and more flat time-action profile[44] than any other product, and early use in clinical cases has resulted in good outcomes.[45] Therefore, Toujeo glargine might provide benefit for cats with excessive glycemic variability.

Treatment and Outcome

- An Abbott Freestyle Libre flash glucose monitoring system was applied to side of the neck to provide more information on glucose excursions overnight and while Mu's owner was at work. The sensor was covered by a loose "scarf" around the neck (**Fig. 8**). Treatment with 1 U every 12 hours Lantus glargine insulin was continued. The owner compared interstitial and BG measurements whenever convenient. Marked glycemic variability was confirmed with glucose ranging less than 40 to greater than 400 mg/dL (<2.2 to >27.8 mmol/L) over the first 4 days (**Fig. 9**). No clinical signs caused by hypoglycemia were observed during this period.

- After 4 days, treatment was changed to 1 U every 12 hour of glargine 300 U/mL insulin administered with the prefilled Toujeo SoloStar pen (**Fig. 10**). Gradual smoothing out of the interstitial glucose curve was observed over the next 4 days (**Fig. 11**).

- Mu improved with resolution of PUPD and polyphagia over the first week. On two occasions during the first 6 weeks of treatment with Toujeo insulin, hypoglycemia with mild clinical signs occurred. The signs were much less severe than the owner was accustomed to so the episodes initially went unrecognized. The dose of Toujeo insulin was decreased first to 1 U every 24 hours and then to 1 U every 48 hours, and Mu then maintained good diabetic control on the latter dose with no further clinical signs of hypoglycemia for many months.

SUMMARY

Flash glucose monitoring allows frequent glucose monitoring in diabetic cats while avoiding patient discomfort, and therefore provides a useful tool in the management of diabetic cats, especially those with glycemic variability and/or in which glucose regulation is changing rapidly.

DISCLOSURE

The authors have nothing to disclose.

REFERENCES

1. Zeugswetter F, Handl S, Iben C, et al. Efficacy of plasma beta-hydroxybutyrate concentration as a marker for diabetes mellitus in acutely sick cats. J Feline Med Surg 2010;12(4):300–5.
2. Zeugswetter F, Pagitz M. Ketone measurements using dipstick methodology in cats with diabetes mellitus. J Small Anim Pract 2009;50(1):4–8.
3. Chong SK, Reineke EL. Point-of-care glucose and ketone monitoring. Top Companion Anim Med 2016;31(1):18–26.
4. Di Tommaso M, Aste G, Rocconi F, et al. Evaluation of a portable meter to measure ketonemia and comparison with ketonuria for the diagnosis of canine diabetic ketoacidosis. J Vet Intern Med 2009;23(3):466–71.
5. ESVE. Project ALIVE. Available at: https://www.esve.org/alive/search.aspx. Accessed January 4, 2020.
6. Davison LJ. Diabetic ketoacidosis, ketoacidosis, and the hyperosmolar syndrome. In: Feldman EC, Fracassi F, Peterson ME, editors. Feline endocrinology. Milano (Italy): Edra; 2019. p. 454–67.
7. Callegari C, Mercuriali E, Hafner M, et al. Survival time and prognostic factors in cats with newly diagnosed diabetes mellitus: 114 cases (2000-2009). J Am Vet Med Assoc 2013;243(1):91–5.
8. Sieber-Ruckstuhl NS, Kley S, Tschuor F, et al. Remission of diabetes mellitus in cats with diabetic ketoacidosis. J Vet Intern Med 2008;22(6):1326–32.
9. Zini E, Benali S, Coppola L, et al. Renal morphology in cats with diabetes mellitus. Vet Pathol 2014;51(6):1143–50.
10. Rudloff E. Diabetic ketoacidosis in the cat: recognition and essential treatment. J Feline Med Surg 2018;19(11):1167–74.
11. Thomovsky E. Fluid and electrolyte therapy in diabetic ketoacidosis. Vet Clin North Am Small Anim Pract 2017;47(2):491–503.
12. Jayashree M, Williams V, Iyer R. Fluid therapy for pediatric patients with diabetic ketoacidosis: current perspectives. Diabetes Metab Syndr Obes 2019;12:2355–61.
13. DiFazio J, Fletcher DJ. Retrospective comparison of early- versus late-insulin therapy regarding effect on time to resolution of diabetic ketosis and ketoacidosis in dogs and cats: 60 cases (2003-2013). J Vet Emerg Crit Care (San Antonio) 2016;26(1):108–15.
14. Cooper RL, Drobatz KJ, Lennon EM, et al. Retrospective evaluation of risk factors and outcome predictors in cats with diabetic ketoacidosis (1997-2007): 93 cases. J Vet Emerg Crit Care (San Antonio) 2015;25(2):263–72.
15. Malerba E, Mazzarino M, Del Baldo F, et al. Use of lispro insulin for treatment of diabetic ketoacidosis in cats. J Feline Med Surg 2019;21(2):115–23.
16. Pipe-Martin HN, Fletcher JM, Gilor C, et al. Pharmacodynamics and pharmacokinetics of insulin aspart assessed by use of the isoglycemic clamp method in healthy cats. Domest Anim Endocrinol 2018;62:60–6.
17. Scholtz HE, Pretorius SG, Wessels DH, et al. Equipotency of insulin glargine and regular human insulin on glucose disposal in healthy subjects following intravenous infusion. Acta Diabetol 2003;40(4):156–62.
18. Feldman EC, Nelson RW, Reusch C. Scott-Moncrieff. Canine and feline endocrinology. 4th edition. St. Louis (MO): Saunders; 2014.

19. Marshall RD, Rand JS, Gunew MN, et al. Intramuscular glargine with or without concurrent subcutaneous administration for treatment of feline diabetic ketoacidosis. J Vet Emerg Crit Care (San Antonio) 2013;23(3):286–90.
20. Gallagher BR, Mahoney OM, Rozanski EA, et al. A pilot study comparing a protocol using intermittent administration of glargine and regular insulin to a continuous rate infusion of regular insulin in cats with naturally occurring diabetic ketoacidosis. J Vet Emerg Crit Care (San Antonio) 2015;25(2):234–9.
21. Kang MH, Kim DH, Jeong IS, et al. Evaluation of four portable blood glucose meters in diabetic and non-diabetic dogs and cats. Vet Q 2016;36(1):2–9.
22. Zini E, Moretti S, Tschuor F, et al. Evaluation of a new portable glucose meter designed for the use in cats. Schweiz Arch Tierheilkd 2009;151(9):448–51.
23. Cohen TA, Nelson RW, Kass PH, et al. Evaluation of six portable blood glucose meters for measuring blood glucose concentration in dogs. J Am Vet Med Assoc 2009;235(3):276–80.
24. Reineke EL, Fletcher DJ, King LG, et al. Accuracy of a continuous glucose monitoring system in dogs and cats with diabetic ketoacidosis. J Vet Emerg Crit Care (San Antonio) 2010;20(3):303–12.
25. Moretti S, Tschuor F, Osto M, et al. Evaluation of a novel real-time continuous glucose-monitoring system for use in cats. J Vet Intern Med 2010;24(1):120–6.
26. Dietiker-Moretti S, Muller C, Sieber-Ruckstuhl N, et al. Comparison of a continuous glucose monitoring system with a portable blood glucose meter to determine insulin dose in cats with diabetes mellitus. J Vet Intern Med 2011;25(5): 1084–8.
27. Fleeman LM. Flash glucose monitoring in diabetic dogs and cats. Paper presented at: American College of Veterinary Internal medicine Forum 2019; Phoenix AZ, June 6-8, 2019.
28. Feldman EC, Church DB. Electrolyte disorders: potassium (hyper/hypokalemia). In: Ettinger SJ, Feldman EC, editors. The textbook of veterinary internal medicine. 7th edition. St. Louis (MO): Saunders Elsevier; 2010. p. 303–7.
29. Dow SW, Fettman MJ. Management of potassium-depleted cats. Compend Contin Educ Vet 1990;12:1612–5.
30. Niessen SJ, Forcada Y, Mantis P, et al. Studying cat (Felis catus) diabetes: beware of the acromegalic imposter. PLoS One 2015;10(5):e0127794.
31. Lamb CR, Ciasca TC, Mantis P, et al. Computed tomographic signs of acromegaly in 68 diabetic cats with hypersomatotropism. J Feline Med Surg 2014; 16(2):99–108.
32. Schaefer S, Kooistra HS, Riond B, et al. Evaluation of insulin-like growth factor-1, total thyroxine, feline pancreas-specific lipase and urinary corticoid-to-creatinine ratio in cats with diabetes mellitus in Switzerland and the Netherlands. J Feline Med Surg 2017;19(8):888–96.
33. Tyson R, Graham JP, Bermingham E, et al. Dynamic computed tomography of the normal feline hypophysis cerebri (Glandula pituitaria). Vet Radiol Ultrasound 2005;46(1):33–8.
34. Meij BP, Voorhout G, Van Den Ingh TS, et al. Transsphenoidal hypophysectomy for treatment of pituitary-dependent hyperadrenocorticism in 7 cats. Vet Surg 2001;30(1):72–86.
35. Owen TJ, Martin LG, Chen AV. Transsphenoidal surgery for pituitary tumors and other sellar masses. Vet Clin North Am Small Anim Pract 2018;48(1):129–51.
36. Zini E, Salesov E, Dupont P, et al. Glucose concentrations after insulin-induced hypoglycemia and glycemic variability in healthy and diabetic cats. J Vet Intern Med 2018;32(3):978–85.

37. Service FJ. Glucose variability. Diabetes 2013;62(5):1398–404.
38. Gilor C, Fleeman LM. The Somogyi effect: is it clinically significant? National Harbor (MD): American College of Veterinary Internal Medicine Forum; 2017.
39. McMillan FD, Feldman EC. Rebound hyperglycemia following overdosing of insulin in cats with diabetes mellitus. J Am Vet Med Assoc 1986;188(12):1426–31.
40. Fanelli CG, Porcellati F, Pampanelli S, et al. Insulin therapy and hypoglycaemia: the size of the problem. Diabetes Metab Res Rev 2004;20(Suppl 2):S32–42.
41. Sparkes AH, Cannon M, Church D, et al. ISFM consensus guidelines on the practical management of diabetes mellitus in cats. J Feline Med Surg 2015;17(3): 235–50.
42. Behrend E, Holford A, Lathan P, et al. 2018 AAHA diabetes management guidelines for dogs and cats. J Am Anim Hosp Assoc 2018;54(1):1–21.
43. Thompson A, Lathan P, Fleeman L. Update on insulin treatment for dogs and cats: insulin dosing pens and more. Vet Med (Auckl) 2015;6:129–42.
44. Gilor C, Culp W, Ghandi S, et al. Comparison of pharmacodynamics and pharmacokinetics of insulin degludec and insulin glargine 300 U/mL in healthy cats. Domest Anim Endocrinol 2019;69:19–29.
45. Linari G, Gilor C, Fleeman LM, et al. Insulin glargine 300U/mL for the treatment of diabetes mellitus in cats [abstract]. 30th ECVIM-CA Congress. Online, September 2-5, 2020.
46. Wormhoudt TL, Boss MK, Lunn K, et al. Stereotactic radiation therapy for the treatment of functional pituitary adenomas associated with feline acromegaly. J Vet Intern Med 2018;32(4):1383–91.
47. Dunning MD, Lowrie CS, Bexfield NH, et al. Exogenous insulin treatment after hypofractionated radiotherapy in cats with diabetes mellitus and acromegaly. J Vet Intern Med 2009;23(2):243–9.
48. Mayer MN, Greco DS, LaRue SM. Outcomes of pituitary tumor irradiation in cats. J Vet Intern Med 2006;20(5):1151–4.
49. Kenny P, Scudder CJ, Keyte S, et al. Treatment of feline hypersomatotropism: efficacy, morbidity and mortality of hypophysectomy [abstract]. J Vet Intern Med 2015;29:1271.
50. Abrams-Ogg AC, Holmberg DL, Stewart WA, et al. Acromegaly in a cat: diagnosis by magnetic resonance imaging and treatment by cryohypophysectomy. Can Vet J 1993;34(11):682–5.
51. Blois SL, Holmberg DL. Cryohypophysectomy used in the treatment of a case of feline acromegaly. J Small Anim Pract 2008;49(11):596–600.
52. Gostelow R, Scudder C, Keyte S, et al. Pasireotide long-acting release treatment for diabetic cats with underlying hypersomatotropism. J Vet Intern Med 2017; 31(2):355–64.
53. Scudder C, Hazuchova K, Gostelow R, et al. Pilot study assessing the use of cabergoline in the management of diabetic acromegalic cats [abstract]. J Vet Intern Med 2018;32:552.

Is It Being Overdiagnosed?
Feline Pancreatitis

Julien Bazelle, DVM, MRCVS[a],*, Penny Watson, MA, VetMD, CertVR, DSAM, FRCVS[b]

KEYWORDS

• Cat • Pancreatitis • Sensitivity • Specificity • Diagnosis

KEY POINTS

• Clinical signs of feline pancreatitis are vague, increasing the risks of both false-positive and false-negative results.
• The common finding of concurrent gut and/or liver disease complicates the diagnosis.
• Available diagnostic tests have a higher sensitivity to detect severe acute pancreatic inflammation than chronic, and/or low-grade, inflammation.
• Histopathology is rarely performed and the clinical significance of mild inflammation in patients with no typical signs is of unclear.
• At present, the evidence suggests that the risk of overdiagnosing pancreatitis is less than the risk of underdiagnosis.

INTRODUCTION

Chronic inflammation of the pancreas is common in cats: 1 study reported inflammatory lesions in up to 60% of pancreases on postmortem regardless of the cat's cause of death,[1] despite a much lower prevalence (<1%) having been previously reported.[2] There is some evidence that acute pancreatitis might also be more common than is recognized. However, until recently, pancreatitis was uncommonly diagnosed in cats because of a combination of mild and nonspecific clinical signs and a lack of sensitive and specific diagnostic tests. With improvement of both clinicopathologic tests and diagnostic imaging, accuracy of the diagnosis has improved but the concern remains that clinicians may be overdiagnosing the disease, especially overinterpreting normal reactive or aging changes. This opinion article analyzes the evidence for clinically significant pancreatitis in cats and critically evaluates whether the disease is being overdiagnosed or underdiagnosed using the diagnostic tests currently available.

[a] Manor Farm Business Park, Higham Gobion, Hitchin, Hertfordshire SG53HR, UK; [b] Queen's Veterinary School Hospital, University of Cambridge, Madingley Road, Cambridge CB30ES, UK
* Corresponding author.
E-mail address: julien.bazelle@vetspecialists.co.uk

Vet Clin Small Anim 50 (2020) 1107–1121
https://doi.org/10.1016/j.cvsm.2020.06.006
0195-5616/20/© 2020 Elsevier Inc. All rights reserved.

DEFINITIONS

Pancreatitis is the inflammation of the exocrine pancreatic tissue secondary to multiple conditions and insults. Some investigators have separated acute pancreatitis (AP) and chronic pancreatitis (CP) forms, based on the severity and longevity of the clinical signs and on histopathologic findings.[1-3] There is no consensus in the literature on whether diagnostic criteria of AP and CP are clinical or histologic. The authors of this article prefer the standard histologic definition used in human medicine but acknowledge that pancreatitis is often diagnosed clinically without histology. On histology, AP is characterized by neutrophilic inflammation and edema (**Fig. 1**A). This condition is different from CP, in which fibrosis is a prominent histologic finding with permanent structural and functional impairment (**Fig. 1**B).[1] Although AP and CP may have different clinical presentations, some overlap occurs and AP and CP may represent different points on a disease continuum in some cats.[3] In humans, the relationship between recurrent AP and CP is complex, and progression to fibrosis depends on multiple environmental and genetic factors.[4] No studies have investigated this in cats.

The typical clinical presentation of AP is considered more severe and of more sudden onset than for CP.[2,3,5] In the aforementioned postmortem study of feline pancreatitis, AP was characterized by neutrophilic inflammation and varying amounts of pancreatic acinar cell and peripancreatic fat necrosis.[1] Earlier descriptions of AP had defined 2 distinct forms: acute necrotizing, where there was significant fat necrosis, and acute suppurative, where fat necrosis was not a common feature.[2] Because some of these patients considered to have AP also had evidence of fibrosis on histopathology, it remains unclear whether they had AP or CP with an acute exacerbation.

At the other end of the spectrum, patients with CP often present with milder signs. Histopathology is characterized by mononuclear or mixed mononuclear and granulocytic inflammation, fibrosis, and acinar atrophy.[1] This form of pancreatitis was most prevalent, with 60% of the pancreases showing signs of CP.[1] This finding could suggest possible age-related changes in some of the patients with mild inflammation, but

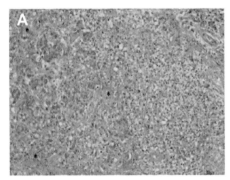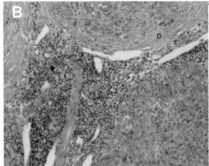

Fig. 1. (A) Histopathologic section of pancreatic biopsy from a cat with AP. Parts of the pancreatic parenchyma are replaced by amorphous material devoid of nuclei (liquefactive necrosis) (*asterisks*) and there are moderate numbers of neutrophils (hematoxylin-eosin, original magnification ×40). (B) Histopathologic section of the pancreas of a cat with CP. Note the extensive fibrous tissue (o) surrounding and the acinar tissue and clumps of lymphoplasmacytic inflammation (♦) (hematoxylin-eosin, original magnification ×40). (*From* Bazelle J, Watson P. Pancreatitis in cats: Is it acute, is it chronic, is it significant? J Feline Med Surg. 2014; 16(5):395-406; with permission.)

nonetheless suggests chronic inflammation is common in cats. Typically, a continuous, progressively worsening condition, with possible extension of the inflammation into the endocrine tissue of the pancreas, leading to destruction of the islets and impaired β-cell function can occur. As a consequence, both diabetes mellitus and exocrine pancreatic insufficiency (EPI) have been linked to CP.[6,7]

Studies assessing pancreatic histopathology are scarce. Moreover, the differentiation between AP and CP is not always well defined even in recent articles on feline pancreatitis. This lack of definition introduces uncertainties when interpreting the performance of the available diagnostic tools.

DIFFICULTIES IN ACHIEVING A DEFINITIVE DIAGNOSIS
Ambiguous Clinical Presentation

Cats with pancreatitis, even severe acute disease, often display vague clinical signs (mainly anorexia and lethargy), and gastrointestinal signs are frequently absent or not observed.[2,3,5,8] The prevalence of vomiting is reported to be 35% to 90% (although most studies report a prevalence of <67%), of diarrhea 11% to 57%, and of abdominal pain 19% to 48%. The secretive nature of feline patients may explain this low prevalence because the signs may be missed by the owners. Findings on physical examination are also nonspecific and may include abdominal discomfort (19%–29%) or fever (19%–25%). Cats are known for hiding pain, even when severe, making recognition of severe acute disease and peritonitis much more difficult than in dogs. Icterus can increase the index of suspicion of a cholestatic condition secondary to extrahepatic biliary obstruction with pancreatitis or concurrent cholangitis (discussed later) but remains uncommon (31%–37%).[5]

A study comparing AP and CP in 63 cats did not reveal any difference in the prevalence or severity of the clinical signs.[3] The clinical presentation therefore does not help in differentiating AP from CP.

This combination of nonspecific signs and rarely severe clinical presentation has historically been associated with underdiagnosis.[1] With the current increased awareness of the veterinary profession about feline pancreatitis, diagnosis should become more frequent and it is possible that the disease may be overdiagnosed.

Common Comorbidities of Pancreatitis

Another issue complicating diagnosis of pancreatitis in cats is the presence of concurrent inflammation in the gut (inflammatory bowel disease [IBD]) and liver (cholangitis) in a subset of cats[9–12] (discussed Jonathan A. Lidbury and colleagues' article, "Triaditis: Truth and Consequences," elsewhere in this issue). IBD and cholangitis share similar clinical signs to pancreatitis. Minimally invasive diagnosis of IBD and cholangitis is facilitated by the availability of endoscopic and ultrasonography-guided biopsies, respectively, making it easier to diagnose these conditions compared with pancreatitis, which can then be overlooked. Other reported comorbidities include hepatic lipidosis and hemolytic anemia. EPI is an end stage of CP when enough parenchyma is destroyed, although this is only occasionally confirmed histopathologically in cats. In addition, diabetes mellitus has a complex cause-and-effect relationship with pancreatitis. These disease associations are detailed in **Table 1** and may all complicate the recognition of pancreatitis or its management.

Poor Performance of the Diagnostic Investigations

Laboratory investigations
The gold standard for diagnosis of feline pancreatitis remains histopathology, but this is rarely performed because it is invasive and usually does not alter treatment or

Table 1
Other disease associations in feline acute and chronic pancreatitis

Disease/Diseases	Potential Reason for Associations	Evidence in the Literature	References

Triaditis: concurrent IBD and cholangitis	• Cause still uncertain but suspected:
	  ○ Ascending bacterial infection
	  ○ Pancreaticobiliary reflux caused by increased pressure during vomiting
	  ○ Autoimmune disease also suspected
	  ○ Common channel theory (junction of the pancreatic and bile ducts before their entry within the duodenum)
	  ○ Sphincter of Oddi dysfunction in some cats
		Strong evidence
		• Pancreatitis in 50%–60% of cats with cholangitis
		• ↑ Spec fPL 16 out of 23 cats with IBD (no histology)
		• Eight out of 10 cats had both pancreatitis and cholangitis confirmed via histology in MRI study
		• When reviewing 27 symptomatic and 20 healthy cats, 57.4% of cats had inflammation in more than 1 organ on histology. In symptomatic cats, 11 had pancreatitis, of which 2 had IBD and 8 had cholangitis
			9–18

Hepatic lipidosis	• Consequence of anorexia and weight loss • Metabolic disturbances induced by hepatic lipidosis can trigger pancreatitis (eg, hypotension, metabolic acidosis, or reactive inflammation)	Strong evidence • In triaditis study, 36% of cats with pancreatitis also had hepatic lipidosis • Prevalence of pancreatitis in patients diagnosed with hepatic lipidosis varies between 5% and 38%	3,10,12,19–21
Diabetes mellitus	• End-stage CP and tissue destruction induces diabetes mellitus • Sustained hyperglycemia induces increased pancreatic neutrophil count	Moderate evidence • 44% and 83% of diabetic cats have increased PLI • But there is a high prevalence of ↑ ↑PLI in nondiabetic cats too • No difference in the severity of pancreatic lesions in cats with diabetes mellitus compared with control or any difference between cats with diabetes with or without ketoacidosis	3,6,22–26

EPI	• End-stage CP and tissue destruction induces diabetes mellitus	Moderate evidence [7,10,27,28] • In 16 cats with EPI, only 1 cat had pancreatic histology reported as pancreatic acinar atrophy (limited investigations because retrospective study) • In 150 cats with EPI, no pathology reported but 13 had concurrent diabetes mellitus (suggestive of loss of pancreatic mass) and 11% had evidence of pancreatitis • Histologic evidence of end-stage chronic pancreatitis with marked loss of tissue mass in 1 cat with concurrent EPI and diabetes mellitus. Likely more common but histology rarely reported in studies

IMHA	• Unclear:
	  ◦ IMHA-induced proinflammatory status, hypoxemia
	  ◦ Pancreatitis triggering secondary IMHA
	  ◦ Common autoimmune origin
		Weak evidence [29]
		• In a population of 155 cats, 9 had pancreatitis, 11 had IMHA, and 3 had both diseases

Abbreviations: fPLI, feline pancreatic lipase immunoreactivity test; IMHA, immune-mediated hemolytic anemia; PLI, pancreatic lipase immunoreactivity.
Data from Refs.[3,6,7,9–19,21–29]

outcome. The diagnosis is therefore often presumptive after ruling out other conditions, based on a combination of clinical suspicion, imaging, serum biochemical and hematological changes, along with assessment of more specific pancreatic tests.

Hematology and biochemistry are only helpful to rule out other conditions because abnormal findings are often mild and nonspecific (**Table 2**). The wide ranges of prevalence for these abnormalities most likely reflect the variable severity of the pancreatitis, concurrent unrecognized cholangitis, IBD, or hepatic lipidosis in some cases, and nonstandardized reference ranges.

At present, the feline pancreatic lipase immunoreactivity test (fPLI) is widely thought to be the most useful laboratory test for diagnosis of feline pancreatitis. This test is an enzyme-linked immunosorbent assay (ELISA) assay developed against the lipase molecule, both organ (pancreas) and species specific. There are 2 commercially available tests for measurement of fPLI, both marketed by the same laboratory: Spec fPL (IDEXX Laboratories Inc, Westbrook, ME) and SNAP fPL (IDEXX Laboratories Inc, Westbrook, ME). The Spec fPL is a quantitative ELISA with a cutoff value for diagnosis of pancreatitis of greater than or equal to 5.4 μg/L, and gray zone of 3.6 to 5.3 μg/L. The use of Spec fPL has only been evaluated in a small number of articles,[31–33] and 1 unpublished abstract.[34] Its sensitivity and specificity vary respectively between 42% and 100% and between 69% and 100% compared with histopathology.[31,33] Sensitivity is higher in AP than in CP and varies depending on whether none or as much as 10% lymphocytic inflammation was considered a normal histopathologic finding,[33] suggesting that increase of Spec fPL is linked to the degree of pancreatic inflammation. In studies of cats in which pancreatitis was suspected clinically and on ultrasonography, the sensitivity and specificity of Spec fPL have been assessed, although it remains to be determined whether fPLI or ultrasonography is the better surrogate marker.[32,34] In these studies, the sensitivity was 61% to 79%, whereas specificity was 35% to 82%. In Oppliger and colleagues[32] (2014), the agreement between ultrasonography findings and Spec fPL greater than or equal to 5.4 μg/L was only fair and was improved when pancreases were hypoechoic and mixed echoic and enlarged. The specificity of Spec fPL has not been studied extensively in the clinical setting. There are currently no studies evaluating the duration of increased Spec fPL

Table 2	
Hematology and biochemistry findings in cats with pancreatitis	
Finding	**Prevalence (%)**
Anemia (normocytic normochromic regenerative or nonregenerative)	20–55
Lymphopenia	57–69
Leukocytosis	27–62
Leukopenia	5–13
Thrombocytopenia	8–33
Increased activity ALP	50
Increased activity ALT	24–68
Hyperbilirubinemia	56–69
Hyperglycemia	10–86
Hypokalemia	56–69
Hypocalcemia	8–61

Abbreviations: ALP, alkaline phosphatase; ALT, alanine transaminase.
Data from Refs.[2,3,5,8,30]

results after an episode of pancreatitis. In dogs, increased SNAP or Spec cPL was found in up to 40% of dogs with conditions such as septic peritonitis or abdominal neoplasia.[35] Similar findings have not been investigated in cats, but it would not be surprising if fPLI was increased with other conditions such as lymphoma or feline infectious peritonitis because these conditions can also involve the pancreas. Overall, these studies highlight variable performance of Spec fPL: the possibility of false-positives and false-negatives should always be considered, especially because this test is frequently used as the main, or even the sole, criterion for diagnosing pancreatitis in studies and in practice.

The SNAP fPL is a semiquantitative assay available as a bedside patient diagnostic tool in veterinary practice. A positive SNAP fPL test should indicate that fPLI is greater than or equal to 3.5 µg/L but does not differentiate between patients with fPLI between 3.6 and 5.3 µg/L (gray zone) and patients with fPLI greater than or equal to 5.4µg/L (considered consistent with pancreatitis), prompting the recommendation to assess a Spec fPL. In 1 recent study, SNAP fPL was in agreement with Spec fPL.[8] When all 111 patients in that study were assessed, including 16 cats with no or unclear clinical suspicion of pancreatitis, SNAP fPL correctly identified that Spec fPLI was within normal limits in 97.5% of the cases and the Spec fPLI was greater than or equal to 5.4 µg/L in 90% of the cases. For the patients with Spec fPL in the gray zone, SNAP fPL was normal in 8 and abnormal in 3 cats. It is yet to be determined whether SNAP fPL correlates with clinical signs, ultrasonography findings, or histopathology.

Standard catalytic lipase and amylase assays have classically been considered of little clinical value, carrying both a poor sensitivity and specificity.[1,5] However, a recent unpublished study, when pancreatitis was diagnosed from increased fPLI, revealed that high lipase level associated with suggestive ultrasonography findings had a sensitivity of 100% and a low lipase level with negative ultrasonography findings reliably predicted an fPLI within the reference range.[36] These results should be interpreted cautiously given the low numbers of cases evaluated, the absence of histology, and that these results have not been published in a peer-reviewed journal. The authors of this article do not recommend the use of traditional lipase assays in cats.

Catalytic assays such as lipase are not organ specific: the test measures a reaction catalyzed by lipase in vitro and thus also measures activity of hormone sensitive lipase, gastric lipase, and other lipases. Recent assays using alternative substrates and conditions of reaction, such as 1,2-o-dilauryl-rac-glycero glutaric acid-(6′-methyl-resorufin) ester (DGGR) and triolein, have been developed to try to increase the specificity. DGGR-lipase is the most studied and showed good agreement with fPLI.[32,37] However, DGGR-lipase had only a fair agreement with ultrasonography,[32] and only a limited agreement with histology,[33] although it performed similarly to Spec fPLI. Given the uncertain significance of a mild lymphocytic inflammation in the pancreas of cats with no apparent clinical signs, Oppliger and colleagues[33] reported that the sensitivity increased from 36.8% to 66.7% but that the specificity decreased from 100% to 78.6% if lymphocytic inflammation in up to 10% of a transverse section of the pancreas was considered normal. These results were similar to Spec fPLI. The DGGR-lipase assay seems clinically useful but risks of underdiagnosis remain, whereas overdiagnosis may be less likely.

Lipase activity assay using triolein has also been investigated in 1 study in cats.[38] The triolein assay correlated poorly with the results of Spec fPLI but this was not compared with other diagnostic tests and the diseased patients were not primarily suspected of pancreatitis, limiting the conclusions regarding its clinical use. In this population, if Spec fPLI was considered the gold standard, the triolein assay had good specificity (93.2%) and negative predictive value (94.0%) but poor sensitivity (66.7%) and positive predictive value (63.6%).

Measurement of increased serum feline trypsinlike immunoreactivity (fTLI) has been evaluated in the context of pancreatitis in a few studies, showing poor sensitivity but moderate to high specificity.[10,30,31,39] Using fTLI to confirm or rule out pancreatitis is therefore not recommended in cats, although using a low value of fTLI to diagnose EPI has a high specificity and good sensitivity.

There is a paucity of investigation of other potential clinicopathologic tests for diagnosing feline pancreatitis. A study evaluating the plasma and urine concentrations of trypsinogen-activation peptide (TAP), and its ratio with creatinine, showed no difference between healthy cats and those with AP.[40] Lipase activity in peritoneal fluid has not yet been evaluated in cats but may be a promising diagnostic tool based on findings in dogs.[41]

Imaging

Abdominal radiographs are generally low yield but may identify signs of peritonitis or a mass effect.[1,2,30] Ultrasonography is the most useful imaging modality in cats and can reveal pancreatic enlargement, changes in echogenicity, mass effect, peripancreatic hyperechogenicity, and free fluid (**Fig. 2**).[2,5,31,32,42,43] It also helps detect other significant abdominal disease, such as neoplasia, and identify concurrent changes in the bile duct and intestine when present. In a study of cats with cholangitis, 17 had concurrent abnormalities of the gut wall and 7 had concurrent pancreatic abnormalities on ultrasonography.[44] Some changes, such as increased diameter of the pancreatic duct, occur normally with aging and should not be overinterpreted as reflecting pancreatitis.[45,46] Sensitivity of ultrasonography compared with histology was poor to moderate (24%–56%) in early studies.[3,30,42] Improved technology and clinician experience have likely significantly improved sensitivity in the 16 or more years since these studies. In a recent article,[43] when increased Spec fPLI was considered diagnostic for pancreatitis, abdominal ultrasonography sensitivity was 84%, with the most sensitive single ultrasonography finding being hyperechoic peripancreatic fat. Similarly, abdominal ultrasonography and Spec fPLI correlated well for the diagnosis of traumatic pancreatitis.[47] The specificity of ultrasonography was rarely evaluated in cats. Williams and colleagues[43] reported an overall specificity of 75%, but, when each ultrasonography parameter (increased pancreatic thickness, abnormal pancreatic margin, and hyperechoic peripancreatic fat) was taken individually, specificity

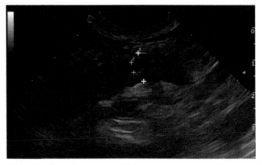

Fig. 2. Ultrasonographic findings in a cat with acute pancreatitis. Note the hypoechoic and enlarged pancreas and the surrounding mesentery hyperechogenicity. The pancreatic duct (delineated by the 2 crosses) was enlarged but this remains a nonspecific finding.

increased to greater than 90%. Providing that this is representative, underdiagnosis is more likely than overdiagnosis when ultrasonography is the sole diagnostic test.

Other imaging modalities that may have potential in the diagnosis of feline pancreatitis include contrast-enhanced ultrasonography,[48,49] endosonography,[50] endoscopic retrograde cholangiopancreatography,[51] contrast-enhanced computed tomography (CT),[30,31] and MRI with cholangiopancreatography.[18,52] The sensitivity for contrast-enhanced CT scan was poor (~20%) and specificity was not reported.[30,31]

Cytology

Cytology of the pancreas was previously mainly evaluated in the context of pancreatic carcinoma.[53] Although trauma of the pancreas can induce pancreatitis, a recent pilot study suggests that fine-needle aspiration of the pancreas is safe.[54] In this pilot study, cytology correlated well with histology.

Overall, diagnostic tests are associated with variable, but often poor to moderate, sensitivity for diagnosis of pancreatitis in cats (**Table 3**). Specificity was not always assessed because of the absence of control groups in many studies but is highly variable. This finding shows that the diagnosis of pancreatitis in cats cannot rely solely on a single investigation but requires a combination of tests while ruling out other conditions.

FACTORS INVOLVED IN VARIATION OF PERFORMANCE OF DIAGNOSTIC TESTS
Acute Versus Chronic Pancreatitis

Most studies have focused on AP despite the higher prevalence of CP.[1] There is a concern that CP may be overdiagnosed, because lymphocytic inflammation in pancreatic biopsies of less than 10% of the tissue may potentially be normal.[33] CP is more frequently associated with a less severe inflammatory reaction and more chronic changes such as fibrosis and atrophy. The consequent loss of tissue mass would be expected to reduce pancreatic enzyme production, and some cats do develop overt EPI as an end stage of CP. Forman and colleagues[31,34] reported that, although the sensitivity of fPLI was 100% for moderate and severe pancreatitis, it decreased to 54% for mild pancreatitis, such as is found in CP.[36] Similarly, Oppliger and colleagues[33] found that the sensitivity of both DGGR-lipase and Spec fPL improved if 10% of lymphocytic inflammation was considered normal, whereas specificity decreased concurrently. The sensitivity of ultrasonography was significantly lower in mild than in moderate and severe disease (62% vs 80%).[31] These imaging

Table 3
Reported sensitivity and specificity of the diagnostic tests for feline pancreatitis

Tests	Sensitivity (%)	Specificity (%)	Studies References
DGGR-lipase	36.8–66.7	78.6–100	CP/AP: 31, 32
Triolein assay	66.7	93.2	Any disease, comparison with Spec fPL: 37
Spec fPL	42–100	35–100	CP/AP: 30–32. Uncertain: 33
fTLI	33–86	50–80	CP/AP: 10, 30, 38
AUS	24–84	75–90	CP/AP: 3, 5, 30, 31, 38. AP: 39, 42
CT scan	20.0	?	CP/AP: 30, 38

Abbreviation: AUS, abdominal ultrasonography scan.
Data from Refs.[3,5,10,30–34,38,39,42]

studies focused on criteria more frequently detected in acute forms, such as hyperechogenic mesentery, free fluid, and hypoechoic parenchyma, and less on criteria that are considered more typical for CP, such as irregular margins, hyperechogenicity, or nodular changes, although Ferreri and colleagues[3] reported no difference between AP and CP. Because most studies evaluated sensitivity and specificity of tests for patients with AP, the sensitivity of the same tests is likely to be overestimated, whereas the specificity may be underestimated for CP, resulting in underdiagnosis of chronic disease.

Intraindividual and Interindividual Variation

There is a paucity of information on biological variation of the laboratory tests, with only 2 articles reviewing variation in Spec fPLI in healthy cats.[55,56] In the original study, the investigators reported that the coefficients of variation for intra-assay and interassay variability were 2.2% to 10.1% and 15.8% to 24.4%, respectively.[55] Cohn-Urbach and colleagues[56] report that both intraindividual and interindividual variations were significantly higher, respectively 33% and 99%. They concluded that individual reference ranges constructed by serial measurement of fPLI may be preferable to population-based reference ranges, although, based on the high interassay variation, this may have limited use for monitoring the progression of the disease.

Histology: a Gold Standard?

Histology is considered the gold standard for diagnosis of pancreatitis, but antemortem diagnosis remains difficult because inflammation may have a multifocal distribution.[1,2,42] When comparing left limb, right limb, and body of the pancreas, only half of the cats had lesions identified in every section.[1] This finding limits the sensitivity of pancreatic biopsies.

In addition, the specificity of lymphocytic inflammation in pancreatic histology has been questioned.[33] Lymphocytic inflammation has been reported in 67% overall and 45% in healthy necropsied patients,[1] raising the concern this may reflect normal response to antigenic stimulation. In another study, focal small nests of lymphocytes were considered normal.[31] The clinical relevance of mild lymphocytic inflammation in the absence of significant concurrent fibrosis is therefore undetermined and standardization would be needed to determine what can be considered normal for this species.

These limitations of histology make it a poor gold standard for diagnosing feline pancreatitis and conclusions regarding the diagnostic power of each diagnostic test should always be interpreted cautiously.

Influence of Renal Function, Dehydration, Corticosteroid Use

The specificity of fPLI measurement is assumed to be high but some factors have emerged as possibly contributing to false-positive results. Like amylase, lipase undergoes renal clearance and renal dysfunction is associated with significant increase of lipase serum level.[57] One unpublished study suggested no effect of azotemia on fPLI,[58] but another revealed increased pancreatic-specific lipase levels in cats with chronic kidney disease.[59]

Dogs with hyperadrenocorticism and no evident signs of pancreatitis have higher SNAP cPL and Spec cPL than patients without hyperadrenocorticism.[60] Although this might represent an increased risk of pancreatitis in patients with hyperadrenocorticism, it is probably caused by steroid-induced effects and can probably be generalized to exogenous steroids. A similar effect on fPLI has not been investigated, but it is conceivable that the effects of steroids may be similar in cats.

Pancreatic Conditions Mimicking Pancreatitis

Like pancreatitis, exocrine pancreatic carcinoma may appear normal in some cats on ultrasonography, whereas in others hyperechoic and coarse pancreatic parenchyma are seen.[61] Another study showed variably sized neoplastic pancreatic nodules on all of the 34 cats that underwent ultrasonography, but abdominal effusion was also present in 16 of them, which could be incorrectly interpreted as being secondary to pancreatitis.[62] Interestingly, fPLI was measured in the abdominal fluid of 1 of these patients and was found to be increased, although, as mentioned previously, the clinical relevance of this has not been evaluated in cats.

In contrast, patients with pancreatitis may have nodular hyperplastic changes that can be mistaken for neoplasia.[32,42,63] Similarly, and unsurprisingly, another study revealed increase of Spec fPL in both cats with pancreatic carcinoma and pancreatitis.[64] Because there is significant overlap of the findings in these 2 conditions, it is difficult to rule out pancreatic carcinoma in feline patients suspected of having pancreatitis.

Pancreatic cysts, pseudocysts, and abscesses are uncommonly described in cats, other than as isolated case reports. These findings are associated with inflammation of the surrounding pancreatic tissue. Increase of Spec fPL was described in 2 case reports of pancreatic abscess[65,66]; this was not evaluated in cats with cysts or pseudocysts. It is also unknown whether cysts without associated pancreatitis have increases of fPLI.

SUMMARY

Diagnosing feline pancreatitis remains a challenge and relies on a combination of history, physical examination, ultrasonographic, and laboratory findings because no single finding is sufficient. The frequent association with other medical conditions, particularly IBD and cholangitis, further complicates diagnosis. The absence of a gold standard, or even consensus, regarding a definition of normal pancreatic histopathology makes it difficult to evaluate other tests. Because fPLI, DGGR-lipase, and ultrasonography are considered to have overall higher specificity than sensitivity, although this article also highlights factors of variation that may affect their specificity, the main concern for clinicians is to avoid underdiagnosis rather than worrying about the risk of false-positive results, particularly with CP.

Pancreatitis is now increasingly recognized in cats, owing to increased awareness of the disease. This increased recognition will inevitably increase the risk of false-positive diagnoses. A consensus on the histopathologic definition of pancreatitis and further large cohort studies are required to improve knowledge and avoid diagnostic pitfalls.

DISCLOSURE

The authors declare no potential commercial or financial conflicts of interest. P. Watson has received funding from the Petplan Charitable Trust and has undertaken consultancies for Mars (Waltham) and VetPlus.

REFERENCES

1. De Cock HE, Forman MA, Farver TB, et al. Prevalence and histopathologic characteristics of pancreatitis in cats. Vet Pathol 2007;44:39–49.
2. Hill RC, Van Winkle TJ. Acute necrotizing pancreatitis and acute suppurative pancreatitis in the cat. A retrospective study of 40 cases (1976–1989). J Vet Intern Med 1993;7:25–33.

3. Ferreri JA, Hardam E, Kimmel SE, et al. Clinical differentiation of acute necrotizing from chronic nonsuppurative pancreatitis in cats: 63 cases (1996-2001). J Am Vet Med Assoc 2003;223:469–74.

4. LaRusch J, Whitcomb DC. Genetics of pancreatitis. Curr Opin Gastroenterol 2011;27:467–74.

5. Nivy R, Kaplanov A, Kuzi S, et al. A retrospective study of 157 hospitalized cats with pancreatitis in a tertiary care center: Clinical, imaging and laboratory findings, potential prognostic markers and outcome. J Vet Intern Med 2018;32: 1874–85.

6. Davison LJ. Diabetes mellitus and pancreatitis–cause or effect? J Small Anim Pract 2015;56:50–9.

7. Xenoulis PG, Zoran DL, Fosgate GT, et al. Feline exocrine pancreatic insufficiency: a retrospective study of 150 cases. J Vet Intern Med 2016;30:1790–7.

8. Schnauß F, Hanisch F, Burgener IA. Diagnosis of feline pancreatitis with SNAP fPL and Spec fPL. J Feline Med Surg 2019;21:700–7.

9. Weiss DJ, Gagne JM, Armstrong PJ. Relationship between inflammatory hepatic disease and inflammatory bowel disease, pancreatitis, and nephritis in cats. J Am Vet Med Assoc 1996;209:1114–6.

10. Swift NC, Marks SL, MacLachlan NJ, et al. Evaluation of serum feline trypsin-like immunoreactivity for the diagnosis of pancreatitis in cats. J Am Vet Med Assoc 2000;217:37–42.

11. Callahan Clark JE, Haddad JL, Brown DC, et al. Feline cholangitis: a necropsy study of 44 cats (1986-2008). J Feline Med Surg 2011;13:570–6.

12. Fragkou FC, Adamama-Moraitou KK, Poutahidis T, et al. Prevalence and clinico-pathological features of triaditis in a prospective case series of symptomatic and asymptomatic cats. J Vet Intern Med 2016;30:1031–45.

13. Arendt T. Bile-induced acute pancreatitis in cats. Roles of bile, bacteria, and pancreatic duct pressure. Dig Dis Sci 1993;38(1):39–44.

14. Widdison AL, Karanjia ND, Reber HA. Routes of spread of pathogens into the pancreas in a feline model of acute pancreatitis. Gut 1994;35:1306–10.

15. Simpson KW, Twedt DC, McDonough SP, et al: Culture-independent detection of bacteria in feline pancreatitis. Proceedings of the Forum of the American College of Veterinary Internal Medicine. Denver, Colorado, June 15-18, 2011.

16. Furneaux RW. A series of six cases of sphincter of Oddi pathology in the cat (2008-2009). J Feline Med Surg 2010;12:794–801.

17. Bailey S, Benigni L, Eastwood J, et al. Comparisons between cats with normal and increased fPLI concentrations in cats diagnosed with inflammatory bowel disease. J Small Anim Pract 2010;51:484–9.

18. Marolf AJ, Kraft SL, Dunphy TR, et al. Magnetic resonance (MR) imaging and MR cholangiopancreatography findings in cats with cholangitis and pancreatitis. J Feline Med Surg 2013;15:285–94.

19. Akol KG, Washabau RJ, Saunders HM, et al. Acute pancreatitis in cats with hepatic lipidosis. J Vet Intern Med 1993;7(4):205–9.

20. Center SA, Crawford MA, Guida L, et al. A retrospective study of 77 cats with severe hepatic lipidosis: 1975-1990. J Vet Intern Med 1993;7:349–59.

21. Kuzi S, Segev G, Kedar S, et al. Prognostic markers in feline hepatic lipidosis: a retrospective study of 71 cats. Vet Rec 2017;181:512.

22. Goossens MM, Nelson RW, Feldman EC, et al. Response to insulin treatment and survival in 104 cats with diabetes mellitus (1985-1995). J Vet Intern Med 1998; 12:1–6.

23. Forcada Y, German AJ, Noble PJ, et al. Determination of serum fPLI concentrations in cats with diabetes mellitus. J Feline Med Surg 2008;10:480–7.

24. Schaefer S, Kooistra HS, Riond B, et al. Evaluation of insulin-like growth factor-1, total thyroxine, feline pancreas-specific lipase and urinary corticoid-to-creatinine ratio in cats with diabetes mellitus in Switzerland and the Netherlands. J Feline Med Surg 2017;19:888–96.

25. Zini E, Osto M, Moretti S, et al. Hyperglycaemia but not hyperlipidaemia decreases serum amylase and increases neutrophils in the exocrine pancreas of cats. Res Vet Sci 2010;89:20–6.

26. Zini E, Ferro S, Lunardi F, et al. Exocrine pancreas in cats with diabetes mellitus. Vet Pathol 2016;53:145–52.

27. Holzworth J, Coffin DL. Pancreatic insufficiency and diabetes mellitus in a cat. Cornell Vet 1953;43(4):502–12.

28. Thompson KA, Parnell NK, Hohenhaus AE, et al. Feline exocrine pancreatic insufficiency: 16 cases (1992-2007). J Feline Med Surg 2009;11:935–40.

29. Zoia A, Drigo M. Association between pancreatitis and immune-mediated haemolytic anaemia in cats: a cross-sectional study. J Comp Pathol 2017;156:384–8.

30. Gerhardt A, Steiner JM, Williams DA, et al. Comparison of the sensitivity of different diagnostic tests for pancreatitis in cats. J Vet Intern Med 2001;15(4):329–33.

31. Forman MA, Marks SL, Cock H, et al. Evaluation of serum feline pancreatic lipase immunoreactivity and helical computed tomography versus conventional testing for the diagnosis of feline pancreatitis. J Vet Intern Med 2004;18:807–15.

32. Oppliger S, Hartnack S, Reusch CE, et al. Agreement of serum feline pancreas-specific lipase and colorimetric lipase assays with pancreatic ultrasonographic findings in cats with suspicion of pancreatitis: 161 cases (2008-2012). J Am Vet Med Assoc 2014;244:1060–5.

33. Oppliger S, Hilbe M, Hartnack S. Comparison of Serum Spec fPL(™) and 1,2-o-dilauryl-rac-glycero-3-glutaric acid-(6'-methylresorufin) ester assay in 60 cats using standardized assessment of pancreatic histology. J Vet Intern Med 2016;30:764–70.

34. Forman MA, Shiroma JT, Robertson JE. Evaluation of feline pancreas-specific lipase (Spec fPL) for the diagnosis of feline pancreatitis. JVIM 2009;23:733–4. ACVIM abstract 165, [abstract].

35. Haworth MD, Hosgood G, Swindells KL, et al. Diagnostic accuracy of the SNAP and Spec canine pancreatic lipase tests for pancreatitis in dogs presenting with clinical signs of acute abdominal disease. J Vet Emerg Crit Care (San Antonio) 2014;24:135–43.

36. Abrams-Ogg A, Ruotsalo K, Kocmarek H, et al. Total serum lipase activity for the antemortem diagnosis of feline pancreatitis. J Vet Intern Med 2013;27(3):708 [Abstract].

37. Oppliger S, Hartnack S, Riond B, et al. Agreement of the serum Spec fPL™ and 1,2-o-dilauryl-rac-glycero-3-glutaric acid-(6'-methylresorufin) ester lipase assay for the determination of serum lipase in cats with suspicion of pancreatitis. J Vet Intern Med 2013;27:1077–82.

38. Oishi M, Ohno K, Sato T, et al. Measurement of feline lipase activity using a dry-chemistry assay with a triolein substrate and comparison with pancreas-specific lipase (Spec fPL(™)). J Vet Med Sci 2015;77:1495–7.

39. Williams DA, Steiner JM, Ruaux CG, et al. Increases in serum pancreatic lipase immunoreactivity (PLI) are greater and of longer duration than those of trypsin-

like immunoreactivity (TLI) in cats with experimental pancreatitis. J Vet Intern Med 2003;17:445–6.

40. Allen HS, Steiner J, Broussard J, et al. Serum and urine concentrations of trypsinogen-activation peptide as markers for acute pancreatitis in cats. Can J Vet Res 2006;70:313–6.

41. Guija de Arespacochaga A, Hittmair KM, Schwendenwein I. Comparison of lipase activity in peritoneal fluid of dogs with different pathologies–a complementary diagnostic tool in acute pancreatitis? J Vet Med A Physiol Pathol Clin Med 2006;53:119–22.

42. Saunders HM, VanWinkle TJ, Drobatz K, et al. Ultrasonographic findings in cats with clinical, gross pathologic, and histologic evidence of acute pancreatic necrosis: 20 cases (1994-2001). J Am Vet Med Assoc 2002;221:1724–30.

43. Williams JM, Panciera DL, Larson MM, et al. Ultrasonographic findings of the pancreas in cats with elevated serum pancreatic lipase immunoreactivity. J Vet Intern Med 2013;27:913–8.

44. Marolf AJ, Leach L, Gibbons DS, et al. Ultrasonographic findings of feline cholangitis. J Am Anim Hosp Assoc 2012;48:36–42.

45. Larson MM, Panciera DL, Ward DL, et al. Age-related changes in the ultrasound appearance of the normal feline pancreas. Vet Radiol Ultrasound 2005;46:238–42.

46. Hecht S, Penninck DG, Mahony OM, et al. Relationship of pancreatic duct dilation to age and clinical findings in cats. Vet Radiol Ultrasound 2006;47:287–94.

47. Zimmermann E, Hittmair KM, Suchodolski JS, et al. Serum feline-specific pancreatic lipase immunoreactivity concentrations and abdominal ultrasonographic findings in cats with trauma resulting from high-rise syndrome. J Am Vet Med Assoc 2013;242:1238–43.

48. Rademacher N, Ohlerth S, Scharf G, et al. Contrast-enhanced power and color Doppler ultrasonography of the pancreas in healthy and diseased cats. J Vet Intern Med 2008;22:1310–6.

49. Leinonen MR, Raekallio MR, Vainio OM, et al. Quantitative contrast-enhanced ultrasonographic analysis of perfusion in the kidneys, liver, pancreas, small intestine, and mesenteric lymph nodes in healthy cats. Am J Vet Res 2010;71:1305–11.

50. Schweighauser A, Gaschen F, Steiner J, et al. Evaluation of endosonography as a new diagnostic tool for feline pancreatitis. J Feline Med Surg 2009;11:492–8.

51. Spillmann T, Willard MD, Ruhnke I, et al. Feasibility of endoscopic retrograde cholangiopancreatography in healthy cats. Vet Radiol Ultrasound 2014;55:85–91.

52. Zhang TT, Wang L, Wang DB, et al. Correlation between secretin-enhanced MRCP findings and histopathologic severity of chronic pancreatitis in a cat model. Pancreatology 2013;13:491–7.

53. Bennett PF, Hahn KA, Toal RL, et al. Ultrasonographic and cytopathological diagnosis of exocrine pancreatic carcinoma in the dog and cat. J Am Anim Hosp Assoc 2001;37:466–73.

54. Crain SK, Sharkey LC, Cordner AP, et al. Safety of ultrasound-guided fine-needle aspiration of the feline pancreas: a case-control study. J Feline Med Surg 2015;17:858–63.

55. Steiner JM, Wilson BG, Williams DA. Development and analytical validation of a radioimmunoassay for the measurement of feline pancreatic lipase immunoreactivity in serum. Can J Vet Res 2004;68:309–14.

56. Cohn-Urbach M, Ruaux CG, Nemanic S. Estimates of biologic variation in specific feline pancreatic lipase concentrations in cats without clinical or ultrasonographic evidence of pancreatitis. Vet Clin Pathol 2017;46:615–9.

57. Stogdale L. Correlation of changes in blood chemistry with pathological changes in the animal's body - II Electrolytes, kidney function tests, serum enzymes, and liver function tests. J S Afr Vet Assoc 1981;52:155–64.

58. Xenoulis PG, Finco DR, Suchodolski JS, et al. Serum fPLI and Spec fPL concentrations in cats with experimentally induced chronic renal failure. J Vet Intern Med 2009;23:758 [Abstract].

59. Jaensch S. The effect of naturally occurring renal insufficiency on serum pancreatic-specific lipase in cats. Comp Clin Path 2013;22:801–2.

60. Mawby DI, Whittemore JC, Fecteau KA. Canine pancreatic-specific lipase concentrations in clinically healthy dogs and dogs with naturally occurring hyperadrenocorticism. J Vet Intern Med 2014;28:1244–50.

61. Nicoletti R, Chun R, Curran KM, et al. Postsurgical outcome in cats with exocrine pancreatic carcinoma: nine cases (2007-2016). J Am Anim Hosp Assoc 2018;54:291–5.

62. Linderman MJ, Brodsky EM, de Lorimier LP, et al. Feline exocrine pancreatic carcinoma: a retrospective study of 34 cases. Vet Comp Oncol 2013;11:208–18.

63. Hecht S, Penninck DG, Keating JH. Imaging findings in pancreatic neoplasia and nodular hyperplasia in 19 cats. Vet Radiol Ultrasound 2007;48:45–50.

64. Meachem MD, Snead ER, Kidney BA, et al. A comparative proteomic study of plasma in feline pancreatitis and pancreatic carcinoma using 2-dimensional gel electrophoresis to identify diagnostic biomarkers: A pilot study. Can J Vet Res 2015;79:184–9.

65. Nemoto Y, Haraguchi T, Shimokawa Miyama T, et al. Pancreatic Abscess in a cat due to Staphylococcus aureus infection. J Vet Med Sci 2017;79:1146–50.

66. Lee M, Kang JH, Chang D, et al. Pancreatic abscess in a cat with diabetes mellitus. J Am Anim Hosp Assoc 2015;51:180–4.

Evidence-Based Medicine
Ultrasound-Guided Percutaneous Cholecystocentesis in the Cat

Craig B. Webb, PhD, DVM

KEYWORDS

- PUC • Cholecystocentesis • Cholangitis • Hepatobiliary • Feline
- Hyperbilirubinemia

KEY POINTS

- Cholangitis is one of the most prevalent hepatobiliary diseases of cats.
- Causes of feline cholangitis include flukes, infection, and immune-mediated processes.
- The therapeutic plan for feline cholangitis would ideally be based on identification of a specific underlying cause.
- Percutaneous ultrasound-guided cholecystocentesis (PUC) is performed to obtain a sample of bile.
- Current literature is reviewed to determine the safety and usefulness of PUC in the diagnosis of feline cholangitis.

From a collection of studies published in 2003 and summarized in 2009, the World Small Animal Veterinary Association Liver Standardization Group changed the nomenclature of feline hepatobiliary disease, and in doing so, focused clinical effort on the biliary system and diagnostic effort on the gallbladder (GB) of felines; this is where the cause and the answer would lie in cats presenting for "liver disease."[1–4] The cat had once again strived to disassociate itself from the dog, as it so often has: carnivore versus omnivore, type 2 versus type 1 diabetes mellitus, cholangitis versus hepatic parenchymal disease, and so forth. It was actually a decade earlier that Center[5] adeptly summarized the peculiarities of the feline hepatobiliary system and highlighted distinct disease differences between cats and dogs.

Cholangitis and cholangiohepatitis are more common in the cat than the dog. The anatomic difference in the biliary duct/pancreatic duct anatomy has long been considered an important predisposing factor in this species difference.

Clinical Sciences Department, Colorado State University Veterinary Teaching Hospital, 300 West Drake Road, Fort Collins, CO 80523, USA
E-mail address: cbwebb@colostate.edu

Vet Clin Small Anim 50 (2020) 1123–1134
https://doi.org/10.1016/j.cvsm.2020.06.007
0195-5616/20/© 2020 Elsevier Inc. All rights reserved.

vetsmall.theclinics.com

This same year, Weiss and colleagues[6] recognized the common occurrence of cholangitis, pancreatitis, and inflammatory bowel disease as comorbidities, a phenomenon that would soon be termed feline triaditis (discussed elsewhere in this issue).

Cats do not present to veterinarians for liver disease, they present for vague, variable, nonspecific signs of illness. Clinical signs that have appeared in publications and proceedings as being consistent with feline liver disease are shown in **Table 1**.

Physical examination may be equally nonspecific, although hepatomegaly, ascites, and jaundice might prompt the clinician to bypass several differentials and quickly hone in on the hepatobiliary system. With the presence of jaundice (a yellow cat) the urge to focus first and foremost on the liver is particularly strong, but that is a mistake. Differentials for the hyperbilirubinemia in a cat include prehepatic, hepatic, and posthepatic causes (**Table 2**).

Following assessment of the signalment, history, and physical examination, the diagnostic work-up of a jaundiced cat starts with a minimum database: complete blood count, chemistry panel, and urinalysis. Not surprisingly, these laboratory results may still be equivocal, or consistent with a variety of conditions other than primary liver disease. The diagnostic work-up for the effective and efficient identification of prehepatic and posthepatic causes of hyperbilirubinemia is beyond the scope of this article but includes critical steps before narrowing the search and excluding those important differentials. The column of prehepatic causes of hyperbilirubinemia is extensive and varied, including infectious agents; infiltrative and inflammatory conditions; drugs, toxins, and adverse reactions; and inherited defects (see **Table 2**). Common causes of posthepatic hyperbilirubinemia are intraluminal and extraluminal masses or inflammatory processes that result in extrahepatic biliary obstruction. Many of these conditions are appreciated as abnormal ultrasonographic images (see **Table 2**).

Regarding hepatic causes of hyperbilirubinemia, cholangitis is reported to be the most common cause of diffuse intrahepatic and extrahepatic cholestasis in cats,[13] and the second most common liver condition (after hepatic lipidosis) that result in an owner bringing a cat to a veterinary clinic. Feline cholangitis (ie, inflammation of the GB and biliary system) is categorized as follows: chronic cholangitis associated with liver flukes (*Platynosomum* spp) (**Box 1**), neutrophilic/suppurative cholangitis (acute and chronic, nonseptic, rarely septic), and lymphocytic cholangitis (generally chronic).

Although there may be subtle differences in the clinical presentation of cats with neutrophilic cholangitis compared with lymphocytic cholangitis, distinguishing between the two is diagnostically challenging (**Table 3**).

Table 1 Clinical signs reported to be consistent with feline liver disease	
Clinical Signs	**Source**
Weight loss, loss of lean muscle mass, unkempt hair coat, weakness	Kerl[7]
Icterus	Twedt[8]
Inappetence, vomiting, malaise, fever, abdominal pain	Cannon[9]
Diarrhea, ascites	Gordon[10]
Ptyalism, constipation, dehydration	Webb,[11] Boland & Beatty[12]
Nausea, PU/PD, acholic feces (research cats)	Otte et al[13]

Abbreviations: PD, polydipsia; PU, polyuria.
Data from Refs.[7–13]

Table 2
Differentials for feline hyperbilirubinemia

Prehepatic	Hepatic	Posthepatic
Primary IMHA	Neutrophilic cholangitis	Choleliths/choledocholithiasis
Mycoplasma hemofelis	Lymphocytic cholangitis	Inspissated bile
Mycoplasma hemominutum	Liver flukes	Biliary foreign body
Mycoplasma turisensis	Neoplasia, infiltrative disease	Biliary mucocele
FeLV/FIV, FIP	Hepatic lipidosis	Common bile duct avulsion
Babesia felis	Hepatic amyloidosis	Helminth parasites
Cytauxzoon felis	Histoplasmosis	Pancreatitis, pancreatic abscess
Dirofilaria	Toxoplasmosis	Neoplasia
Lymphosarcoma or leukemia	FIP	Diaphragmatic hernia
Myeloproliferative disease	Cirrhosis, fibrosis	Congenital
Pancreatitis, abscessation	Drugs, toxins	Cholangitis
Cholangitis	Sepsis, SIRS	Cholecystitis
Pyothorax		Duodenitis
Hypophosphatemia		Gallbladder dysmotility
Vaccine reaction		Liver flukes
Transfusion reaction		
Neonatal isoerythrolysis		
Zinc, toxins		
Methimazole, acetaminophen, other drugs		
Increased osmotic fragility		
Pyruvate kinase deficiency		
Heinz body anemia		

Abbreviations: FeLV, feline leukemia virus; FIP, feline infectious peritonitis; FIV, feline immunodeficiency virus; IMHA, immune-mediated hemolytic anemia; SIRS, systemic inflammatory response syndrome.
Data from Webb CB. How I approach the cat with cholangitis. Vet Focus 2020; 29(3); May 2020 and Webb CB. The yellow cat: Diagnostic & therapeutic strategies. Today's Vet Pract 2016; Sept/Oct:38-49.

Furthermore, a presumptive diagnosis of neutrophilic cholangitis still leaves the etiologic agent, and therefore the most appropriate and effective treatment, in question. Bile has been shown to be the sample of choice for culture in the diagnosis of cholangitis in the cat.[14,15] Hence, the argument for performing cholecystocentesis in cats presenting for clinical signs consistent with a diagnosis of liver disease.

That argument raises a key question: Is ultrasound-guided cholecystocentesis a safe and useful diagnostic test for the diagnosis of cholangitis in cats?

Although the category of chronic cholangitis associated with liver flukes is not featured in this paper, Köster and colleagues[16] used percutaneous ultrasound-guided cholecystocentesis (PUC) to collect bile for the analysis and successful detection of *Platynosomum* spp–induced cholangitis in 27 feral cats. The PUC procedure (**Box 2**) was performed with the cats under short duration anesthesia (ketamine hydrochloride, buprenorphine hydrochloride, and dexmedetomidine hydrochloride given intramuscularly) and were euthanized for postmortem examination immediately after

> **Box 1**
> **Chronic cholangitis associated with liver flukes**
>
> Etiology: *Platynosomum* spp
>   Tropical environment
>   Lethargy, vomiting, anorexia
>   Jaundice
>
> Diagnosis
>   Histopathology: identify organisms
>   Cholecystocentesis: identify eggs
>
> Treatment[14,15]
>   Praziquantel 20 to 30 mg/kg PO every 24 hours
>   3 to 10 days
>   ± express gallbladder
>   ± cannulate common bile duct

the procedure, so post-procedure follow-up is unavailable. Bile was examined micro-scopically for egg quantification. *Escherichia coli* was cultured from the bile of 6 of 13 cats where PUC was performed. Ultrasound of the GB was reported as normal in 12 cats, whereas wall thickness was increased (>2 mm) in seven cats. Common bile duct abnormalities, including diameter, echogenicity, and tortuosity, was reported in 12, 13, and 16 cats, respectively. PUC was performed successfully in 100% of attempts (in two cats it was deemed too difficult to attempt), yielding a mean of 3 mL of bile, although the GB was rarely seen as empty at the conclusion of the procedure.[16] No complications (ie, bleeding from the liver, bile leakage, free peritoneal fluid accumula-tion) were reported in any of the 27 cats where PUC was performed.[16] Although this publication suggests that PUC can be safely performed and provide an informative sample, the study population consisted of feral cats from a geographic area endemic for *Playtnosomum* spp. The prevalence of the specific agent being investigated would be expected to be extremely high, which would certainly impact the positive predictive value of the diagnostic effort. Hence, the question as to the safety and usefulness of PUC as a diagnostic tool in cats presenting for clinical signs consistent with cholangi-tis, where liver flukes are not an issue, remains unresolved.

The remainder of the discussion draws heavily from the references in **Table 4**. These papers came from a PubMed search using the phrases "cholecystocentesis AND fe-line," "percutaneous ultrasound guided cholecystocentesis AND feline," and "cholan-gitis AND feline," and an examination of the references cited within the PubMed publications identified by that search.

SAFETY OF PERCUTANEOUS ULTRASOUND-GUIDED CHOLECYSTOCENTESIS

In all of these studies it seems that the PUC procedure was performed on cats that were either heavily sedated or under anesthesia.

It was the Savary-Bataille and colleagues[17] study of PUC in healthy cats that set the foundation for future diagnostic efforts using this technique (see **Box 2**). PUC was per-formed using a 22-gauge 1.5-inch needle attached to 12-mL syringe, retrieving approximately 2 mL of bile. The authors targeted the GB using a right ventral abdom-inal approach in most cases; in one cat the approach was right-sided transhepatic. It was in this cat that a small amount of abdominal effusion appeared post-procedure, otherwise there was no ultrasound evidence of complications in any of the other 11 cats. During the 2 days after the procedure, four cats demonstrated a decrease in appetite or mild abdominal pain; in no case did this persist.[17]

Table 3
Characterization of neutrophilic and lymphocytic cholangitis in cats

	Neutrophilic (N) Acute and Chronic	Lymphocytic (L)
Signalment	Younger males	Older, chronic, progressive (European breeds)
Clinical signs	Acute, febrile, icteric, lethargic, abdominal pain, ± vomiting or diarrhea	Variable appetite, vomiting, weight loss, icterus, ascites
Serum biochemistry abnormalities	Total bilirubin, ALP, GGT are all variable, ↑ALT (although can be normal)	↑Globulins, total bilirubin, ALT, ALP, GGT are all variable
CBC abnormalities	CBC shows left shift with toxic neutrophils	CBC may be unremarkable or lymphocytosis
Abdominal US changes	Extrahepatic biliary obstruction, lipidosis	Bile duct distention, hepatomegaly, mixed echogenicity
GB US changes	US reveals thickened GB wall	US may reveal GB sludge, thickening, or normal

Abbreviations: Abd, abdominal; ALP, alkaline phosphatase; ALT, alanine aminotransferase; CBC, complete blood count; GGT, γ-glutamyltransferase; US, ultrasound.

In the report of Brain and colleagues[18] PUC was performed in four of six cats presenting for some combination of clinical signs including lethargy, inappetence, fever, jaundice, and cranial abdominal pain. A ventral abdominal approach was chosen, and 1 to 2 mL of bile was aspirated using a 23-gauge hypodermic needle. In one case PUC resulted in GB rupture and bile peritonitis.[18]

The Peters and colleagues[19] publication on the diagnostic utility of cytologic assessment of bile aspirates included 78 cats that underwent cholecystocentesis. This retrospective study included cases where the GB was aspirated by PUC or during

Box 2
Technique for percutaneous ultrasound-guided cholecystocentesis in cats

Adequate sedation

Percutaneous

Ultrasound-guided

22-gauge 1.5-inch needle

Attached to a 12-mL syringe

Right-sided transhepatic approach *OR*

Right ventral abdominal approach

Fundus of the gallbladder

Empty gallbladder contents

Submit sample for cytology

Submit sample for aerobic and anaerobic culture

Data from Savary-Bataille KC, Bunch SE, Spaulding KA, et al. Percutaneous ultrasound-guided cholecystocentesis in healthy cats. J Vet Intern Med 2003; 17:298-303.

Table 4
References used as evidence-based medicine to address the safety of PUC

First Author, Ref #	Citation	# of Cats
Savary-Bataille et al,[17] 2003	PUC in healthy cats	12
Brain et al,[18] 2006	Feline cholecystitis and acute neutrophilic cholangitis: clinical findings, bacterial isolates, and response to treatment in 6 cases	4
Peters et al,[19] 2006	Cytologic findings of 140 bile samples from dogs and cats and associated clinical pathologic data	78
Byfield et al,[20] 2017	Percutaneous cholecystocentesis in cats with suspected hepatobiliary disease	83
Schiborra et al,[21] 2017	PUC: complications and association of ultrasonographic findings with bile culture results	51
Smith et al,[22] 2017	Association between gallbladder ultrasound findings and bacterial culture of bile in 70 cats and 202 dogs	70

Abbreviation: #, number of cats in which PUC was performed.
Data from Refs.[17–22]

either laparoscopy or laparotomy. Only one cat (and 4 of 78 dogs) experienced a complication, namely bile leakage, but that cat's GB was aspirated during laparotomy, not a PUC procedure.[19]

In a large retrospective report by Byfield and colleagues,[20] 83 cats presenting with clinical signs consistent with hepatobiliary disease underwent PUC. The PUC was performed with a 22-gauge needle attached to a 10-mL syringe via an extension set, through the ventral approach or through the ventrolateral portion of the liver. Complications were reported in 14 cases (17%), of which two were procedural (failed first attempt and plugged aspiration needle). In 11 cases there was an accumulation of abdominal fluid post-procedure, and in one case the cat developed a pneumoperitoneum.[20] It is difficult to draw a direct cause-and-effect relationship between PUC and these complications, because many of these cats also underwent additional procedures, usually involving the liver or spleen (ie, aspiration or biopsy). None of the cats experienced GB rupture or bile peritonitis.

Shiborra and colleagues[21] performed a retrospective analysis of complications in 51 cats (and 202 dogs) presented for PUC. Major complications occurred in three cats (8 of 300 total PUC procedures in dogs and cats, some number of which had PUC more than once). Two of these cats suffered cardiorespiratory arrest during anesthesia and one cat developed acute kidney failure and was euthanized shortly after the procedure. An important clinical note is that there were cases where the decision was made not to attempt the PUC procedure. In particular, if the diagnostic work-up or ultrasonography identified certain GB changes (eg, emphysematous cholecystitis) or other concurrent conditions (eg, severe coagulopathies), PUC was not performed, and these cases were therefore not included in this study. The authors suggest that there was no predictable relationship between the severity of GB wall changes and the risk of complications.[21]

USEFULNESS OF PERCUTANEOUS ULTRASOUND-GUIDED CHOLECYSTOCENTESIS FOR BACTERIAL ISOLATION

Table 5 shows the yield of PUC in terms of bacteria identified from cultured samples of collected bile. Although the study was performed in healthy cats, Savary-Bataille and

Table 5
Bacterial isolates identified by PUC

Ref #	Isolate	# of Cats
Brain et al,[18] 2006	Escherichia coli	4
	Streptococcus spp	1
	Clostridium spp	1
	Salmonella enterica serovar Typhimurium	1
Peters et al,[19] 2006	E coli	14
	Enterococcus spp	4
	Clostridium spp	2
	Proteus spp	1
	Peptostreptococcus spp	1
	α-Hemolytic Streptococcus	1
Byfield et al,[20] 2017	E coli	7
	Streptococcus spp	2
	Klebsiella pneumoniae	1
	Pseudomonas aeruginosa	1
	Enterococcus faecalis	1
Shiborra et al,[21] 2017	E coli	65%[a]
	Enterococcus spp	34%
	Clostridium perfringens	8%
	Bacteroides spp	3%
	Actinomyces spp	3%
Smith et al,[22] 2017	E coli	25
	Enterococcus spp	10
	Streptococcus spp	2
	Staphylococcus sp	1
	Clostridium sp	1
	Bacillus sp	1
	Enterobacter cloacae	1

Abbreviation: #, number of cats from Ref in which bile culture produced growth of specified bacterial isolate.
[a] Percent of 64 positive cultures. The paper did not distinguish between cats and dogs.
Data from Refs.[18–22]

colleagues[17] found acellular cytology in 11 of 12 cats and no bacterial culture growth in 12 of 12 cats.

In the Brain and colleagues[18] report, bacterial culture of the bile collected by PUC identified *E coli* as the most common bacterial isolate in these cases. Only cats with antemortem identification of bacteria cultured from bile were included in this paper, so nothing can be said about the likelihood of a positive culture from a population of cats suspected of having bacterial cholangitis. Culture media and conditions were tailored to the cytology and Gram staining of the bile collected by PUC in each individual cat.[18]

Peters and colleagues[19] obtained positive culture results in 21% of the cats sampled, and also identified *E coli* as the most common bacterial isolate followed by a variety of enteric organisms. Inclusion criteria included clinical, biochemical, or ultrasonographic findings suggestive of liver or biliary disease.

Byfield and colleagues[20] selected medical records of cats that underwent PUC, presumably because they were being worked up for suspected hepatobiliary disease. In that study bacteria were identified in 10 of 71 samples (14%) on cytology, all 10 of which then had growth on bacterial culture. Only one cat had cytologic evidence of bacteria but not growth on culture and there was one false-negative bile cytology. Although cytology was predictive of growth, it was not useful in the identification of the organism that was eventually cultured.[20]

In the Shiborra and colleagues[21] study, culturing the bile produced growth of bacteria in 21% of the cases, with *E coli* again being the most prevalent bacteria isolate. In 81% of cases where cytology and bacterial culture results were available, cytology revealed bacteria. These results were not broken down by cats and dogs, and there was no description of what these patients had actually presented for, although PUC was obviously deemed a potentially useful diagnostic endeavor.[21]

The pattern of bacterial growth was similar in the 70 cats described by Smith and colleagues.[22] The inclusion criteria for this retrospective study did not include clinical data, but again, it is presumed that cholecystocentesis was performed as part of the diagnostic work-up of cats whose presentation was consistent with hepatobiliary disease.

THE IMPACT OF ULTRASOUND

Because abdominal ultrasound is required to perform PUC, a question of direct clinical relevance is whether or not the ultrasonographic appearance of the GB or biliary tree helps predict the likelihood of obtaining important information by performing PUC. Unfortunately, there are surprisingly few studies in veterinary medicine that are specifically designed to answer this question.

As early as 1998, Newell and colleagues[23] looked for correlations between ultrasound imaging and liver disease in cats. Cats with hepatic lipidosis were not included in the survey, otherwise the specific hepatic disease was confirmed with histopathology. It was determined that using ultrasonographic findings as part of a classification tree resulted in a sensitivity between 70% and 90% and specificity between 86% and 98% for distinguishing among various feline liver diseases.[23]

Hittmair and colleagues[24] used ultrasound to compare GB wall thickness between healthy cats and cats with postmortem confirmation of GB abnormalities. The study identified a myriad of GB abnormalities in cats with hepatobiliary disease, including: shape, distention, obstruction, wall thickening, tortuosity, polyps, and sludge. It was this study that determined that a GB wall thickness greater than 1 mm is an accurate predictor of significant GB disease in cats.[24]

Center's[25] algorithm for feline cholestatic disease identifies a GB wall greater than 2 mm as abnormal, although the review states that in healthy cats the wall thickness is less than 1 mm. The only observation directed at the predictive value of ultrasound is that "ultrasonographic assessment may fail to detect abnormalities" in cases of feline cholangitis.

Neutrophilic and lymphocytic cholangitis cannot be distinguished by ultrasonography.[26] Both forms of feline cholangitis may include a thickened GB wall or "double" layering, and dilation of the biliary tree. Gaschen[26] also states that "bile duct dilation and gallbladder wall changes may not occur in cats that have neutrophilic cholecystitis."

In the Brian and colleagues[18] study four of four cats in which there was a positive culture result following PUC had GB abnormalities, including: thickened GB wall (1.3–2.6 mm) in all four and tortuous and dilated ducts in three of the four.

Marolf and colleagues[27] specifically set out to answer the question of whether or not it was possible to use ultrasonographic changes to diagnose cholangitis in cats and distinguish between the neutrophilic and lymphocytic forms. The study evaluated a large number of parameters (discussed previously) including a GB wall thickness greater than 1 mm. Histopathology was used to determine the final diagnosis. Most of these cats had normal sonographic findings, and there were no parameters that could be used to distinguish between the two forms of cholangitis. For those cats with cholangitis that did have sonographic changes, the most common were an enlarged, hyperechoic liver; dilated common bile ducts; and echogenic GB contents. The authors also emphasize the potential importance of ultrasonographic changes in the pancreas of these cats, seemingly found more frequently in cats with neutrophilic cholangitis.[27]

Byfield and coworkers[20] reported that 71% of the cats investigated for suspected cholangitis had GB or biliary tract abnormalities, including: sediment, distention or dilation, choleliths, thickening, or a hyperechogenic wall.

Shiborra and colleagues[21] found that the GB was considered ultrasonographically abnormal in 52% of the cats and dogs presented for PUC, and, when evaluated for predicting a positive bile culture, ultrasound had a sensitivity, specificity, and accuracy of 82%, 55.7%, and 61.5%, respectively. Maximum GB wall thickness, irregular GB wall thickness, irregular GB luminal surface, hyperechoic GB wall, and GB contents all demonstrated some association with a positive culture on univariable analysis, with only maximum wall thickness and an irregular luminal surface remaining significantly associated on multivariable analysis.[21]

The association between ultrasound findings and bacterial culture results was addressed specifically by Smith and colleagues.[22] An abnormal GB was found by ultrasound (eg, wall thickening or sludge) in 66% of the cases and had a 96% sensitivity and 49% specificity with positive and negative culture results from bile obtained by PUC, laparotomy, or laparoscopy. Cats that had one or more abnormal GB ultrasound findings were 21-times more likely to have bacterial growth on cultured bile. Perhaps the most important finding was that the negative predictive value of ultrasound was 96%; if a cat had a normal GB on ultrasound it was highly unlikely that culturing bile would yield bacterial growth.

Griffin[28] provides a superb review of the ultrasonography of the feline biliary tree, including description and pictures of PUC. The author also observes that the feline liver and biliary tree may be normal in cases of cholangitis.

SUMMARY

Although hepatic lipidosis is considered the most common hepatobiliary disease in cats, it develops secondary to some other underlying condition in up to 95% of cases.[29] Cholangitis is the next most prevalent feline hepatobiliary disorder, and although it may present concurrently with other conditions (ie, inflammatory bowel disease, pancreatitis), its cause is a specific etiologic agent targeting the feline biliary system (ie, flukes, bacteria, deleterious immune-mediated process). If the cause can be identified, then it can be targeted with appropriate and specific treatments (ie, antiparasiticides, antibiotics, immunomodulators). With the World Small Animal Veterinary Association recognition of neutrophilic (acute and chronic) and lymphocytic cholangitis being the categories of most interest, and the demonstration that bile is the sample of choice for culture-positive growth of a causative infectious agent, PUC became a potentially critical, even standard, diagnostic procedure in the work-up of these cases. This review provides an evidence-based assessment of the safety and usefulness of PUC in the diagnosis of cholangitis in cats.

The Veterinarian's Oath states, "at first do no harm." The literature shows that PUC is performed safely, with few reported complications. In fact, it seems likely that the complications that are reported may be the result of other interventions and procedures that were performed on the same patient at the same time. This also seems to be the case for some post-procedure interventions that were not discussed in this review, such as blood transfusions or the administration of plasma. It is critical to remember that all of the literature that was reviewed was based on client-owned cats brought for veterinary care. It seems reasonable to presume that one reason for the low complication rate was the preprocedure clinical acumen that led to a decision as to whether or not any specific patient was a good candidate for PUC. Unfortunately, that number, and the clinical process leading up to the "no go" decision, is rarely reported, despite the impact it could have on future case selection.

That these studies were looking at client-owned cats also impacts the answer to the second part of the question, namely, how useful is the PUC procedure in the diagnosis of cholangitis. The positive predictive value of a diagnostic test is a function of the prevalence of the disease in the population being tested. Most of the studies reviewed clearly stated that PUC was being performed in cat for whom cholangitis was determined to be a top differential based on the clinical assessment of the cat. Within that population, PUC provided a sample of bile that produced bacterial growth in approximately 20% of the cases presented for culture. This is an approximation, because in some studies the inclusion criterium was just that, a positive culture result from bile.[18] Not surprisingly, every study reviewed found E coli to be the most prevalent bacteria cultured from bile, alone or in combination, in those cases that produced a positive culture. The other organisms cultured to a lesser degree were enteric bacteria, organisms likely to be found within the feline gastrointestinal tract. This is consistent with the theory that bacterial cholangitis is caused by gastrointestinal bacteria that manage to migrate through the duodenal papilla and up the biliary tree. It is, however, equally plausible that commensal or pathogenic bacteria from the gut have translocated across the intestinal barrier and their appearance in the bile of the GB is caused by hematogenous spread. Identification of the most common bacteria responsible for neutrophilic cholangitis in cats is impactful because it gives practitioners a "best-guess" target for therapy when, for whatever reason, they are not able to use the PUC procedure as part of their diagnostic work-up.

The impact of ultrasound in the diagnostic work-up of cases of suspected feline cholangitis awaits further directed examination. What can or does ultrasound do in the evaluation of these cases beyond providing the vehicle for the PUC procedure? Although the prevailing opinion is that ultrasound cannot distinguish between lymphocytic and neutrophilic cholangitis in cats, the Shiborra and colleagues[21] study suggested that maximal GB wall thickness and irregularity might be predictive of a positive culture result. Smith and colleagues[22] provided the most direct and quantitative answer, with the most powerful result being the negative predictive value of a normal GB on ultrasound; in those cases it was highly unlikely that PUC would provide a sample that produced a positive bacterial culture result. Contrary to these finding, several reviews conclude that feline cholangitis (not divided into neutrophilic or lymphocytic) may occur, even frequently, in the absence of notable changes on abdominal ultrasound.

Many aspects of feline cholangitis and cholecystocentesis were not covered in this review. Not only can PUC help identify the organisms involved in bacterial cholangitis, but protozoal infections, such as toxoplasmosis, coccidiosis, and hepatozoonosis, have been diagnosed through inspection of bile obtained with PUC. One article on the importance of bile cytology was presented, but much remains to be learned from that modality.[19] Treatment of feline cholangitis is beyond the scope of this article but is best based on the results of PUC sample evaluation. Molecular techniques, such as fluorescent in situ hybridization, DNA extraction, and polymerase chain reaction tests of clonality, are applied to samples from the biliary system to better define and differentiate between disease entities. There were a significant number of feline hepatobiliary cases that did not produce bacterial growth from the culture of bile. In what category do those cats belong?

When performed carefully following thoughtful case selection, the evidence supports the use of PUC as a safe way to obtain samples of bile for cytology and culture, results that may impact the diagnosis and treatment recommendations in this patient population.

DISCLOSURE

The authors have nothing to disclose.

REFERENCES

1. Cullen JM. Summary of the World Small Animal Veterinary Association standardization committee guide to classification of liver disease in dogs and cats. Vet Clin North Am Small Anim Pract 2009;39:395–418.

2. Charles JA. Histologic classification of cholangitis in cats. In: Neiger R, Rutgers HC, editors, Proceedings of the 12th ECVIM-CA/ESVIM Congress 2003. Utrecht (The Netherlands): The European Society of Veterinary Internal Medicine, pp.113–6. Available at: https://beta.vin.com/members/cms/project/defaultadv1.aspx?pid=0&id=3845772. Accessed July 3, 2020.

3. Van den Ingh T. Morphologic classification of biliary disorders of the canine and feline liver. In: Proceedings of the American College of Veterinary Internal Medicine 21st Congress. Charlotte, NC, p. 763. Available at: https://beta.vin.com/members/cms/project/defaultadv1.aspx?id=3847596&pid=8874&.   Accessed July 3, 2020.

4. Rothuizen J. Infectious agents in feline cholangiohepatitis. In: Neiger R, Rutgers HC (eds), Proceedings of the 12th ECVIM-CA/ESVIM Congress 2003. Utrecht, The Netherlands: The European Society of Veterinary Internal Medicine, p.39. Available   at: https://beta.vin.com/members/cms/project/defaultadv1.aspx?pid=0&id=3845771. Accessed July 3, 2020.

5. Center SA. Diseases of the gallbladder and biliary tree. In: Guilford, Center, Strombeck, Williams, Meyer, editors. Strombeck's small animal gastroenterology. 3rd. Philadelphia: W.B. Saunders Co, Center SA. Diseases of the Gallbladder and Biliary Tree; 1996. p. 860–88. Chapter 37.

6. Weiss DJ, Gagne JM, Armstrong PJ. Relationship between inflammatory hepatic disease and inflammatory bowel disease, pancreatitis, and nephritis in cats. J Am Vet Med Assoc 1996;209:1114–6.

7. Kerl ME. Feline liver disease: it's not all lipidosis. Int Vet Emerg Crit Care Symposium 2018. Available at: https://beta.vin.com/members/cms/project/defaultadv1.aspx?id=8688827&pid=22106&. Accessed July 3, 2020.

8. Twedt DC. Update on feline liver disease. Atlantic Coast Vet Conf 2017. Available at: https://beta.vin.com/members/cms/project/defaultadv1.aspx?id=8207615&pid=19448&. Accessed July 3, 2020.

9. Cannon M. Unravelling the causes of inflammatory liver disease in cats. Int Soc Feline Med Asia Pacific Cong 2014. Available at: https://beta.vin.com/members/cms/project/defaultadv1.aspx?id=6717837&pid=11538&.   Accessed July 3, 2020.

10. Gordon J. Not another yellow cat: inflammatory liver disease in the cat. Wild West Vet Conf 2009. Available at: https://beta.vin.com/members/cms/project/defaultadv1.aspx?id=5672089&pid=8870&. Accessed July 3, 2020.

11. Webb CB. Hepatic lipidosis: clinical review drawn from collective effort. J Feline Med Surg 2018;20:217–27.

12. Boland L, Beatty J. Feline cholangitis. Vet Clin North Am Small Anim Pract 2017; 47:703–24.

13. Otte CM, Penning LC, Rothuizen J. Feline biliary tree and gallbladder disease: aetiology, diagnosis and treatment. J Feline Med Surg 2017;19:514–28.

14. Wagner KA, Hartmann FA, Trepanier LA. Bacterial culture results from liver, gallbladder, or bile in 248 dogs and cats evaluated for hepatobiliary disease: 1998-2003. J Vet Intern Med 2007;21:417424.

15. Morgan M, Rankin S, Berent A, et al. Prospective evaluation for bacterial infection in hepatic tissue and bile of cats with diffuse hepatobiliary disease. J Vet Intern Med 2008;22:806.

16. Köster L, Shell L, Illanes O, et al. Percutaneous ultrasound-guided cholecystocentesis and bile analysis for the detection of *Platynosomum* spp.-induced cholangitis in cats. J Vet Intern Med 2016;30:787–93.

17. Savary-Bataille KC, Bunch SE, Spaulding KA, et al. Percutaneous ultrasoundguided cholecystocentesis in healthy cats. J Vet Intern Med 2003;17:298–303.

18. Brain PH, Barrs VR, Martin P, et al. Feline cholecystitis and acute neutrophilic cholangitis: clinical findings, bacterial isolates and response to treatment in six cases. J Feline Med Surg 2006;8:91–103.

19. Peters LM, Glanemann B, Garden OA, et al. Cytological findings of 140 bile samples from dogs and cats and associated clinical pathological data. J Vet Intern Med 2006;30:123–31.

20. Byfield VL, Clark JEC, Turek B, et al. Percutaneous cholecystocentesis in cats with suspected hepatobiliary disease. J Feline Med Surg 2017;19:1254–60.

21. Shiborra F, McConnell JF, Maddox TW. Percutaneous ultrasound-guided cholecystocentesis: complications and association of ultrasonographic findings with bile culture results. J Small Anim Pract 2017;58:389–94.

22. Smith RP, Gookin JL, Smolski W, et al. Association between gallbladder ultrasound findings and bacterial culture of bile in 70 cats and 202 dogs. J Vet Intern Med 2017;31:1451–8.

23. Newell SM, Selcer BA, Girard E, et al. Correlations between ultra-sonographic findings and specific hepatic diseases in cats: 72 cases (1985–1997). J Am Vet Med Assoc 1998;213(1):94–8.

24. Hittmair KM, Vielgrader HD, Loupal G. Ultrasonographic evaluation of gallbladder wall thickness in cats. Vet Radiol Ultrasound 2001;42:149–55.

25. Center SA. Diseases of the gallbladder and biliary tree. Vet Clin North Am Small Anim Pract 2009;39:543–98.

26. Gaschen L. Update on hepatobiliary imaging. Vet Clin North Am Small Anim Pract 2009;39:439–67.

27. Marolf AJ, Leach L, Gibbons DS, et al. Ultrasonographic findings of feline cholangitis. J Am Anim Hosp Assoc 2012;48:36–42.

28. Griffin S. Feline abdominal ultrasonography: what's normal? what's abnormal? The biliary tree. J Feline Med Surg 2019;21:429–41.

29. Valtolina C, Favier RP. Feline hepatic lipidosis. Vet Clin North Am Small Anim Pract 2017;47:68–702.

Triaditis: Truth and Consequences

Jonathan A. Lidbury, BVMS, MRCVS, PhD[a],
Shankumar Mooyottu, DVM, PhD[b], Albert E. Jergens, DVM, PhD[c],*

KEYWORDS

- Pancreatitis • Cholangitis • Inflammatory bowel disease • Cat • Histopathologic
- Prognosis

KEY POINTS

- Clinical findings with triaditis as well as the individual disease components overlap and may include hyporexia, weight loss, lethargy, vomiting, diarrhea, dehydration, icterus, abdominal pain, thickened bowel loops, pyrexia, dyspnea, and shock.
- A definitive diagnosis of triaditis requires histologic confirmation of inflammation in each organ, but this may not be possible because of financial or patient-related constraints.
- Evidence-based data indicate that histologic lesions of triaditis are present in 30% to 50% of cats diagnosed with pancreatitis and cholangitis/inflammatory liver disease.
- How inflammation in 1 organ contributes to inflammation in other gastrointestinal organs is not fully known but likely involves either a bacterial- or an immune-mediated process.
- Treatment of triaditis is based on the overall health status of the patient and the type and severity of disease in component organs.

INTRODUCTION

"*Triaditis*" is a term applied to feline inflammatory gastrointestinal (GI) disease describing concurrent inflammation of the small intestines, pancreas, and hepatobiliary system.[1,2] Anecdotally, multiorgan GI inflammation in cats would appear to be a clinically prevalent disorder that complicates treatment strategies and impacts outcome for affected cats versus cats having single-organ inflammation alone. However, there is a paucity of evidence-based data on the etiopathogenesis, diagnosis, and treatment of triaditis in cats. This article provides a thorough overview of the putative causes of simultaneous multiorgan inflammatory disease in cats as well as how to diagnose and treat these disorders, and whether inflammation in multiple organs affects long-term outcome.

[a] Department of Small Animal Clinical Sciences, College of Veterinary Medicine & Biomedical Sciences, Texas A&M University, 4474 TAMU, College Station, Texas 77843, USA; [b] Department of Veterinary Pathology, College of Veterinary Medicine, Iowa State University, 2716 Vet Med, 1800 Christensen Drive, Ames, IA 50011, USA; [c] Department of Veterinary Clinical Sciences, College of Veterinary Medicine, Iowa State University, L2565 Lloyd, 1809 South Riverside Drive, Ames, IA 50011, USA
* Corresponding author.
E-mail address: ajergens@iastate.edu

Vet Clin Small Anim 50 (2020) 1135–1156
https://doi.org/10.1016/j.cvsm.2020.06.008
0195-5616/20/© 2020 Elsevier Inc. All rights reserved.

TRIADITIS: PAST AND CURRENT PERSPECTIVE

A definitive diagnosis of triaditis requires histologic confirmation of inflammation in each organ.[3] However, triaditis, or inflammation of more than 1 GI organ, is often clinically suspected in cats based on salient clinical, laboratory, imaging, and fine needle aspiration (FNA) findings. Kelly and colleagues[4] were the first to report an association between cholecystitis, cholangitis, and pancreatitis in a cat with intermittent vomiting and weight loss, closely followed by a series of reports in the mid-1990s from different investigative groups evaluating multiorgan inflammation in cats (**Table 1**).[2,5–12] Collectively, these data report histologic lesions of triaditis in 30% to 50% of cats diagnosed with pancreatitis and cholangitis/inflammatory liver disease (ILD). Caution is advised when drawing conclusions about specific multiorgan inflammatory conditions from these earlier reports for several reasons (**Box 1**). In a recent prospective study, inflammatory bowel disease (IBD) with cholangitis was noted to occur in 6 of 27 (22%) cats with GI signs, IBD with pancreatitis in 2 of 27 (7%), and triaditis in 8 of 27 (30%), suggesting that triaditis or inflammation of two-thirds of these organs is relatively common. However, some combination of histopathological changes of 2 or more of these organs was also found in 20 of 39 (51%) asymptomatic cats undergoing ovariohysterectomy, although interestingly none of the cats in this group had histologic inflammation in 3 or more organs.[12] This finding may truly reflect subclinical disease or be due to the inability to histologically appreciate the spectrum of normal morphology for the small intestine, liver, and pancreas.

DOES INFLAMMATION IN ONE COMPONENT ORGAN CONTRIBUTE TO TRIADITIS?
Pancreatitis

Even with comprehensive diagnostic evaluation, the cause for acute and chronic pancreatitis in most cats remains unknown (**Box 2**). Following a triggering event, pancreatic enzymes are activated within the pancreatic parenchyma, and cytokines and other inflammatory mediators are released causing cell injury resulting in both pancreatitis and systemic effects.[13,14] The spectrum of acute inflammation varies from acute necrotizing pancreatitis with necrosis predominating (>50% of pathologic condition) compared with suppurative pancreatitis with neutrophilic inflammation accounting for greater than 50% of pathologic condition.[7] Acute pancreatic necrosis is more common than suppurative inflammation and is a well-recognized GI disorder causing significant morbidity and mortality in cats.[7,10] However, because pancreatic biopsy is seldom performed in the acute setting, these histologic distinctions are rarely made antemortem.

Acute pancreatitis may progress to chronic pancreatitis characterized by lymphocytic inflammation, variable fibrosis, and acinar atrophy, potentially resulting in exocrine pancreatic insufficiency. Bacterial infection and biliary tract obstruction may exacerbate pancreatic injury. Fluorescence in situ hybridization (FISH) has revealed the presence of bacteria in pancreata of 13 of 46 cats with pancreatitis.[3] Bacterial colonization was more frequent in cats having moderate to severe pancreatitis (13/46) versus cats with mild pancreatitis (2/15) with bacteria visualized in diverse tissues, including connective/periductal regions (n = 9), within glandular parenchyma (n = 6), saponified fat (n = 5), ducts (n = 3), and in areas of necrosis (n = 3). Obstruction of the pancreatic and/or bile duct may also cause intrahepatic cholestasis and impaired clearance of bacteria that translocate across the inflamed intestines. It remains unclear whether enteric bacteria are a primary cause or a secondary consequence on pancreatitis and whether this may vary between individual cats.

Table 1

Evidence-based literature describing multi-organ (pancreas, liver and/or intestines) histopathologic inflammation

Study	Study Design	# Cats	Pancreatitis	ILD	IBD	Triaditis
Kelly et al	Necropsy	1	1	1		ND
Weiss et al	Retrospective, necropsy	18	9/18 (50%)	18/18 (100%)	15/18 (83%)	7/18 (39%) CIN 6/33
Callahan et al	Retrospective, necropsy	44	22/34 (65%)	44/44 (100%) CNC - 33/44 ANC - 7/44	17/37 (46%)	10/31 (32%) CIN 30/37 HL 14/44
Ferreri et al	Retrospective, necropsy	63	ANP - 30/63 CP - 33/63			ND
Hill and Van Winkle	Retrospective, necropsy	40	ANP - 32/40 ASP - 8/40	5/40 (12%)	13/40 (32%) IC	ND CIN 14/40 HL 19/40
Twedt et al	Retrospective, biopsy - 27, necropsy - 12	39	15/23 CP - 12/15	39/39 (100%) NC - 12/39 LC - 7/39 RH - 12/39	11/24 LPE - 8/11 LSA - 5/24	7/14 (50%)
Brain et al	Prospective, biopsy - 3	6	2/6	NC - 3/6 CC - 3/6	LSA - 1/6	ND
Marolf et al	Prospective, biopsy	10	8/10 (80%) CP - 6/8	9/10 (90%) Cholangitis		ND
Swift et al	Prospective, biopsy, necropsy	28	18/28 (64%)	15/18 (83%) HL, CH	11/18 (61%)	10/28 (36%)

(continued on next page)

Table 1 (continued)						
Study	Study Design	# Cats	Pancreatitis	ILD	IBD	Triaditis
Forman et al	Prospective, biopsy, necropsy	21	18/21 (86%) M - 5/18 M-S - 13/18	11/18 (61%) Cholangitis HL - 3/18	10/18 (56%) LSA - 3/18	ND
Fragkou et al	Prospective, biopsy	47[a]	1/47 (2%)	6/47 (13%)	13/47 (28%)	8/27 (30%)

Abbreviations: ANC, acute neutrophilic cholangitis; ANP, acute necrotizing pancreatitis; ASP, acute suppurative pancreatitis; CC, cholecystitis; CIN, chronic interstitial nephritis; CNC, chronic neutrophilic cholangitis; CP, chronic pancreatitis; HL, hepatic lipidosis; IC, intestinal changes; LC, lymphocytic cholangitis; LSA, lymphosarcoma; M, mild; M-S, moderate-severe; NC, neutrophilic cholangitis; ND, not determined; RH, reactive hepatopathy.

[a] Includes cats with (n = 27) and without (n = 20) chronic GI signs.

Box 1

Reasons for caution when estimating the prevalence of triaditis from the available evidence

- Early studies were retrospective and necropsy based.

- Most publications focused on subsets of cats having different GI diseases rather than triaditis.

- Early studies used less sophisticated diagnostic indices for diagnosing tissue inflammation.
  - Even with standardized templates for histopathological evaluation of the GI tract, agreement between pathologists is suboptimal.

- Most studies failed to confirm active inflammation of all 3 organs.

- In necropsy studies, severe inflammatory disorders, such as neutrophilic cholangitis and suppurative pancreatitis, may be overrepresented compared with less severe disease.

- Direct comparison between studies is difficult due to differences in study design.

Data from Refs.[5,7,19,29,39,58]

Inflammatory Liver Disease

Feline ILD is a group of acquired disorders that are centered on the biliary tract (cholangitis) with secondary involvement of the hepatic parenchyma (cholangiohepatitis).[8,15–17] Morphologically, this group of heterogeneous inflammatory hepatic disorders has arbitrarily been classified as being suppurative or nonsuppurative based on the predominant inflammatory cell type (neutrophils, lymphocytes, and/or plasma cells), and by the extent of bile duct hyperplasia and fibrosis.[18] A refined

---

Box 2

Proposed causes of feline acute or chronic pancreatitis

- Pancreatic ischemia
  - Hypotension
  - Cardiac disease

- Concurrent biliary or GI tract disease

- Pancreatic ductal obstruction
  - Neoplasia, choleliths, flukes

- Infectious agents
  - *Toxoplasma gondi*
  - Enteric bacteria
  - Feline herpes virus
  - Feline infectious peritonitis virus
  - Virulent feline calicivirus infection

- Liver or pancreatic flukes
  - *Platynosomum fastosum*
  - *Eurytrema procyonis*

- Trauma

- Metabolic
  - Lipodystrophy
  - Hypercalcemia

- Immune-mediated disease

- Organophosphate intoxication (experimental)

Data from Refs.[2,3,6,8,20,21,24,28,42].

histopathological classification scheme by the World Small Animal Veterinary Association has now divided cholangitis into 4 major types: neutrophilic cholangitis, lymphocytic cholangitis, chronic cholangitis caused by liver fluke infestation, and destructive cholangitis.[19] To the authors' knowledge, destructive cholangitis has been described in dogs but not cats and therefore will not be discussed further. Similarly, chronic cholangitis caused by liver fluke infestation will not be discussed. Infectious causes (ie, toxoplasmosis, feline infectious peritonitis [FIP]) for inflammatory hepatobiliary disease remain much less common (~15% prevalence for ILD) but are important differential diagnoses for ILD.

There is no clear understanding of the steps leading to ILD and its different phenotypes (including neutrophilic and lymphocytic cholangitis), but it is generally accepted that infectious agents (eg, enteric bacteria) and immune mechanisms contribute to inflammatory lesions.[19–21]

Bacteria are frequently cultured from the bile and/or liver of cats with neutrophilic cholangitis, with isolation of a single bacterial species in 80% of cats; these cats often respond well to appropriate antimicrobial therapy.[2,8,22–25] Thus, there is compelling evidence that bacteria are the primary etiologic agent in this form of feline ILD. The bacteria isolated are often those expected to be present in the intestinal tract, with Escherichia coli being the most frequently isolated species followed by Enterococcus spp, Bacteroides spp, Clostridium spp, and Streptococcus spp.[2,8,22–25] Some controversy exists as to the most likely mechanism by which these organism reach the liver. In about 80% of cats, the common bile duct and pancreatic duct both enter the duodenum together at the major duodenal papilla. It has long been suspected that this "common channel" creates a route via which bacteria can ascend from the duodenum into the liver (and pancreas).[3,22] However, more recent work suggests that bacterial translocation across the intestinal wall and hematogenous spread via the portal circulation are more likely routes for hepatic colonization.[2] The role of Helicobacter spp in causing neutrophilic cholangitis (and pancreatitis) in cats is questionable. Although Helicobacter spp DNA has been found in the liver and bile of cats with ILD, it has also been found in the livers of cats with non-ILD, and the livers of healthy cats.[2,21,26]

Lymphocytic cholangitis is thought to occur because of loss of immune tolerance resulting in an adaptive immune response targeting the bile ducts and is typically treated with immunomodulatory agents, such as prednisolone.[3,22,27] Interestingly, an association between ILD, pancreatitis, and nephritis has been found in cats, suggesting a possible common immune-mediated cause.[1] It is possible that bacteria also play a role in the development of this form of feline ILD. Transient bacterial infection of the liver (or another organ) could lead to an aberrant host immune response that persists once infection has cleared.[22] Using molecular techniques, such as FISH or polymerase chain reaction (PCR), a variety of bacteria, including E coli, Enterococcus spp, Helicobacter spp, Micrococcus spp, and Streptococcus spp, have been found in the livers of cats with lymphocytic cholangitis. However, it is hard to determine if these organisms are the primary cause of this disease or a secondary consequence because they can occur in mixed microbe populations as well as in liver tissue of healthy control cats.[2,20,28] In 1 recent study, the presence and distribution of bacteria within the livers of 39 cats with ILD (both neutrophilic and lymphocytic cholangitis) and 19 control cats with histologically normal livers were evaluated with eubacterial FISH.[2] Although bacteria were observed in 21 of 39 ILD and 3 of 19 control hepatic sections, the prevalence of intrahepatic bacteria was higher in ILD (13/31; 41%) versus control (1/17; 6%) tissues. Moreover, bacteria in cats with ILD were primarily localized to portal vessels, venous sinusoids, and parenchyma (12/13) than bile ducts (1/13). The spatial distribution of bacteria in liver tissue of cats with ILD supports the hypothesis that colonization likely occurs by enteric translocation or by hematogenous means rather than ascending infection of the bile duct. Concurrent pancreatic and intestinal disease was frequent in all 13 cats with intrahepatic bacteria, suggesting a possible link between hepatic bacterial colonization and GI or pancreatic diseases that reduce intestinal barrier function and promote hematogenous seeding of the liver with enteric bacteria.

It is also possible that the bile ducts are injured because of loss of immune tolerance to components of the GI microbiota or dietary constituents in cats with IBD. Possible mechanisms are discussed later.

Inflammatory Bowel Disease

IBD denotes 1 form of chronic enteropathy characterized by persistent or intermittent GI signs associated with histologic inflammation of the GI tract.[29,30] Current hypotheses support the notion that feline IBD results from interactions between host genetics, intestinal environment (gut microbiome, dietary constituents), and mucosal immunity.[29,31] It is noteworthy that cats with IBD show an expanded and intensified expression of major histocompatibility complex class II, which may contribute to antigen presentation and aberrant host responses.[32] What the triggers are that drive chronic intestinal inflammation and the variable phenotypic expression and individual response to treatment remain unknown. As observed in humans[33,34] and dogs with IBD,[35–37] shifts in gut bacterial populations (ie, reduced overall microbial diversity with decreased beneficial species but increased harmful species, including the Enterobacteriaceae) are found in cats with active disease. Mucosal bacteria have been linked to both clinical signs and histopathologic lesions in cats with IBD. Using FISH, increased total numbers of Enterobacteriaceae correlated to chronic duodenal histopathologic lesions (ie, villus atrophy, fusion), number of GI signs, and upregulated proinflammatory cytokine messenger RNA expression (ie, interleukin-1 [IL-1], -8, and -12) in cats with IBD as compared with healthy cats. It is possible that these shifts occur as a consequence of a primary insult rather than being the inciting cause of IBD. Growing evidence also supports the importance of diet in the development of feline IBD. In 1 study investigating 55 cats with variable signs of chronic enteropathy, 49% responded to dietary modification using an elimination diet alone.[38] Upon challenge with the original diet, signs recurred in 16 of 55 (29%) of these cats but not in the remaining 11 of 55 (20%) responders.

Histologically, IBD in cats is characterized by variable degrees of cellular infiltration (most commonly lymphocytic-plasmacytic enteritis) and architectural alterations causing mucosal disruption and increased intestinal permeability.[29,30,39,40] Because cats have high numbers of bacteria in their proximal small intestines, translocation of enteric bacteria can occur across the inflamed intestines into the portal circulation potentially seeding the liver and/or pancreas. Alternatively, reflux of enteric contents into the pancreaticobiliary duct causing ascending infection in the liver and pancreas could occur.[41] Duodenal reflux may occur in response to an increase in duodenal pressure during vomiting associated with IBD.

Interplay of Pancreatitis, Inflammatory Liver Disease, and Inflammatory Bowel Disease

How inflammation in 1 organ contributes to inflammation in other GI organs is not fully known. Different scenarios are proposed with current hypotheses supporting either a bacterial- or an immune-mediated pathogenesis.

The first model proposed by Simpson[3] (**Fig. 1**A) relates to the development of acute (suppurative) pancreatitis and neutrophilic cholangitis. One variant of this is that the

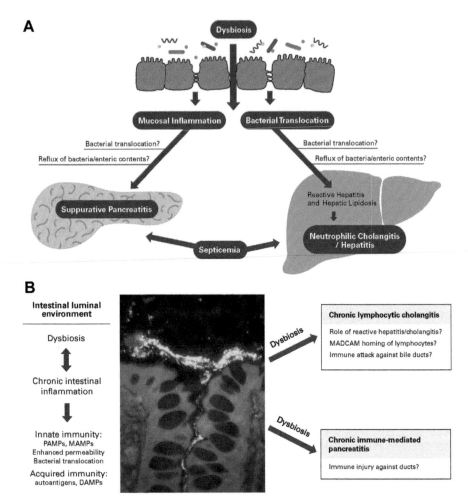

Fig. 1. (A) Proposed pathogenesis for triaditis emphasizing the roles of dysbiosis, enteric inflammation (IBD), bacterial translocation, and secondary seeding of the liver and pancreas causing neutrophilic cholangitis and acute pancreatitis, respectively. (B) Proposed pathogenesis for triaditis emphasizing the roles of dysbiosis, chronic intestinal inflammation, and autoimmunity as stimuli for chronic lymphocytic cholangitis and chronic immune-mediated pancreatitis. DAMPs, damage-associated molecular patterns; MAdCAM, mucosal addressin cell adhesion molecule-1; MAMPs, microbe-associated molecular patterns; PAMPs, pathogen-associated molecular patterns. (*Modified from* Ref.[3])

inciting event is intestinal disease that results in enteritis and dysbiosis with enteric translocation of bacteria across the inflamed intestinal mucosa. Translocation of bacteria could cause septicemia, resulting in hematogenous infection of the liver and/or the pancreas. An alternative model suggests that the inciting event is acute pancreatitis that secondarily leads to acute enteritis and/or neutrophilic cholangitis, possibly because of the proximity of these 3 organs. In this scenario, enteritis favors secondary dysbiosis with potential sequelae of bacterial translocation, septicemia, and microbial seeding of the liver and/or pancreas. In an experimental model of induced feline acute pancreatitis, seeding of the pancreas with enterically translocated *E coli* has been shown to occur supporting the hypothesis that acute pancreatitis could be the initial event in the pathogenesis of triaditis.[42–44]

The other proposed mechanism (**Fig. 1**B) hinges on chronic intestinal inflammation and the development of secondary immune mechanisms as a cause for triaditis.[3] Genetic and environmental factors are suggested to play a role in decreasing immune tolerance to components of the GI microbiota and/or diet, resulting in chronic IBD. In this scenario, dysbiosis, increased intestinal permeability, low-grade bacterial translocation, and activation of innate and/or adaptive immunity contribute to immune-mediated injury to the liver and pancreas. Chronic intestinal disease is often associated with nonspecific reactive hepatitis in dogs and cats.[45] Moreover, loss of immune tolerance in the intestines could secondarily affect the liver and pancreas causing lymphocytic cholangitis and/or chronic pancreatitis, respectively. In humans, autoimmune pancreatitis[46] and primary sclerosing cholangitis (PSC)[47] may occur in association with IBD. In PSC, 1 mechanism for targeting of bile ducts is "gut lymphocyte homing" of activated T cells generated in the intestine. Homing is mediated by mucosal addressin-cell adhesion molecule I and chemokine (C-C motif) ligand 25, which are normally expressed in the intestine but can also be aberrantly expressed by the liver in this disease.[3,48,49] In addition, in PSC, cholangiocytes can produce inflammatory cytokines in response to pathogen-associated molecular patterns and other stimuli.[50] Another potential mechanism is that in response to gut-derived microbial molecules from the portal circulation, cholangiocytes become senescent and secrete inflammatory cytokines and other molecules.[48] It is likely that the GI tract and the liver also communicate via bile acids and the host-microbiota metabolome.[47] In humans, autoimmune pancreatitis can be part of a multisystemic condition that often occurs in association with IBD and/or PSC.[46,51] A variety of autoantibodies, including those against carbonic anhydrase type II and pancreatic secretory trypsin inhibitors, have been identified in people with autoimmune pancreatitis. It has been proposed that molecular mimicry between microbial and host proteins could lead to autoimmunity.[52] For example, significant homology between human carbonic anhydrase-II and α-carbonic anhydrase of *Helicobacter pylori* has been shown. Therefore, in a genetically susceptible person it is possible the *H pylori* infection could lead to autoimmune pancreatitis.[53] It is possible that similar mechanisms could lead to loss of immune tolerance and the development of triaditis in cats.

It is important to note that because triaditis is a syndrome with variation in the combinations of organs affected, the type, severity, and duration of clinical signs, and the type of inflammatory infiltrates present, different mechanisms may be at play in individual cats. It is also clear that there is still much unknown about the pathogenesis of this syndrome.

HOW TO DIAGNOSE TRIADITIS
General Diagnostic Overview

Definitive diagnosis of triaditis requires integration of the patient's history, clinical examination, results of laboratory testing, diagnostic imaging findings, and tissue biopsies confirming histologic inflammation (**Table 2**). Sometimes because of financial or patient-related constraints, a presumptive diagnosis is made based on the patient's history, clinical examination, results of laboratory testing, diagnostic imaging findings, and cytologic evaluation of the liver/pancreas. However, this approach hinders the clinician's ability to make an accurate diagnosis. Ultrasound-guided FNA of hepatic parenchyma and bile may be useful for confirming active bacterial infection causing ILD[8,25] (see Craig B. Webb's article, "Evidence-Based Medicine: Ultrasound-guided

Table 2
Diagnostic testing options for triaditis

Diagnostic Test	Pancreatitis	ILD	IBD
Clinical signs	Decreased appetite, lethargy, vomiting, weight loss, diarrhea	Decreased appetite, lethargy, vomiting, weight loss, icterus	Decreased appetite, lethargy, vomiting, weight loss, diarrhea
Physical examination	Abdominal pain, mass or effusion	Icterus, hepatomegaly, ± fever	Thickened bowel loops, mesenteric lymphadenopathy
Laboratory tests			
CBC	Neutrophilia, neutropenia, thrombocytopenia	Anemia, leukocytosis, neutrophilia ± left shift	Anemia, neutrophilia
Biochemistry	Low calcium and albumin	Increased ALT, AST, ALP, total bilirubin, globulins[5,8,71]	Low phosphorous ± low albumin[40]
Specialized serology/biomarkers	Elevated feline pancreatic lipase immunoreactivity, fPL[6,11,67]	Bile acid test	Low cobalamin ± low folate[29,74]
Diagnostic imaging			
Radiographs	Loss of serosal detail, abdominal effusion	± Mild hepatomegaly, choleliths	Fluid-distended bowel loops
Ultrasound	Increased pancreatic size, hypoechoic parenchyma, hyperechoic mesenteric fat, abdominal effusion,[9,13]	Hepatomegaly, hyperechoic liver, enlarged common bile duct, choleliths, gall bladder wall abnormalities[5,9,71]	Thickened intestinal wall, ± normal wall layering, muscularis thickening, mesenteric lymphadenopathy[29]
US interventions	FNA of pancreas for cytology and culture	FNA of liver ± gall bladder for cytology and culture, needle (Tru-Cut) biopsy[8,25]	Possible FNA of mesenteric lymph nodes
Tissue diagnosis	Biopsy by laparoscopy, laparotomy	Biopsy by US guidance (needle), laparoscopy, laparotomy	Biopsy by GI endoscopy, laparotomy

Data from Refs.[5,6,8,9,11,13,25,29,40,67,71,74]

Percutaneous Cholecystocentesis in the Cat," in this issue). The presence of neutrophils or lymphocytes on cytologic evaluation of hepatic aspirates is suggestive of neutrophilic or lymphocytic cholangitis (or small cell lymphoma), respectively. However, hepatic FNA cytology has significant diagnostic limitations, and results should be cautiously interpreted.[54] Tissue biopsy by GI endoscopy, laparoscopy, or exploratory laparotomy with histopathology confirms inflammation in the liver, pancreas, and/or intestines.

Histopathologic Features of Tissue Inflammation

Histopathologic evaluation of liver, intestine, and pancreas is required for a definitive diagnosis of triaditis in cats. However, many veterinary pathologists do not recognize this as a distinct disease complex in cats.

Chronic interstitial pancreatitis is the most common histologic type seen in cats with triaditis (**Fig. 2**).[3,12] A multifocal distribution, with interlobular, intralobular, or dissecting fibrosis, is a prominent feature of chronic pancreatitis. The interstitium is infiltrated with lymphocytes, plasma cells, and occasionally, macrophages.[55] When a neutrophilic component is seen, it is described as chronic *active* pancreatitis, and cholangitis and/or IBD are commonly present.[12] Additional features of chronic pancreatitis include cystic dilatation of acini, ductal ectasia, ductal epithelial hyperplasia, and acinar atrophy in severely fibrosed areas.[55]

Histologically, hepatic inflammation in cats with triaditis can be broadly divided into neutrophilic cholangitis and lymphocytic cholangitis.[5,12]

- In the acute form of neutrophilic cholangitis, the portal region is generally edematous and populated with neutrophils. Inflammatory cells often infiltrate the bile ducts and transmigrate through the degenerating or viable biliary epithelium to the ductular lumen. Based on the severity and disease progression, the inflammatory infiltrate may cross the limiting plate and cause hepatocellular necrosis in the periportal regions (cholangiohepatitis).

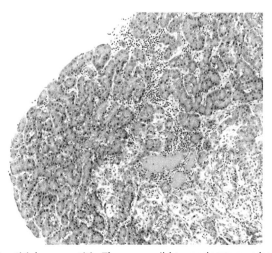

Fig. 2. Chronic interstitial pancreatitis. There are mild to moderate numbers of lymphocytes expanding the interstitium between pancreatic exocrine acini and between pancreatic lobules. There is a modest degree of fibrosis expanding the pancreatic interstitium. Hematoxylin-eosin [HE] stained sections, original magnification ×200.

- In chronic neutrophilic cholangitis, the inflammatory infiltrate is mixed with lymphocytes and plasma cells, and the portal region is expanded with biliary hyperplasia and portal to bridging fibrosis (**Fig. 3**).
- Lymphocytic cholangitis is characterized by infiltration of lymphocytes in the portal region accompanied with bile duct proliferation, bile duct epithelial degeneration, bile duct loss (ductopenia), and periportal to bridging fibrosis.[5,15,20,22] Occasionally, lipogranulomas may be present in the portal regions that are helpful in differentiating lymphocytic cholangitis from hepatic lymphomas.[20] Other features of lymphocytic cholangitis that can help differentiate it from small cell lymphoma include bile duct targeting, ductopenia, peribiliary fibrosis, and portal B-cell aggregates.[20]

Because IBD is a diagnosis of exclusion, the histologic changes indicative of this condition are interpreted cautiously and in a contextual manner.[39,56,57] Despite the standardization attempts made to characterize the GI inflammation, inconsistencies associated with interobserver variability and specimen quality are of real concern.[58] In some cases, differentiating between IBD and feline small intestinal lymphoma can be challenging and may require specialized testing (eg, immunophenotyping or clonality testing with PCR for antigen receptor rearrangement [PARR]).[59] It should be noted that there is evidence that clonality testing with PARR has a low diagnostic specificity for feline intestinal small cell alimentary lymphoma, so results must be interpreted in conjunction with histologic findings and immunophenotyping results.[60,61] Histologically, the extent of mucosal architectural changes, and to a lesser degree, the type and degree of inflammatory infiltration are used to assess intestinal inflammation. An increased number of inflammatory cells (lymphocytes, plasma cells, and/or eosinophils) are observed in the lamina propria depending on the subtype, with lymphocytic-plasmacytic enteritis being the most common form of IBD in cats (**Fig. 4**).[30,39] In addition, an increased number of intraepithelial lymphocytes is seen

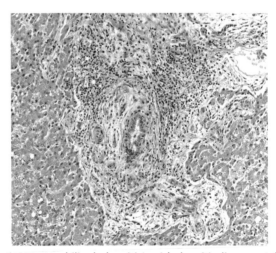

Fig. 3. Chronic-active neutrophilic cholangitis/pericholangitis: liver, portal region. The portal area is expanded by edema, by peribiliary fibrosis, and by moderate numbers of lymphocytes admixed with fewer plasma cells and neutrophils. Multifocally, biliary epithelium is infiltrated by a few neutrophils. There are multiple cross-sectional profiles of bile ducts (biliary reduplication/hyperplasia). HE stained sections, original magnification ×200.

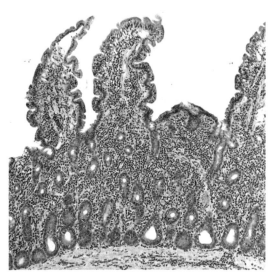

Fig. 4. Chronic lymphocytic enteritis (IBD): small intestine, jejunum. Villi within the section are stumpy and thicker than normal with more than 4 layers (up to 10–12 layers) of lympho-cytes expanding the lamina propria. There is a diffuse infiltrate of lymphocytes and plasma cells in all layers of the mucosa with subjectively increased numbers of intraepithelial lym-phocytes. There are scattered neutrophils admixed with the mononuclear infiltrate. HE stained sections, original magnification ×100 magnification.

in the intestinal mucosa. Architectural changes generally noticed in the intestine (eg, duodenum) include villous blunting, villous epithelial erosion, crypt ectasia, lacteal dilation, and periglandular fibrosis.[39] Architectural changes in the intestinal mucosa are considered a more reliable criterion that correlates best with disease severity.[39,62] In 1 study, the histologic lesions of IBD in cats with triaditis were found to be more se-vere compared with cats with IBD alone.[12]

TREATMENT STRATEGIES FOR TRIADITIS
General Considerations

Treatment of triaditis is based on the overall health status of the patient and the type and severity of disease in component organs. Global treatment recommendations are found in **Table 3**. Because histopathologic confirmation of multiorgan inflammation is often unavailable, therapy is often directed to the organ thought to be primarily responsible for the clinical signs. When using this approach, the clinician should avoid or use care when prescribing treatments that could adversely affect another compo-nent or possible component of the cat's disease. For example, in a cat with histolog-ically confirmed IBD that has suspected but not histologically confirmed ILD, empiric antibiotic therapy is often initiated before starting corticosteroids in case neutrophilic cholangitis with an active bacterial infection is present. Integrating clinical findings, laboratory testing, diagnostic imaging, and targeted FNA or biopsy results (if possible) serve to prioritize treatment decisions. Immediate supportive care is required in cats with persistent vomiting, abdominal pain, icterus, prolonged anorexia, severe hypovo-lemia, hypotension, signs of sepsis, and/or pyrexia. These general nonspecific treat-ments include hospitalization with intravenous (IV) fluid therapy for rehydration and electrolyte correction, analgesics for abdominal discomfort, and antiemetics to control

Table 3
Treatment of pancreatitis, inflammatory liver disease, and inflammatory bowel disease

Treatment	Pancreatitis[3,67]	ILD[3,24,69-72]	IBD[29,38,40,57,63,74]
Fluid therapy	Parenteral crystalloids Colloid fluids Plasma?	Parenteral crystalloids	Uncommon
Analgesia	*Buprenorphine*: 0.02 mg/kg IV, IM q6h *Fentanyl*: transdermal patch 25 μg/h as required	Uncommon	Uncommon
Antibiotics	For confirmed bacterial infection, sepsis, severe neutrophilia ± left shift or suspicion of bacterial translocation; target *E coli* and other enteric bacteria: *Enrofloxacin*: 2.5 mg/kg SC or PO q12h *Ticarcillin-clavulanate*: 40 mg/kg IV q6h	For confirmed bacterial infection (liver ± bile) seen with neutrophilic cholangitis; suspicion of bacterial translocation; targets *E coli* and other enteric bacteria: *Enrofloxacin* *Amoxicillin-clavulanate* *Ticarcillin-clavulanate*	For neutrophilic inflammation or abundant mucosal bacteria (FISH)
Antiemetics	*Maropitant*: 1 mg/kg SC q24h *Ondansetron*: 0.5–1.0 mg/kg PO q24h Combination therapy has additive effects	*Maropitant* *Ondansetron*	*Maropitant* *Ondansetron*
Immunosuppressive drugs	*Prednisolone* for chronic pancreatitis: 1–2 mg/kg PO q24h	Lymphocytic cholangitis: *Prednisolone*: 1–2 mg/kg PO q12h	LPE: *Prednisolone* *Chlorambucil* for severe IBD or LSA: 2 mg/cat PO 2–3 times/wk
Nutrition	Naso-esophageal tube Esophagostomy tube *Mirtazapine*: 2 mg PO q24 h	Naso-esophageal tube Esophagostomy tube *Mirtazapine*	Hydrolyzed/restricted antigen diet Soluble fiber for colitis *Mirtazapine*

Vitamins	Cobalamin if deficient	Vitamin K_1 for coagulopathy: 0.5–1.5 mg/kg SQ q12 h for 3 doses +/– cobalamin if deficient Vitamin E?	Cobalamin: 250 µg SC weekly x 6 wk +/– folate if deficient
Nutraceuticals	Uncommon	SAMe: 20 mg/kg PO q24 h Ursodiol: 10–15 mg/kg PO q24 h with food	Probiotics/prebiotics? n-3 fatty acids?
Surgery	Biopsy (rarely performed) EHBO ± biliary stent or cholecystoduodenostomy	Biopsy with culture of liver ± bile	Full-thickness biopsy uncommon except to rule out LSA GI endoscopy (always obtain ileal biopsies)
Co-morbidities	ILD, IBD and/or diabetes mellitus EPI with severe disease	IBD and/or pancreatitis	ILD and/or pancreatitis

Abbreviations: EHBO, extrahepatic biliary obstruction; IM, intramuscularly; LC, lymphocytic cholangitis; LPE, lymphocytic-plasmacytic enteritis; LSA, low-grade alimentary lymphoma; NC, neutrophilic cholangitis; SC, subcutaneously.
Data from Refs.[3,24,29,38,40,57,63,69–72,74,78]

vomiting. Cats with hypocobalaminemia can be supplemented by parenteral means, although recent work suggests that daily oral administration is also effective.[63] Nutrition is provided in persistently anorexic cats by use of nasoesophageal, esophageal, or gastric feeding tubes.[64–66]

Treatment of Pancreatitis

Treatment of pancreatitis is mainly symptomatic and supportive. IV fluid therapy, analgesics, antiemetics, and enteral nutrition are the cornerstones of therapy. Fluid therapy corrects the circulating fluid volume, restores and maintains microcirculation of the pancreas (important because pancreatic ischemia can contribute to the development of necrotizing pancreatitis), and restores and maintains plasma oncotic pressure, especially if used with a synthetic colloid. Antiemetics (eg, maropitant and ondansetron) control vomiting and continued fluid and electrolyte loss. The combination of maropitant and ondansetron provides an effective control of vomiting and nausea in those patients who fail to respond to single antiemetic treatment alone. Analgesics, including buprenorphine or fentanyl, are typically used for control of abdominal pain during hospitalization. Transdermal fentanyl patches are very effective at maintaining analgesia for longer periods of time (approximately 72 hours); however, it may take up to 12 hours for therapeutic fentanyl concentrations to be achieved.[3] The optimal diet to feed cats with pancreatitis is unknown; however, there is no evidence that dietary fat restriction results in improved outcome. The authors often feed these cats a highly digestible, moderate fat diet designed for intestinal disease, or possibly, if concurrent IBD is present, an elimination diet. Some cats require placement of a feeding tube to provide appropriate enteral nutrition. Antimicrobial therapy is reserved for severe cases, such as those presenting with shock, fever, marked leukocytosis, or suspected/confirmed sepsis.[67] The considerations for selection of antimicrobials are similar to those later discussed for neutrophilic cholangitis. Use of corticosteroids for acute pancreatitis is not recommended. For some cats with chronic pancreatitis, however, especially if neutrophilic cholangitis has been ruled out, treatment with anti-inflammatory doses of prednisolone seems to be beneficial. Whether this is owing to a reduction in pancreatic inflammation or treatment of concurrent IBD is uncertain.

The presence of comorbidities is common but only confirmed if biopsy of the pancreas, liver, and small intestines are evaluated and cultures of the pancreas and liver are performed. Although pancreatic biopsy remains the gold standard for diagnosing pancreatitis, the patchy distribution of histopathologic lesions limits routine performance of this procedure by clinicians, especially in the acute setting.[68] Persistent biliary obstruction secondary to pancreatitis is another potential indication for surgery when biliary stenting or cholecystojejunostomy is required. General anesthesia allows for placement of an enteral feeding tube into the esophagus or stomach for nutritional support.

Treatment of Inflammatory Liver Disease

Vitamin K_1 is typically given to icteric cats before hepatic FNA, cholecystocentesis, or hepatic biopsy. Antibiotics and supportive care are the primary treatments for neutrophilic cholangitis. Antibiotics are ideally chosen based on bacterial culture and susceptibility testing. They should be active against gram-positive and gram-negative aerobic and anaerobic bacteria (especially *E coli* and *Enterococcus* spp because these are isolated most often).[24,69] Bactericidal antibiotics that are active in bile and can be administered IV are most suitable. Empirical first-choice options (these are often given pending culture and susceptibility testing results) include a fluoroquinolone, potentiated penicillin, a fluoroquinolone combined with a potentiated penicillin or clindamycin, or ticarcillin-clavulanate; however, antimicrobial resistance is frequent with Enterobacteriaceae, including *E coli*.[24] Antibiotic therapy is typically continued for 4 to 6 weeks.[8] Other supportive measures are similar for cats with acute pancreatitis and include IV fluid therapy and analgesics for control of abdominal pain. Feline ILD is associated with oxidative stress and depletion of hepatic glutathione.[70] Therefore, there is justification for administering oral antioxidants (ie, S-adenosylmethionine [SAMe], silybin, or vitamin E). There is also rationale for giving cats with cholestasis the synthetic bile acid and choleretic agent, ursodeoxycholic acid (UCDA). Although there are few to no data documenting improved outcomes when these cytoprotective drugs are given, their use is unlikely to be detrimental to the patient. However, it is important to prioritize medications that treat the underlying disease and essential supportive care over them and to be cognizant that giving multiple oral medications places a burden on the cat and its guardian.

The primary treatment of culture-negative lymphocytic cholangitis involves immunosuppressive drug treatment with prednisolone for induction of remission and then tapering over 6 to 8 week to the lowest effective dose. Supportive care, such as feeding tubes, IV fluid therapy, antiemetics, and therapeutic abdominocentesis, may also be indicated.[71] One study showed that cats treated with prednisolone therapy had prolonged survival[27] and greater improvement in histopathologic inflammation compared with cats treated with UCDA, but no difference in hepatic fibrosis was found.[72] Chlorambucil is sometimes used for refractory cases or to reduce the corticosteroid dose needed to maintain remission.[3] Again, there is a rationale to administer antioxidant agents, but no improvement in clinical outcome has been documented with their use. Cats with complete biliary obstruction and some cats with choleliths will require surgery.

Treatment of Inflammatory Bowel Disease

Sequential therapy using specially formulated diets, antimicrobials, and immunosuppressive drugs is the most common strategy used to achieve clinical remission in cats with chronic enteropathies (including IBD), with a final diagnosis made following histopathologic evaluation of intestinal biopsy samples.[73] The type of cellular infiltrate (lymphocytic-plasmacytic, eosinophilic, neutrophilic, or granulomatous) and severity of mucosal epithelial/architectural alterations (erosion/ulceration, villus atrophy/fusion, fibrosis) serve to guide treatment decisions. There is strong evidence from clinical trials to support a recommendation to feed elimination diets to cats with mild IBD.[38,40] Clinical signs in food-responsive cats may resolve quickly within 3 to 5 days on an elimination diet. It is not possible to ascertain which form of diet (eg, antigen-restricted or hydrolyzed) is most effective in modulating GI signs in cats. Cats with more severe mucosal inflammation that fail to achieve remission to diet alone may respond to a combination of diet plus prednisolone.[29,56] Vitamin B_{12} deficiencies are common in cats with chronic GI disease and require parenteral or oral supplementation.[63,74]

Cats failing prednisolone therapy should be investigated further (eg, through immunophenotyping and possibly clonality testing with PARR) to rule out misdiagnosis and the possibility of small cell alimentary lymphoma. Cats with small cell alimentary lymphoma usually respond well to combination therapy with prednisolone and chlorambucil and supplementation with vitamins B12 and folate.[75,76] Cats with neutrophilic or granulomatous infiltrates on intestinal biopsy should be screened for infectious agents (eg, bacterial, viral [FIP, feline leukemia virus, feline immunodeficiency virus], fungal) before initiating immunosuppressive therapy.

Box 3
Risk factors associated with negative outcomes in triaditis or component organ inflammation

- Acute pancreatitis: plasma ionized hypocalcemia; ionized hypocalcemia, lethargy, pleural effusion, hypoglycemia, azotemia, parenteral nutrition administration, and persistent anorexia[67]
- Chronic pancreatitis: development of diabetes mellitus and EPI[3]
- Lymphocytic cholangitis: presence of concurrent illness[71]
- IBD: severe histologic inflammation seen with triaditis?[12]; failed response to dietary trials + prednisolone[76]

Abbreviation: EPI, exocrine pancreatic insufficiency.

Data from Refs.[3,12,67,71,76]

PROGNOSIS FOR CATS WITH TRIADITIS

There is a paucity of information defining prognosis for cats with triaditis. Overall, the prognosis of each patient will depend on the severity of their disease and extent of systemic involvement. For example, cats with severe acute pancreatitis or neutrophilic cholangitis, especially with systemic signs (shock, septicemia, systemic hypotension, disseminated intravascular coagulation), will require aggressive medical therapy to survive the initial period of hospitalization. On the other hand, cats diagnosed with mild to moderate lymphocytic-plasmacytic IBD, accompanied by increased serum pancreas-specific lipase concentrations, typically respond well to treatment of IBD with a hydrolyzed diet and prednisolone.[40,77] Several risk factors linked to prognosis have been identified for cats with triaditis or its inflammatory components (**Box 3**). A compilation of additional evidence-based data, ideally based on clinical trials, will improve the understanding of the complex interactions among inflammation in the pancreas, liver, and/or intestines.

ACKNOWLEDGMENTS

The authors gratefully acknowledge Dr Kenny Simpson, Cornell University for his insight into manuscript preparation and Dr Tyler A. Harm, Iowa State University for histopathologic images.

DISCLOSURE

The authors have no disclosures to report nor was funding required for production of this article.

REFERENCES

1. Weiss DJ, Gagne JM, Armstrong PJ. Relationship between inflammatory hepatic disease and inflammatory bowel disease, pancreatitis, and nephritis in cats. J Am Vet Med Assoc 1996;209:1114–6.
2. Twedt DC, Cullen J, McCord K, et al. Evaluation of fluorescence in situ hybridization for the detection of bacteria in feline inflammatory liver disease. J Feline Med Surg 2014;16:109–17.
3. Simpson KW. Pancreatitis and triaditis in cats: causes and treatment. J Small Anim Pract 2015;56:40–9.

4. Kelly DF, Baggott DG, Gaskell CJ. Jaundice in the cat associated with inflammation of the biliary tract and pancreas. J Small Anim Pract 1975;16:163–72.

5. Callahan Clark JE, Haddad JL, Brown DC, et al. Feline cholangitis: a necropsy study of 44 cats (1986-2008). J Feline Med Surg 2011;13:570–6.

6. Ferreri JA, Hardam E, Kimmel SE, et al. Clinical differentiation of acute necrotizing from chronic nonsuppurative pancreatitis in cats: 63 cases (1996-2001). J Am Vet Med Assoc 2003;223:469–74.

7. Hill RC, Van Winkle TJ. Acute necrotizing pancreatitis and acute suppurative pancreatitis in the cat. A retrospective study of 40 cases (1976-1989). J Vet Intern Med 1993;7:25–33.

8. Brain PH, Barrs VR, Martin P, et al. Feline cholecystitis and acute neutrophilic cholangitis: clinical findings, bacterial isolates and response to treatment in six cases. J Feline Med Surg 2006;8:91–103.

9. Marolf AJ, Kraft SL, Dunphy TR, et al. Magnetic resonance (MR) imaging and MR cholangiopancreatography findings in cats with cholangitis and pancreatitis. J Feline Med Surg 2013;15:285–94.

10. Swift NC, Marks SL, MacLachlan NJ, et al. Evaluation of serum feline trypsin-like immunoreactivity for the diagnosis of pancreatitis in cats. J Am Vet Med Assoc 2000;217:37–42.

11. Forman MA, Marks SL, De Cock HE, et al. Evaluation of serum feline pancreatic lipase immunoreactivity and helical computed tomography versus conventional testing for the diagnosis of feline pancreatitis. J Vet Intern Med 2004;18:807–15.

12. Fragkou FC, Adamama-Moraitou KK, Poutahidis T, et al. Prevalence and clinico-pathological features of triaditis in a prospective case series of symptomatic and asymptomatic cats. J Vet Intern Med 2016;30:1031–45.

13. Simpson KW. Feline pancreatitis. J Feline Med Surg 2002;4:183–4.

14. Rinderknecht H. Activation of pancreatic zymogens. Normal activation, premature intrapancreatic activation, protective mechanisms against inappropriate activation. Dig Dis Sci 1986;31:314–21.

15. Gagne JM, Weiss DJ, Armstrong PJ. Histopathologic evaluation of feline inflammatory liver disease. Vet Pathol 1996;33:521–6.

16. Weiss DJ, Armstrong PJ, Gagne J. Inflammatory liver disease. Semin Vet Med Surg (Small Anim) 1997;12:22–7.

17. Sergeeff JS, Armstrong PJ, Bunch SE. Hepatic abscesses in cats: 14 cases (1985-2002). J Vet Intern Med 2004;18:295–300.

18. Day DG. Feline cholangiohepatitis complex. Vet Clin North Am Small Anim Pract 1995;25:375–85.

19. van den Ingh TSGAM, Cullen JM, Twedt DC, et al. Morphological classification of biliary disorders of the canine and feline liver. In: Rothuizen J, Bunch SE, Charles JA, et al, editors. WSAVA standards for clinical and histological diagnosis of canine and feline liver diseases. Edinburgh (Scotland): W.B. Saunders; 2006. p. 61–76.

20. Warren A, Center S, McDonough S, et al. Histopathologic features, immunophenotyping, clonality, and eubacterial fluorescence in situ hybridization in cats with lymphocytic cholangitis/cholangiohepatitis. Vet Pathol 2011;48:627–41.

21. Greiter-Wilke A, Scanziani E, Soldati S, et al. Association of Helicobacter with cholangiohepatitis in cats. J Vet Intern Med 2006;20:822–7.

22. Boland L, Beatty J, Cholangitis Feline. Vet Clin North Am Small Anim Pract 2017; 47:703–24.

23. Peters LM, Glanemann B, Garden OA, et al. Cytological findings of 140 bile samples from dogs and cats and associated clinical pathological data. J Vet Intern Med 2016;30:123–31.

24. Wagner KA, Hartmann FA, Trepanier LA. Bacterial culture results from liver, gallbladder, or bile in 248 dogs and cats evaluated for hepatobiliary disease: 1998-2003. J Vet Intern Med 2007;21:417–24.

25. Byfield VL, Callahan Clark JE, Turek BJ, et al. Percutaneous cholecystocentesis in cats with suspected hepatobiliary disease. J Feline Med Surg 2017;19:1254–60.

26. Sjodin S, Trowald-Wigh G, Fredriksson M. Identification of Helicobacter DNA in feline pancreas, liver, stomach, and duodenum: comparison between findings in fresh and formalin-fixed paraffin-embedded tissue samples. Res Vet Sci 2011;91:e28–30.

27. Otte CM, Penning LC, Rothuizen J, et al. Retrospective comparison of prednisolone and ursodeoxycholic acid for the treatment of feline lymphocytic cholangitis. Vet J 2013;195:205–9.

28. Otte CM, Gutierrez OP, Favier RP, et al. Detection of bacterial DNA in bile of cats with lymphocytic cholangitis. Vet Microbiol 2012;156:217–21.

29. Simpson KW, Jergens AE. Pitfalls and progress in the diagnosis and management of canine inflammatory bowel disease. Vet Clin North Am Small Anim Pract 2011;41:381–98.

30. Jergens AE, Moore FM, Haynes JS, et al. Idiopathic inflammatory bowel disease in dogs and cats: 84 cases (1987-1990). J Am Vet Med Assoc 1992;201:1603–8.

31. Allenspach K. Clinical immunology and immunopathology of the canine and feline intestine. Vet Clin North Am Small Anim Pract 2011;41:345–60.

32. Waly NE, Stokes CR, Gruffydd-Jones TJ, et al. Immune cell populations in the duodenal mucosa of cats with inflammatory bowel disease. J Vet Intern Med 2004;18:816–25.

33. Frank DN, St Amand AL, Feldman RA, et al. Molecular-phylogenetic characterization of microbial community imbalances in human inflammatory bowel diseases. Proc Natl Acad Sci U S A 2007;104:13780–5.

34. Sartor RB, Wu GD. Roles for intestinal bacteria, viruses, and fungi in pathogenesis of inflammatory bowel diseases and therapeutic approaches. Gastroenterology 2017;152:327–39.e4.

35. Suchodolski JS, Dowd SE, Wilke V, et al. 16S rRNA gene pyrosequencing reveals bacterial dysbiosis in the duodenum of dogs with idiopathic inflammatory bowel disease. PLoS One 2012;7:e39333.

36. Suchodolski JS, Xenoulis PG, Paddock CG, et al. Molecular analysis of the bacterial microbiota in duodenal biopsies from dogs with idiopathic inflammatory bowel disease. Vet Microbiol 2010;142:394–400.

37. Xenoulis PG, Palculict B, Allenspach K, et al. Molecular-phylogenetic characterization of microbial communities imbalances in the small intestine of dogs with inflammatory bowel disease. FEMS Microbiol Ecol 2008;66:579–89.

38. Guilford WG, Jones BR, Markwell PJ, et al. Food sensitivity in cats with chronic idiopathic gastrointestinal problems. J Vet Intern Med 2001;15:7–13.

39. Day MJ, Bilzer T, Mansell J, et al. Histopathological standards for the diagnosis of gastrointestinal inflammation in endoscopic biopsy samples from the dog and cat: a report from the World Small Animal Veterinary Association Gastrointestinal Standardization Group. J Comp Pathol 2008;138(Suppl 1):S1–43.

40. Jergens AE, Crandell JM, Evans R, et al. A clinical index for disease activity in cats with chronic enteropathy. J Vet Intern Med 2010;24:1027–33.

41. Johnston KL, Swift NC, Forster-van Hijfte M, et al. Comparison of the bacterial flora of the duodenum in healthy cats and cats with signs of gastrointestinal tract disease. J Am Vet Med Assoc 2001;218:48–51.

42. Widdison AL, Alvarez C, Chang YB, et al. Sources of pancreatic pathogens in acute pancreatitis in cats. Pancreas 1994;9:536–41.

43. Widdison AL, Karanjia ND, Reber HA. Antimicrobial treatment of pancreatic infection in cats. Br J Surg 1994;81:886–9.

44. Widdison AL, Karanjia ND, Reber HA. Routes of spread of pathogens into the pancreas in a feline model of acute-pancreatitis. Gut 1994;35:1306–10.

45. Cullen J. Liver and biliary system. In: Maxie G, editor. Jubb, Kennedy & Palmer's pathology of domestic animals. 6th edition. Saunders Elsevier; 2015. p. 258–352.

46. Nagpal SJS, Sharma A, Chari ST. Autoimmune pancreatitis. Am J Gastroenterol 2018;113:1301.

47. Lazaridis KN, LaRusso NF. Primary sclerosing cholangitis. N Engl J Med 2016; 375:1161–70.

48. Gupta A, Bowlus CL. Primary sclerosing cholangitis: etiopathogenesis and clinical management. Front Biosci (Elite Ed) 2012;4:1683–705.

49. Eksteen B, Grant AJ, Miles A, et al. Hepatic endothelial CCL25 mediates the recruitment of CCR9+ gut-homing lymphocytes to the liver in primary sclerosing cholangitis. J Exp Med 2004;200:1511–7.

50. O'Hara SP, Splinter PL, Trussoni CE, et al. Cholangiocyte N-Ras protein mediates lipopolysaccharide-induced interleukin 6 secretion and proliferation. J Biol Chem 2011;286:30352–60.

51. Zhang L, Smyrk TC. Autoimmune pancreatitis and IgG4-related systemic diseases. Int J Clin Exp Pathol 2010;3:491–504.

52. Okazaki K, Uchida K, Sumimoto K, et al. Autoimmune pancreatitis: pathogenesis, latest developments and clinical guidance. Ther Adv Chronic Dis 2014;5:104–11.

53. Guarneri F, Guarneri C, Benvenga S. Helicobacter pylori and autoimmune pancreatitis: role of carbonic anhydrase via molecular mimicry? J Cell Mol Med 2005;9:741–4.

54. Wang KY, Panciera DL, Al-Rukibat RK, et al. Accuracy of ultrasound-guided fine-needle aspiration of the liver and cytologic findings in dogs and cats: 97 cases (1990-2000). J Am Vet Med Assoc 2004;224:75–8.

55. De Cock HE, Forman MA, Farver TB, et al. Prevalence and histopathologic characteristics of pancreatitis in cats. Vet Pathol 2007;44:39–49.

56. Jergens AE. Feline idiopathic inflammatory bowel disease: what we know and what remains to be unraveled. J Feline Med Surg 2012;14:445–58.

57. Willard MD, Moore GE, Denton BD, et al. Effect of tissue processing on assessment of endoscopic intestinal biopsies in dogs and cats. J Vet Intern Med 2010; 24:84–9.

58. Willard MD, Jergens AE, Duncan RB, et al. Interobserver variation among histopathologic evaluations of intestinal tissues from dogs and cats. J Am Vet Med Assoc 2002;220:1177–82.

59. Kiupel M, Smedley RC, Pfent C, et al. Diagnostic algorithm to differentiate lymphoma from inflammation in feline small intestinal biopsy samples. Vet Pathol 2011;48:212–22.

60. Marsilio S, Ackermann MR, Lidbury JA, et al. Results of histopathology, immunohistochemistry, and molecular clonality testing of small intestinal biopsy specimens from clinically healthy client-owned cats. J Vet Intern Med 2019;33:551–8.

61. Marsilio S, Newman SJ, Estep JS, et al. Differentiation of lymphocytic-plasmacytic enteropathy and small cell lymphoma in cats using histology-guided mass spectrometry. J Vet Intern Med 2020;34:669–77.

62. Janeczko S, Atwater D, Bogel E, et al. The relationship of mucosal bacteria to duodenal histopathology, cytokine mRNA, and clinical disease activity in cats with inflammatory bowel disease. Vet Microbiol 2008;128:178–93.

63. Toresson L, Steiner JM, Olmedal G, et al. Oral cobalamin supplementation in cats with hypocobalaminaemia: a retrospective study. J Feline Med Surg 2017;19: 1302–6.

64. Jensen KB, Chan DL. Nutritional management of acute pancreatitis in dogs and cats. J Vet Emerg Crit Care (San Antonio) 2014;24:240–50.

65. Fink L, Jennings M, Reiter AM. Esophagostomy feeding tube placement in the dog and cat. J Vet Dent 2014;31:133–8.

66. Abood SK, Buffington CA. Enteral feeding of dogs and cats: 51 cases (1989-1991). J Am Vet Med Assoc 1992;201:619–22.

67. Nivy R, Kaplanov A, Kuzi S, et al. A retrospective study of 157 hospitalized cats with pancreatitis in a tertiary care center: clinical, imaging and laboratory findings, potential prognostic markers and outcome. J Vet Intern Med 2018;32: 1874–85.

68. Pratschke KM, Ryan J, McAlinden A, et al. Pancreatic surgical biopsy in 24 dogs and 19 cats: postoperative complications and clinical relevance of histological findings. J Small Anim Pract 2015;56:60–6.

69. Policelli Smith R, Gookin JL, Smolski W, et al. Association between gallbladder ultrasound findings and bacterial culture of bile in 70 cats and 202 dogs. J Vet Intern Med 2017;31:1451–8.

70. Center SA, Warner KL, Erb HN. Liver glutathione concentrations in dogs and cats with naturally occurring liver disease. Am J Vet Res 2002;63:1187–97.

71. Gagne JM, Armstrong PJ, Weiss DJ, et al. Clinical features of inflammatory liver disease in cats: 41 cases (1983-1993). J Am Vet Med Assoc 1999;214:513–6.

72. Otte CM, Rothuizen J, Favier RP, et al. A morphological and immunohistochemical study of the effects of prednisolone or ursodeoxycholic acid on liver histology in feline lymphocytic cholangitis. J Feline Med Surg 2014;16:796–804.

73. Makielski K, Cullen J, O'Connor A, et al. Narrative review of therapies for chronic enteropathies in dogs and cats. J Vet Intern Med 2019;33:11–22.

74. Simpson KW, Fyfe J, Cornetta A, et al. Subnormal concentrations of serum cobalamin (vitamin B12) in cats with gastrointestinal disease. J Vet Intern Med 2001;15: 26–32.

75. Richter KP. Feline gastrointestinal lymphoma. Vet Clin North Am Small Anim Pract 2003;33:1083–98, vii.

76. Kiselow MA, Rassnick KM, McDonough SP, et al. Outcome of cats with low-grade lymphocytic lymphoma: 41 cases (1995-2005). J Am Vet Med Assoc 2008;232: 405–10.

77. Bailey S, Benigni L, Eastwood J, et al. Comparisons between cats with normal and increased fPLI concentrations in cats diagnosed with inflammatory bowel disease. J Small Anim Pract 2010;51:484–9.

78. VIN veterinary drug handbook website. Available at: https://www.vin.com/members/cms/project/defaultadv1.aspx?pId=13468. Accessed April 29, 2020.

Neurobehavioral Disorders
The Corticolimbic System in Health and Disease

Clare Rusbridge, BVMS, PhD, DECVN, FRCVS[a,b,*]

KEYWORDS

- Feline orofacial pain • Feline hyperaesthesia • Limbic encephalitis • Mutilation
- Neuropathic pain • Neuropathic itch • Trigeminal neuralgia • Temporal lobe epilepsy

KEY POINTS

- The corticolimbic system (prefrontal cortices, amygdala, and hippocampus) integrates emotion with cognition and produces a behavioral output that is flexible based on the environmental circumstances. It also modulates pain, being implicated in pathophysiology of maladaptive pain.
- Feline orofacial pain syndrome is characterized by oral discomfort and tongue mutilation. Genetic factors, oral pain, anxiety, and social stress influence disease expression.
- The pathognomic sign of feline hyperesthesia syndrome is rippling skin, a reflex cutaneous trunci contraction following noxious irritation, but also seen in emotional states of high arousal. Before diagnosing maladaptive pain, all other explanations must be eliminated.
- Feline limbic encephalitis is characterized by behavioral changes and treatment-resistant focal seizures with orofacial involvement. It is an autoimmune encephalitis resulting in hippocampal neuronal hyperexcitability and impaired synaptic plasticity.

 Video content accompanies this article at http://www.vetsmall.theclinics.com.

INTRODUCTION

The corticolimbic system (**Fig. 1**) integrates emotion with cognition and produces a behavioral output that must be flexible based on the environmental circumstances.[1] The corticolimbic system circuitry of the prefrontal cortex, amygdala, and hippocampus is connected to the hypopituitary-pituitary axis, and environmental circumstances such as stress and anxiety input decision making, emotion regulation, and memory.[1] The corticolimbic system is also the modulator for acute pain, a mediator for chronic

[a] Fitzpatrick Referrals, Godalming, Surrey GU7 2QQ, UK; [b] School of Veterinary Medicine, Faculty of Health & Medical Sciences, University of Surrey, Guildford, Surrey GU2 7AL, UK
* School of Veterinary Medicine, Faculty of Health & Medical Sciences, Vet School Main Building (VSM), University of Surrey, Daphne Jackson Road, Guildford, Surrey GU2 7AL, UK.
E-mail address: C.Rusbridge@surrey.ac.uk
Twitter: @neurovet_clare (C.R.)

Vet Clin Small Anim 50 (2020) 1157–1181
https://doi.org/10.1016/j.cvsm.2020.06.009
vetsmall.theclinics.com
0195-5616/20/Crown Copyright © 2020 Published by Elsevier Inc. All rights reserved.

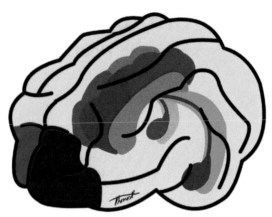

Fig. 1. The corticolimbic system circuitry of the prefrontal cortex, amygdala (*red*), and hippocampus (*orange*). The amygdala and hippocampus lie within the medial temporal lobes and encode and consolidate the emotional memory of events (amygdala), convert short-term to long-term memory and spatial memory (hippocampus), and regulate the fear response by activating the hypothalamic-pituitary-adrenal axis (both). The prefrontal cortex (*purple*) including the cranial cingulate gyrus (*pink*) receives somatosensory, visual, auditory, and emotive inputs and is involved in planning complex cognitive behavior, personality expression, decision making, and moderating social behavior.

pain, and critical for the chronification of pain.[2] There is a high comorbidity of negative affective disorders with chronic pain and vice versa, hypothesized because of similar changes in neuroplasticity and overlapping neurobiological mechanisms.[3] This article discusses 3 feline disorders that affect or are affected by the corticolimbic systems: the maladaptive pain disorder feline orofacial pain syndrome (FOPS) in which disease expression is influenced by environmental stress; feline hyperesthesia syndrome (FHS) in which there is still debate as to whether this is a primary neurobehavioral disorder or a behavioral response to a negative affective state; and limbic encephalitis, an autoimmune encephalitis that results in neurobehavioral signs and seizures. There is a focus on diagnosis and management, which is challenging in all 3 diseases.

FELINE OROFACIAL PAIN SYNDROME

FOPS is a maladaptive pain disorder characterized by episodic behavioral signs, oral discomfort, and tongue mutilation, triggered in many cases by mouth movements. Burmese cats are predisposed, and an inherited disorder affecting processing of nociceptive trigeminal information is suspected. Signs are precipitated by conditions causing oral pain. Anxiety and social stress also influence disease expression. Signs may be poorly responsive to licensed analgesics but managed with adjuvant analgesics. Good dental care and treatment are paramount.

Clinical Signs

FOPS is characterized by signs that suggest oral discomfort, particularly of the tongue. Owners of affected cats describe exaggerated licking and chewing movements, with pawing at the mouth typically to once side only (Video 1). There are 2 presentations: acute-severe and chronic-episodic. The acute disease is characterized by signs of severe and unrelenting discomfort with mutilation of the tongue or buccal mucosa. The tongue can be so badly lacerated that surgical repair may be necessary

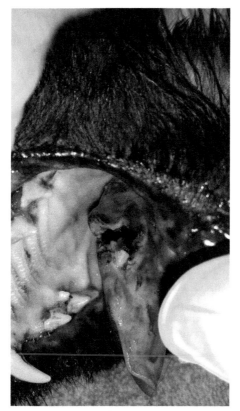

Fig. 2. Tongue laceration and secondary infection in an 11- year-old male Burmese cat with signs of FOPS. (*Courtesy of* P. Andrew, BVSc, MRCVS, Macclesfield, UK.)

(**Fig. 2**). Tongue auto-amputation is even possible. The classic presentation is in young teething kittens. The chronic-episodic form occurs in older cats, that may have had the acute form as kittens. Signs are similar, but in adult cats the pain can be paroxysmal and triggered in many cases by mouth movements such as chewing, drinking, or grooming. Due to the severity of the pain, some cats are anorexic or inappetent.

Pathogenesis

FOPS is seen in a variety of feline populations (including some crossbred cats), although Burmese cats from Europe and Australasia predominate.[4] FOPS is triggered by conditions causing oral pain, but the extent of oral disease may be considered minor and less than what a veterinary surgeon would typically associate with clinical signs.

In young cats, the disease is almost always associated with permanent teeth eruption and is self-limiting, with signs resolving within a few weeks. More rarely signs may be triggered by other oral lesions such as mouth ulceration associated with feline respiratory virus infection.

In adult cats, periodontal disease, especially, upper canine root exposure and tooth resorption (TR) are the more important predisposing cause.

One of the many controversies of FOPS is if the trigger is toothache then why is there mutilation of the tongue? Tongue referred pain (also known as ectopic tongue pain or orofacial dysesthesia) can be associated with tooth pulp inflammation.[5] An inflammatory reaction in the pulp will occur rapidly after exposure of dentin (experimentally, 1–2 weeks in dogs).[6] Dental pulp is densely innervated with fibers that originate from the trigeminal ganglion. Rarely, when injured, neurogenic inflammation and a maladaptive pain syndrome can develop.[7] A neurovascular autonomic phenomenon is also possible via the trigemino-parasympathetic brain stem reflex whereby noxious information from the teeth results in vasodilation in the orofacial area, including the lip, palate, and tongue.[8] This can be inhibited at the level of the brainstem medulla by GABA agonists.[8] Autonomic dysfunction is implicated in migraine and trigeminal neuralgia and pterygopalatine ganglion blockade can be used to manage pain syndromes in humans.[9] FOPS has been compared with various maladaptive pain syndromes in humans, in particular trigeminal neuralgia. These are summarized in **Table 1** and reviewed by Tait and others.[10]

The predominance of affected Burmese cats suggests an inherited predisposition. A genome-wide case-control association study had a suggested association to a genomic region that included the gene low-density lipoprotein receptor-related protein 1 (LRP1).[11] LRP1 is a multifunctional plasma membrane receptor with a myriad of functions. In the central nervous system it influences NMDA receptor functioning, long-term potentiation, and synaptic signaling,[12] and plays a role in neuronal development[13] and may be implicated in development of maladaptive pain states.

Table 1
Maladaptive orofacial pain syndromes in humans

Condition	Notes
Trigeminal neuralgia	Frequent unilateral paroxysmal attacks of pain lasting seconds to minutes described by humans as stabbing, shooting, or electrical lightning and triggered by chewing, light touch, talking, brushing teeth, cold, or occurring spontaneously.
Burning mouth syndrome (glossodynia when confined to tongue)	Burning, stinging, scalding, and numbness of the tongue, lips, and oropharyngeal structures, often in association with taste alterations (dysgeusia) and dry mouth (xerostomia). Pain is typically continuous and bilateral.
Glossopharyngeal neuralgia	Paroxysmal attacks lasting seconds to minutes characterized by stabbing, sharp pain deep in the throat, ear, and pharynx and triggered by swallowing, chewing, talking, coughing, and yawning.
Atypical odontalgia	Continuous or almost continuous tooth pain or pain at the site of a tooth extraction. Initially localized to the tooth region, this is more common in the maxillary molars. It can be triggered by mechanical stimulation or pressure to site of pain and the subject is often hyperalgesic in the facial area near the site of oral discomfort, Important differential for humans with recent endodontic treatment or tooth extraction.

The expression of FOPS is influenced by anxiety and emotional state. A retrospective study found that for 1 in 5 FOPS cases, environmental factors influenced the disease expression.[4] Individuals with poor social coping strategies in multi-cat households appear to be more vulnerable, but other reported events that have triggered FOPS events have included attending cats shows, admission to catteries and veterinary hospitals, home renovations, and death of a primary carer.[4] Maladaptive pain states may be influenced by functional and anatomic differences in corticolimbic circuitry.[3] Structural differences in the hippocampus and medial prefrontal cortex are found in humans suffering from burning mouth syndrome, as well as increased functional connectivity between frontal and limbic regions when the pain intensifies.[14] In humans, the relationship among chronic pain, anxiety, and depression is extremely complex, with extensive overlap making it difficult to determine the cause and effect.[3] A similar mutual maintenance model of negative affective disorders and painful conditions appears to occur in cats, with FOPS and idiopathic cystitis being the classic examples.

Diagnosis

There is no definite diagnostic test for FOPS. Diagnosis is made based on appropriate signalment, elimination of other explanations, and identification of contributory causes (**Box 1**) A diagnosis of FOPS is not appropriate for a cat in discomfort because of dental disease or other oral lesions. Pain associated with dental disease can be under-recognized and undertreated[15] (see Mark Epstein's article, "Feline Neuropathic Pain"; and see Elizabeth Stelow's article, "Behavior as an Illness Indicator," in Part 1). Cats will paw at their mouths, chatter teeth, have bruxism, or be anorexic with dental pain. The quantity of analgesia required for management of dental disease in cats is often underestimated. One study found that cats with severe dental disease required opioids for up to 72 hours after surgery and still had high pain scores 6 days after surgery.[15]

Assessing environmental triggers

Spending time establishing the cat's environment and social interactions, especially with other cats is paramount. Using a questionnaire[16] is a useful means of ensuring the correct information is obtained. Cats have a fundamental need to be in control and to be able to access vital resources freely and immediately without conflict with cats, humans, or other pets.[17] Using modern technology (eg, video) can improve

---

Box 1
Criteria supporting a diagnosis of feline orofacial pain syndrome (FOPS)

- Mutilation of the oral cavity: typically one-sided and directed at the tongue.
- Apparent discomfort/behavior of the cat is disproportion to the associated trigger (eg, teething) or continues after its resolution (successful dental treatment).
- The discomfort can be triggered by tongue movement (drinking, eating, grooming).
- Signalment (Burmese cat or cross).
- No other neurologic deficits especially (in particular, normal facial sensation).
- Failure to response to routine analgesia (nonsteroidal anti-inflammatory drugs and opioid) and dental treatment.
- Possible association to negative affective state.

understanding of the home layout and ascertain if the cat can traverse its territory, obtain water and food, and use the litter tray without running the gauntlet of other cats. Points of entry and exit to rooms containing resources and to the outside world (if appropriate) need to be freely accessible. Cats also need undisturbed access to preferred resting places (see Feline Chronic Pain and Osteoarthritis by Beatriz Monteiro in Part 1). Do not rely solely on the owners' perception of their cats' relationships for determining if social tension is present, as signs of conflict can be subtle and easily missed by owners; for example, cats staring at each other, or one cat blocking access to resources or stealing a resting place.[17] Asking owners to closely observe their cats over a 7-day period to identify social interactions, such as allogrooming, allorubbing, nose touching, and sleep-touching helps to determine if the FOPS-affected cat is part of a social group or subgroup or just coexisting with other cats in the household.[17,18] Information about visual access points from which the resident cat(s) can observe the outdoor environment and neighborhood cats is extremely important because social stress can result from visual as well as actual invasion of the core territory. Questions should be asked to determine whether neighborhood cats are able to lurk within gardens, on top of sheds, fences, or walls, and restrict the resident cat's free access to its outdoor environment.

Clinical examination

Examination focuses on investigation of causes of oral or facial pain. The head should be examined for symmetry (including the masticatory muscles), swellings, and lymph node enlargement. The eyes should be examined for vision, ocular discharge, normal tearing, blepharospasm, discoloration, and normal ability to retro-pulse the globe. Pain or dysfunction of the temporomandibular joint is assessed when opening the mouth. The oral cavity should be inspected; periodontitis is indicated if there is gingival recession or the tooth is mobile on digital palpation. However, a thorough oral examination can be performed only under general anesthesia,[19] especially as on cursory inspection TR may only appear as zone of inflamed gingiva over the lesion. A full neurologic examination should be performed with attention paid to cranial nerve testing, in particular the trigeminal nerve and closely associated structures (**Box 2**). In FOPS, neurologic findings are normal.

Oral examination under general anesthesia

The reader is recommended to review comprehensive guidelines for oral examination published by the World Small Animal Veterinary Association (WSAVA)[19] and to use a dental chart. Signs of FOPS can be worsened or induced by dental work and referral to specialist may be warranted especially if specialist equipment, such as being able to take dental radiographs, is not available. All structures of the oral cavity should be inspected, examining every tooth, evaluating pocket depth and furcation exposure with a periodontal probe. Any irregularity in the tooth surface is suspicious for a pathologic process and intrinsic staining indicates pulpitis and a nonvital tooth, which requires root canal therapy or extraction.[19] TR is characterized by a highly vascular and edematous area of inflammation over the lesion. Introduction of a probe can reveal a depression in the sulcus area and is typically associated with pronounced gingival bleeding. The teeth most commonly affected are the upper fourth premolar, lower molar, and lower third premolar.

Diagnostic imaging

Dental radiographs are an essential part of a diagnostic workup for an adult FOPS case. Protocols, methodology, and interpretation for intraoral radiographs are reviewed by Niemiec[20] and the WSAVA Global Dental Guidelines.[19] The changes

---

Box 2
Most important cranial nerve testing for a cat presented with orofacial pain

Paramount cranial nerve testing in a cat with orofacial pain
  Trigeminal nerve: sensory (facial sensation)
  • Palpebral reflex
  • Corneal reflex
  • Lip sensation
  • Nasal sensation
  • Ear sensation
  Trigeminal nerve: motor (muscles of mastication)
  • Masticatory muscle mass
  • Jaw tone
  Facial nerve: motor (facial muscles)
  • Facial symmetry
  • Palpebral reflex
  • Corneal reflex
  • Lip movement and tone
  • Ear movement and tone
  Facial nerve: parasympathetic (tear production)
  • Schirmer tear test
  Sympathetic supply to the eye (Horner syndrome)
  • Pupil size (miosis)
  • Third eyelid (protruded)
  • Palpebral aperture (narrowed)
  Glossopharyngeal motor (swallowing)
  • Gag reflex

---

associated with TR are characterized by lysis of tooth tissue, typically in the sulcus at the cemento-enamel junction (**Fig. 3**).

Other diagnostic investigation
If there are neurologic deficits, especially of the trigeminal nerve, then MRI is indicated. MRI is unremarkable in the instance of FOPS, but can be useful to rule out other causes of orofacial pain. There are no specific hematological or serum biochemistry abnormalities in the case of FOPS. However, it is important to obtain at least a minimal database to rule out contributory systemic disease and identify if there are any contra-indications to medical management. In addition, determining the cat's retroviral status is recommended.

Treatment and Prognosis

The diagnostic and management approach to FOPS is illustrated in **Fig. 4**. Any other systemic disease should be addressed. Until discomfort can be controlled, mutilation may need to be prevented by using an Elizabethan collar and/or paw bandaging; however, using barrier methods of this nature have a negative welfare impact and consequently stress reduction will be even more important.[21]

Periodontal disease
In an older cat, it is highly likely that periodontal disease has precipitated the disease and therefore examination under general anesthesia, intraoral radiographs, and appropriate management are recommended. It is important to supply appropriate analgesia and for long enough.[15] Referral to a veterinary dental specialist is recommended if the expertise and equipment are not available to extract teeth correctly, especially as alveolar bone compromise can damage trigeminal nerve endings and

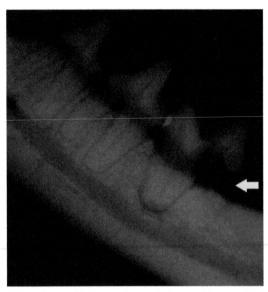

Fig. 3. Section of a lateral mandibular radiograph from a 7-year-old female Burmese cat with signs of FOPS. There is molar resorption (TR; *arrow*) with a periapical abscess of the rostral root. The radiograph also confirms marked gingival recession and horizontal bone loss. Adult cats with signs of FOPS should have full-mouth intraoral radiographs that would include a parallel technique for lateral views of the caudal mandibular dentition; a bisecting angle technique for all maxillary and the rostral mandibular teeth; lateral views of the canines, premolars, and molars; mesio-distal or rostro-caudal views of the incisors and canines; and oblique views of the maxillary fourth premolars. Early TR can be difficult to spot, and the radiograph should be examined carefully against a strong light with a magnifying glass.

precipitate a maladaptive pain state. Some cases of FOPS develop following routine dental treatment and extractions. Early and aggressive therapy for postoperative pain reduces the risk of developing a persistent pain state[22] (see Mark Epstein's article, "Feline Neuropathic Pain," in Part 1). Performing nerve blocks to desensitize the oral cavity completely will reduce the chance of the dental procedure exacerbating the pain. The maxillary nerve block, where an injection of lidocaine and bupivacaine is made in the direction of the maxillary foramen in the pterygopalatine fossa,[23] should block the pterygopalatine ganglion. Long-term analgesia is required after dental extractions in cats with severe oral disease.[15]

Environmental needs
Addressing environmental needs according to the 5 "pillars" framework[17] is an essential rather than an optional part of management of a FOPS-affected cat. The home should be optimized so that the cat feels in control and has free and immediate access to resources (**Box 3**) (see Sarah Heath's article, "Environment and Feline Health: At Home and in the Clinic," in Part 1).

Pharmacologic treatment of feline orofacial pain syndrome
First-line analgesia for FOPS should be with licensed analgesics; however, because FOPS likely involves disordered somatosensory nervous system processing, this therapy is insufficient in many cases. Maladaptive pain is managed with adjunctive drugs that have antihyperalgesic and antinociceptive activities (**Fig. 5**). **Table 2** lists the

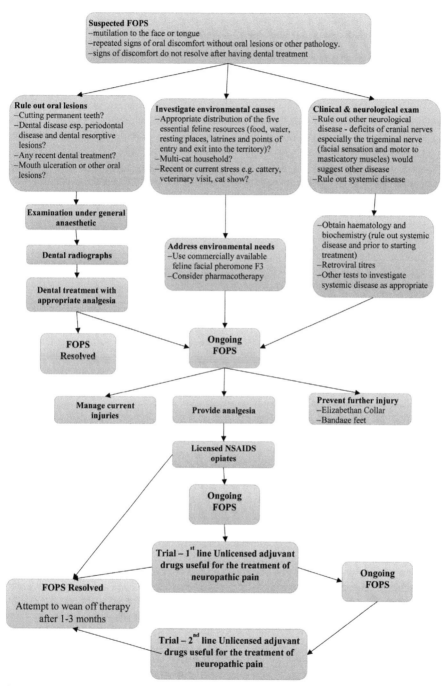

Fig. 4. Management algorithm for feline orofacial pain syndrome. NSAIDS, nonsteroidal anti-inflammatory drugs.

Box 3
Checklist for essential feline resources and environmental needs

- The essential feline resources are food, water, resting places (including elevated perches and individual hiding places), latrines, and points of entry and exit into the territory.
- Use house plans and video to identify and discuss problems associated with the distribution of these resources.
- Separate resource stations are needed for each social group.
- Resource stations should be out of view of other resource locations allowing an individual cat to avoid others and minimize competition, bullying, and stress.
- In multi-cat households there should be as least as many safe places as there are cats, and these should be separated from each other and have more than one entry so that it is more difficult to block.
- In multi-cat neighborhoods, it may be necessary to prevent visual intrusion using blinds or temporary frosting on the windows and to prevent physical intrusion using microchip-operated cat flaps.
- Cats should have free access to safe places outdoors (if possible).
- Cats should be able to engage in pseudo-predatory play and feeding behaviors.
- Cats need positive, consistent, and predictable human–cat social interaction.
- Cats need an environment that respects the importance of their sense of smell.
- Use of commercially available feline facial pheromone F3 within the home environment can increase the sensation of safety but will only be beneficial when used alongside environmental modifications.

For more details, the reader is referred to the American Association of Feline Practitioners and International Society of Feline Medicine Feline Environmental Needs Guidelines.[17]

---

adjuvant drugs used for feline maladaptive pain. Based on anecdotal information, the most useful adjuvant drugs for treating FOPS are gabapentinoids (gabapentin or pregabalin) or phenobarbital. Although the gabapentinoids are generally considered the most useful for management of feline maladaptive pain and can also reduce anxiety,[24] it is the author's experience that phenobarbital can be more effective for FOPS.[4] It is unclear why this might be, if true. Phenobarbital is not considered useful in human trigeminal neuralgia where carbamazepine remains first-line therapy.[25] Potentially, phenobarbital has an activity via increasing activity of inhibitory GABAergic circuits[26]; for example, influencing the trigemino-parasympathetic brain stem reflex[8] or perception of noxious stimuli in the prelimbic region.[27] Phenobarbital has the advantage for FOPS that once-daily dosing may be possible, and tablet sizes are more convenient for dosing. By contrast, gabapentin and pregabalin may need to be compounded. However, adverse effects of sedation, reduced jumping ability and ataxia, may limit use of phenobarbital. Adverse effects such as hematological abnormalities, pseudolymphoma, and liver compromise are rare but even less common with the gabapentinoids. For this reason, the author usually starts treatment with gabapentin and if this is not effective within 2 weeks, switches to phenobarbital. The other drugs listed in **Table 2** are options if phenobarbital cannot be tolerated or is ineffective or for polypharmacy.

For acute management of hospitalized cases, drugs such as parental phenobarbital, benzodiazepines, dexmedetomidine, or constant rate infusions of ketamine can be useful.

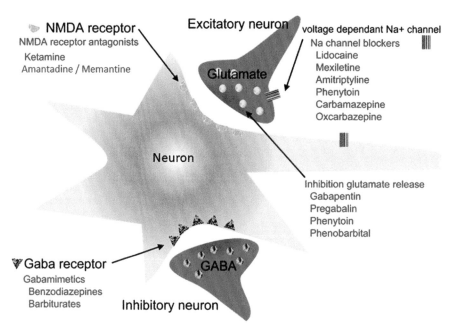

Fig. 5. Adjuvant drugs for neuropathic pain affect a wide range of pharmacologic targets, including glutaminergic and GABAergic systems, sodium and calcium channels, and voltage-dependent potassium currents. Phenytoin is not recommended in cats.

Cats with ongoing anxiety due to environment stress should have their welfare needs addressed (see **Box 3**); however, there may be some cases in which medication with selective serotonin reuptake inhibitors is necessary while environment optimization is achieved.

In kittens, signs resolve spontaneously when "teething" is complete, and it should be possible to withdraw medication over a 4-week to 8-week period. In adults, if periodontal disease is addressed successfully, it may be possible to withdrawal the adjuvant analgesic; however, as healing after dental extraction can be prolonged, it is recommended that this be delayed until after the cat has been free of clinical signs for at least 4 weeks. FOPS may occur in bouts over a period of weeks or months, with subsequent spontaneous remission. Over time, however, the disease can become unremitting, with up to 10% of the cases being euthanized because of the perceived poor quality of life.

FELINE HYPERESTHESIA SYNDROME

FHS is a poorly understood maladaptive pain condition that is a diagnosis of exclusion. Treatment with neuropharmacological agents is indicated in a minority of cases and only after addressing environmental needs according to the 5 "pillars" framework[17] and taking a systematic approach to rule out dermatologic causes and other causes of spinal or tail pain.

Clinical Signs

The classic signs of FHS are lumbar hyperesthesia, rippling skin, vocalization, and episodes of attacking or overgrooming the tail causing soft tissue damage or

Table 2
Unlicensed drugs used in the medical management of maladaptive pain in the cat

Drug	Dose	Notes
Phenobarbital	1–3 mg/kg PO/IM/IV/SID/BID	1st-line monotherapy (FOPS only).
Gabapentin	10 mg/kg PO BID/TID increasing up to 20 mg/kg BID/TID	1st-line monotherapy.
Pregabalin	4–5 mg/kg PO BID/TID increasing up to 10 mg/kg BID/TID	1st-line or 2nd-line monotherapy. Anecdotally more effective than gabapentin.
Topiramate	2.5 mg/kg PO SID/BID increasing up to 10 mg/kg BID	2nd-line therapy, often in polytherapy with pregabalin.
Carbamazepine	25 mg PO BID	3rd-line therapy. Liquid formulation and low cost. Frequent monitoring of hematology recommended.
Amantadine	3–5 mg/kg PO SID	3rd-line therapy. Bitter taste; difficult to administer. Occasionally used in polytherapy.
Amitriptyline	0.25 mg/kg PO SID in polytherapy increasing up to 2 mg/kg BID	3rd line therapy. Bitter taste; difficult to administer.
Tramadol	2–4 mg/kg PO BID/TID	3rd-line therapy. Bitter taste; difficult to administer.
Ketamine	0.5 mg/kg IV loading dose then 0.1–0.6 mg/kg/h IV CRI 24 h	Hospitalized cases.

Abbreviations: BID, twice daily; CRI, constant rate infusion; IM, intramuscular; IV, intravenous; PO, per os; SID, once daily; TID, 3 times daily (every 8 hours).

Important points.
- None of drugs listed in Table 2 are licensed for veterinary medicine.
- Doses are those used by the author. Unless otherwise indicated, start at the low end of the dose range and make increases based on effect and absence of adverse effects.
- All drugs should be prescribed by a veterinary surgeon who should refer to a formulary for drug adverse effects/drug interactions/titration and tapering details.
- Effect assessed over a 2-week to 4-week period except amantadine, tramadol, and amitriptyline, which require at least 4 weeks to assess effectiveness.
- Assess hematology and biochemistry before starting drugs and reassess at a minimum annually for animal receiving long-term medication.
- Gabapentin and pregabalin are Schedule 3 controlled drugs under the Misuse of Drugs Regulations 2001, and Class C of the Misuse of Drugs Act 1971 in the United Kingdom.

mutilation.[28] It is reputedly more common in Siamese, Burmese, Himalayan, and Abyssinian cats, and typically signs appear between 1 to 4 years. Commonly described signs include dilated pupils; appearing to be annoyed with, twitching, or biting at the tail; rippling skin on the back just above the tail; sensitive to touch around the tail and spine; and personality change. Cats may self-mutilate by biting, licking, chewing, and plucking hair and may be difficult to distract during an episode. The personality of the cats is often described as highly aroused (anxious, aggressive, restless, constantly wandering and pacing) and the behavior may be provoked by petting/stroking and may be more likely when anxious or stressed (Video 2).

Pathogenesis

The pathognomic signs of FHS is contraction of the *panniculus carnosus* (cutaneous trunci) muscle, which is intimately attached to the skin and fascia, hence the other monikers of FHS being "rolling skin syndrome," or "twitchy cat disease." The main function of *panniculus carnosus* is to shake off unwarranted foreign bodies or stimuli.[29] In the cat, noxious stimulation of the flank results in reflex contraction with the irregular twitching moving caudocranially to the shoulder region. At the same time the tail raises and is swept in a circular fashion toward the stimulus.[30] Consequently, the most common cause of rippling skin is skin irritation, which induces this reflex; however, rippling and twitching of the skin is also observed when a cat is highly aroused and frustrated[31]; that is, emotionally rather than physically irritated. This emotional expression is possibly mediated from higher centers via a brain stem nucleus.[32] Negative emotional state can also explain the other behavior seen with FHS. For example, brief, intense grooming behavior directed to the shoulder or base of the tail is a typical displacement activity for a frustrated cat.[31] Frustrated cats also rapidly switch between behaviors and thrash their tails. Anxious or very aroused cats may have mydriasis, piloerection, or be hypervigilant.[31]

The suggestion that FHS is a seizure disorder is spurious and likely based on positive response by some cats to anti-epileptic drugs with anxiolytic or analgesic activity. Likewise, an aversion to being touched on the back and "resolution" on medication used to treat neuropathic pain does not confirm spinal pain. FHS is often used as an umbrella term to cover cats with signs of excessively twitchy skin to tail mutilation and this is likely inappropriate; however, it is possible that some cats may be experiencing abnormal sensations and have some sort of neuropathic pain or itch disorder.

Diagnosis

Diagnostic workup of affected cats includes ruling out all other possible explanations, in particular skin disease, assessing environmental triggers, and investigation for spinal pain (**Fig. 6**). Cats with caudal spinal pain typically have behavioral signs of restricted movement; for example, reduced jumping or tail movements. When assessing the environmental triggers (as for FOPS), it is important to ascertain the contextual information: where the behavior occurs; who was there (owner and other animals) and how did they react; and what was happening immediately before. It is especially important to ascertain how the owners react to the behavior (past and present), as for many owners the sight of their cat behaving in an "odd" manner can be very distressing and repeated attempts to interrupt the behavior can inadvertently lead to increasing levels of arousal and a subsequent worsening of the behavioral signs.

Treatment and Prognosis

As for FOPS, addressing environmental needs according to the 5 "pillars" framework[17] is essential (see **Box 3**). A study that used a welfare scoring system to achieve this found that 12 of 13 cats with self-induced wounds and dermatologist diagnosis of idiopathic ulcerative dermatitis (IUD) had healing within 15 days of addressing the welfare needs.[33] IUD has many similarities to FHS. Pruritic skin disease should be ruled out with skin scrapes and cytology; control of ectoparasites; fungal culture; responses to 6-week to 8-week restriction diet; and response to immune-modulating therapy (eg, allergen-specific immunotherapy, glucocorticoids, or ciclosporin).[34] A diagnosis of a maladaptive pain syndrome can be made only after environmental needs and dermatologic causes have been ruled out. In this instance, medication for neuropathic pain can be tried (see **Fig. 5, Table 2**). The author's first-line therapy is gabapentinoids and second-line therapy is topiramate. Prognosis is fair if the preceding systematic approach is taken.

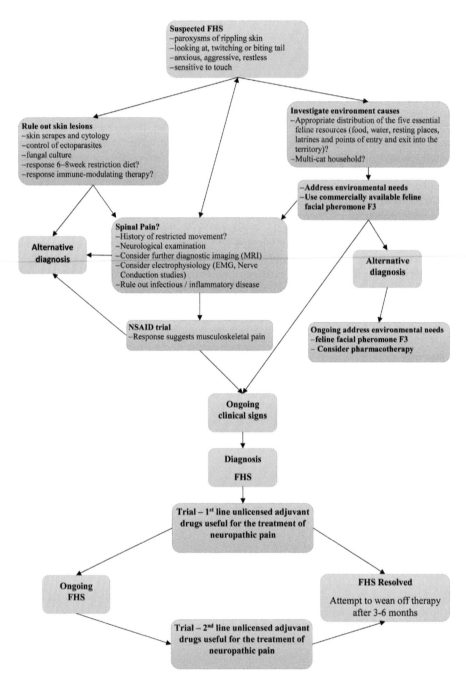

Fig. 6. Management algorithm for FHS. EMG, electromyography; NSAID, nonsteroidal anti-inflammatory drug.

FELINE LIMBIC ENCEPHALITIS

Feline limbic encephalitis (FLE, also known as feline complex partial seizures with orofacial involvement, feline temporal lobe epilepsy, or hippocampal necrosis) is characterized by behavioral changes and focal seizures with orofacial involvement and secondary generalization to tonic-clonic seizures. It is thought to be autoimmune encephalitis resulting in hippocampal neuronal hyperexcitability and impaired synaptic plasticity and memory. Management is with immunosuppression and anti-epilepsy drugs and prognosis is guarded.

Clinical Signs

Initial signs are behavioral changes including increased vocalization, aggression, or signs suggesting anxiety and fear. Pyrexia may be recorded. After a few days to a couple of weeks the affected cat develops focal seizures with orofacial automatism including salivation, facial twitching, lip smacking, chewing, licking, and swallowing (**Fig. 7**, Video 3). Neurologic examination can be difficult because of aggression or agitation. Affected cats may also be observed with mydriatic pupils and behavior as if watching or searching (**Fig. 8**, Video 4). Other reported interictal signs include ataxia, rapid running, circling, apparent blindness and deafness, weakness, polyphagia, and polydipsia.[35] The focal seizures with orofacial automatism become more frequent and are resistant to treatment with standard anti-epilepsy drugs. Signs progress over days, with focal seizures generalizing to tonic-clonic seizure then status epilepticus. Experimental feline temporal lobe epilepsy is useful to understand the signs (**Box 4**).[36]

The signs in FLE have many similarities with human autoimmune limbic encephalitis (LE), which is characterized by acute development of mood changes, anxiety, short-term memory deficit, rapid eye movement–sleep behavior disorders, and seizures.[37] Humans may have a prodrome of fever and headaches, probably representing early signs of blood brain barrier dysfunction.[38] The pathognomic signs of human antibody–leucine-rich glioma inactivated protein 1 (LGI1) LE (LGI1-Ab LE) are faciobrachial dystonic seizures. Humans with LGI1-Ab LE may also have hyponatremia due to hypothalamic dysfunction and inappropriate antidiuretic hormone secretion.[39] This has also been reported in cats.[40] The author has observed hypernatremia with low or low normal serum potassium in 2 affected cats; hypernatremia is rare in human LE. More unusual signs and complications associated with LE observed by the author are (1) neurogenic bladder with overflow requiring manual bladder expression, transient neurogenic urinary retention is reported in cats following severe cluster seizures[41]; and (2) sudden unexpected death.

Pathogenesis

There is a considerable weight of evidence that FLE is an autoimmune epilepsy. In humans, autoimmune LE is associated with antibodies against neuronal cell-surface, synaptic, or onconeural proteins resulting in hippocampal neuronal hyperexcitability (**Fig. 9**). In humans, the most common autoantibody associated with LE is against LGI1, also described in cats.[40,42] The complex of LGI1 and its receptors ADAM22 and ADAM23 forms a transsynaptic complex network that interacts with voltage-gated potassium channel and modulates AMPA receptor-mediated synaptic transmission.[43] FLE associated with netrin-1 receptor antibodies has also been described.[44] Netrin-1 is required for NMDA receptor-dependent synaptic plasticity (learning and memory) in the adult hippocampus.[45]

In humans, autoimmune encephalitis can be triggered by viral encephalitis (especially herpes simples), tumors (paraneoplastic autoantibodies), and biological cancer

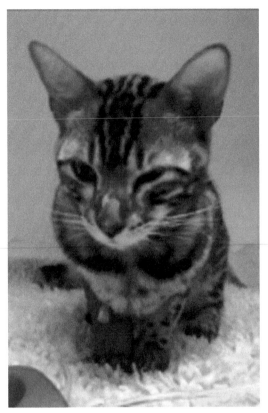

Fig. 7. A 1-year-old male Bengal cat with suspected LE with focal seizures with orofacial automatism. The cat had a 10-day history of behavioral change described as being more vocal and jumpier, urinating outside of the tray, and eating more and faster than usual. He then developed focal seizures with facial twitching that progressed over 3 days to more complex focal seizures that included vocalization, almost continuous facial twitching, and circling to the left.

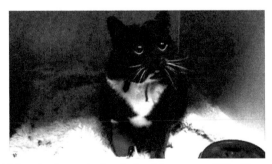

Fig. 8. A 2-year-old female domestic shorthair with suspected LE with mydriatic pupils and behavior as if watching or searching. Slight tongue protrusion is occasionally reported.

Box 4
Six stages of a feline temporal lobe seizure

Stage 1: Attention (looking around and up, sniffing)

Stage 2: Motor arrest (motionless starring)

Stage 3: Autonomic manifestations (salivation, mydriasis)

Stage 4: Orofacial automatisms (lip smacking, facial twitching, chewing, swallowing, eye-blinking)

Stage 5: Tonic extension of contralateral forepaw, head nodding, head turning

Stage 6: Secondary generalization into a tonic-clonic seizures.

Summarizing and combining experimental and clinical studies, 6 stages of feline temporal lobe seizures are recognized and were reviewed by Kitz and others.[36]

therapies.[38] For example, up to 20% of LGI1-Ab LE in humans is triggered by small cell lung carcinoma or thymoma.[38] In 1 feline study, 1 of 5 cats had a papillary adenoma.[46]

Histopathological studies of FLE have demonstrated blood brain barrier disturbance correlating to MRI changes but not to T-cell infiltrates.[40] This suggested that T cells do not directly contribute neurodegeneration and that antibodies transverse the blood brain barrier to affect specific neurons of the limbic system.[40]

Diagnosis

It is suggested that the veterinary profession adopt a similar diagnostic approach to that in humans[47,48]; however the challenge for veterinary medicine is that

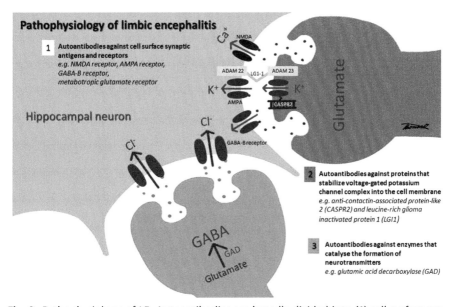

Fig. 9. Pathophysiology of LE. Autoantibodies are broadly divided into (1) cell-surface synaptic antigens and receptors, (2) proteins that stabilize voltage-gated potassium channel complex into the cell membrane, and (3) enzymes that catalyze the formation of neurotransmitters.

electroencephalography and testing for autoantibodies is not widely available.[49] In addition, cerebrospinal fluid (CSF) analysis is often normal and MRI can also be normal early in the disease course. Consequently, a 3-tier confidence level for the premortem diagnosis (based on human guidelines for diagnosis of autoimmune LE) is suggested (**Box 5**). Tier 1 confidence is based on very poor evidence; however, the window for initiating successful immunosuppression and limiting hippocampal necrosis and sclerosis is small, therefore immunosuppressive treatment should be considered if other explanations have been excluded and there is a failure to control the seizures with anti-epileptic drugs.

Magnetic resonance imaging

An epilepsy-specific brain magnetic resonance protocol[50] is recommended to optimize visualization of the medial temporal lobe. LE is characterized by bilateral medial temporal lobe (hippocampal, parahippocampal, and piriform cortex) swelling with T1-weighed hypointensity or isointensity and T2-weighted/fluid-attenuated inversion recovery (FLAIR) hyperintensity with variable and patchy paramagnetic contrast enhancement on postcontrast T1-0weighed images (**Figs. 10** and **11**).[51] Initial swelling of these structures is often followed by atrophy. Although bilateral involvement is typical, it is not always symmetric (see **Fig. 11**). Unilateral temporal lobe changes would be suspicious for another pathology, especially neoplasia (**Table 3**). One of the greatest controversies for making a diagnosis of LE is that repetitive or prolonged seizures, can also cause bilateral T2-weighted/FLAIR hyperintensity because of temporal lobe edema or necrosis.[52] Cats with seizures that have orofacial involvement due to any cause are more likely to have cluster seizures and status epilepticus[53] and the hippocampus is more vulnerable to convulsion-induced excitotoxic damage because is it rich in kainate and NMDA receptors and lacks protection against calcium overload.[54] A guide to distinguish hippocampal pathology using MRI is suggested in **Table 3**.

Laboratory testing and other investigation

CSF analysis should be performed, and in the instance of LE is either normal (majority) or demonstrates a mild pleocytosis.[35] Testing of the CSF and serum for central nervous system autoantibodies (antibodies against cell-surface, synaptic, or onconeural proteins) is not widely available in veterinary medicine, although Pakozdy and others[42] have validated voltage-gated potassium channel complex (LGI1 and VGKC-Ak) serum antibody testing. Other diagnostic investigation is detailed in **Table 4**.

Treatment and Prognosis

The human literature suggests that early suspicion of and treatment for LE is associated with reduced seizure frequency, recovery of cognition, and improved survival.[55] In humans, first-line therapy is 3 to 5 days of high-dose intravenous steroids followed by intravenous immunoglobulin. If there is no response after 4 weeks, then second-line therapy is plasmapheresis or immunotherapeutics, such as rituximab (monoclonal antibody) or cyclophosphamide. Third-line treatment options are bortezomib (a proteasome inhibitor) or tocilizumab (an interleukin-6 receptor antagonist). If possible, tumors should be removed.[38,55] Because of the paucity of case studies, there is little information on treatment regimens in cats. Most clinicians use prednisolone dosed initially at 1 to 2 mg/kg twice daily then tapered over variable time periods.[35] Of the preceding listed agents, cyclophosphamide is the only one previously used in cats. Although normally reserved for neoplastic disease, this could be an option in refractory cases.

Box 5
Three-tier confidence level for the premortem diagnosis of limbic encephalitis

Tier I confidence level for diagnosis
1. Prodromal behavioral changes.
2. Acute-onset frequent treatment-resistant focal seizures with orofacial involvement (including motionless staring, mydriasis, vocalization, facial twitching, salivation, lip smacking, chewing, licking, swallowing) with or without secondary generalization with interictal behavioral changes.
3. Reasonable exclusion of alternatives, including unremarkable MRI of the brain (epilepsy-specific brain MRI protocol).

Tier II level of confidence
1. Prodromal behavioral changes.
2. Acute-onset frequent treatment-resistant focal seizures with orofacial involvement (including motionless staring, mydriasis, vocalization, facial twitching, salivation, lip smacking, chewing, licking, swallowing) with or without secondary generalization with interictal behavioral changes.
3. Bilateral medial temporal lobe (hippocampal) T1 hypointensity and isointensity and T2 hyperintensity with variable paramagnetic contrast enhancement.
4. Reasonable exclusion of alternatives.

Tier III level of confidence[47,48]

Diagnosis made when all 4 of the following criteria have been met:
1. Acute-onset frequent treatment-resistant focal seizures with orofacial involvement (including motionless staring, mydriasis, vocalization, facial twitching, salivation, lip smacking, chewing, licking, swallowing) with or without secondary generalization.
2. Bilateral medial temporal lobe (hippocampal) T1 hypointensity and isointensity and T2 hyperintensity with variable paramagnetic contrast enhancement.
3. At least 1 of the following:
   • Cerebrospinal fluid pleocytosis
   • Electroencephalography with epileptic or slow-wave activity involving the temporal lobes
4. Reasonable exclusion of alternatives.

If 1 of the first 3 criteria is not met, a diagnosis of definite limbic encephalitis can be made only with the detection of antibodies against cell-surface, synaptic, or onconeural proteins.

Data from Budhram A, Leung A, Nicolle MW, et al. Diagnosing autoimmune limbic encephalitis. *CMAJ.*2019;191(19):E529-e534 and Graus F, Titulaer MJ, Balu R, et al. A clinical approach to diagnosis of autoimmune encephalitis. *Lancet neurology.* 2016;15(4):391-404.

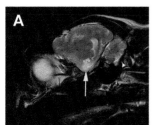 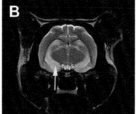 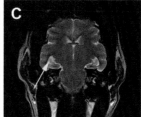

Fig. 10. Suspected LE in a 6-year-old female domestic shorthair. T2-weighted images of the brain (*A*). Parasagittal at the level of the right medial temporal lobe (*B*). Transverse at the level of the sella turcica (*C*). Dorsal at the level of the ventral medial temporal lobe. There is bilateral hyperintensity of the hippocampus and surrounding piriform cortex (*arrows*).

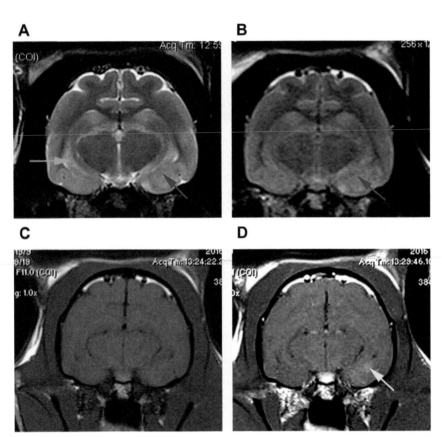

Fig. 11. Suspected LE in a 14-year-old male domestic shorthair. Brain MRI at the level of the medial temporal lobe (A). T2 -weighted (B). FLAIR (C). T1-weighted (D). T1-weighted following paramagnetic contrast enhancement. There are bilateral changes of the medial temporal lobe that are hyperintense on T2-weighting and FLAIR, isointense and hypointense on T1-weighting with subtle paramagnetic contrast enhancement (*yellow arrow*). The changes are asymmetrical, being more obvious and with swelling on the left (*red arrow*) and subtle on the right (*green arrow*).

Anti-epileptic drugs should be used to control and limit damage from seizures and again there is no consensus option. Controlling the repetitive seizures and status epilepticus is challenging, and polytherapy is likely to be necessary and continued over several days. The reader is referred to a review on management of status epilepticus.[56] First-line therapy for the author is phenobarbital combined with levetiracetam, then sequentially adding, as necessary, ketamine constant rate infusion, propofol, and dexmedetomidine. For maintenance therapy of seizures, the author typically uses a combination of phenobarbital and levetiracetam. It may be possible to withdraw therapy eventually.[35] In refractory epilepsy, likely related to hippocampal atrophy, the author uses polytherapy, adding topiramate or zonisamide and rarely clonazepam.[57] Prognosis is considered guarded; however, if the cat can be supported in the acute phase and started on immunosuppressive therapy, then the prognosis is improved.

Table 3
A guide to distinguish hippocampal pathology using MRI

Distinguishing Limbic Encephalitis from Other Hippocampal Pathology by MRI

Features Suggestive Limbic Encephalopathy	Features Suggestive of Post-Ictal Hippocampal Edema/Necrosis	Features Suggestive Other Pathology

• Bilateral medial temporal lobe T2-weighted/FLAIR hyperintensity
• Medial temporal lobe swelling
• Medial temporal lobe paramagnetic contrast enhancement
	• Bilateral medial temporal lobe swelling and T2-weighted/FLAIR hyperintensity
	• Lateral temporal lobe involvement
	• Other cortical involvement
	• DWI increased signal intensity and reduced ADC at the same location as T2 hyperintensity (reflects restricted diffusion from cytotoxic cell swelling and vasogenic edema)
	• Changes transient
		• Unilateral medial temporal lobe pathology
		  ○ swelling
		  ○ T2-weighted/FLAIR) hyperintensity
		  ○ +/− paramagnetic contrast enhancement
		• Lateral temporal lobe or other brain involvement

Abbreviations: ADC, apparent diffusion coefficient; DWI, diffusion-weighted imaging; FLAIR, fluid attenuated inversion recovery.

Table 4
Diagnostic investigation for suspected feline limbic encephalitis

Diagnostic Test	Notes
Hematology and serum biochemistry	As part of workup for encephalopathy or repetitive seizures.
MRI	See **Table 3**
CSF analysis	Typically normal or a mild pleocytosis
Autoantibody panel	If facilities exist. In humans, serum and CSF testing for the most commonly identified antibodies (anti-LGI1, GABABR, AMPAR, CASPR2, Hu, Ma2, and GAD) is recommended to maximize diagnostic yield. Some antibodies (eg, anti-LGI1) are more sensitive in serum and others (eg, anti-GABABR) may be identified only in CSF.
Thoracic and abdominal diagnostic imaging	Although paraneoplastic and infectious triggers of feline limbic encephalitis appear uncommon, it is important to rule these out, as these may adversely affect prognosis or have a specific treatment.
Screening for infectious disease	FeLV, FIV, toxoplasma, coronavirus, and in appropriate geographic regions Borna virus. Although herpes simplex is associated with limbic encephalitis in humans, there is no evidence (yet) that there is a similar association with feline herpes virus.

Abbreviations: CSF, cerebrospinal fluid; FeLV, feline leukemia virus; FIV, feline immunodeficiency virus; GABABR, gamma-aminobutyric acid B receptor; LGI1, leucine-rich glioma inactivated protein 1.

SUMMARY

When presented with neurobehavioral disorders, the corticolimbic system may be implicated either because of direct pathology, such as LE, because it modulates the response to pain such as in FOPS, or because it coordinates the behavioral output according to the emotional and environmental circumstances as FHS. Because of the anatomic and function overlap between corticolimbic circuitry for pain and emotion, the pathophysiology for maladaptive pain conditions is extremely complex. Addressing environmental needs and underlying triggers is more important than pharmacotherapy when dealing with FOPS or FHS. By contrast, autoimmune LE requires prompt diagnosis and management with immunosuppression and seizure control.

ACKNOWLEDGMENTS

The author is grateful to Thomas Rusbridge for his artistic talents in creating **Figs. 1** and **9**.

DISCLOSURE

None.

SUPPLEMENTARY DATA

Supplementary data related to this article can be found online at https://doi.org/10.1016/j.cvsm.2020.06.009.

REFERENCES

1. Bergstrom HC, Pinard CR. Corticolimbic circuits in learning, memory, and disease. J Neurosci Res 2017;95(3):795–6.
2. Vachon-Presseau E, Centeno MV, Ren W, et al. The emotional brain as a predictor and amplifier of chronic pain. J Dent Res 2016;95(6):605–12.
3. Yang S, Chang MC. Chronic pain: structural and functional changes in brain structures and associated negative affective states. Int J Mol Sci 2019;20(13):3130.
4. Rusbridge C, Heath S, Gunn-Moore DA, et al. Feline orofacial pain syndrome (FOPS): a retrospective study of 113 cases. J Feline Med Surg 2010;12(6):498–508.
5. Ohara K, Shimizu K, Matsuura S, et al. Toll-like receptor 4 signaling in trigeminal ganglion neurons contributes tongue-referred pain associated with tooth pulp inflammation. J Neuroinflammation 2013;10(1):139.
6. Hirvonen T, Ngassapa D, Narhi M. Relation of dentin sensitivity to histological changes in dog teeth with exposed and stimulated dentin. Proc Finn Dent Soc 1992;88(Suppl 1):133–41.
7. Narhi M, Yamamoto H, Ngassapa D, et al. The neurophysiological basis and the role of inflammatory reactions in dentine hypersensitivity. Arch Oral Biol 1994;39(Suppl):23S–30S.
8. Kawakami S, Izumi H, Masaki E, et al. Role of medullary GABA signal transduction on parasympathetic reflex vasodilatation in the lower lip. Brain Res 2012;1437:26–37.
9. Piagkou M, Demesticha T, Troupis T, et al. The pterygopalatine ganglion and its role in various pain syndromes: from anatomy to clinical practice. Pain Pract 2012;12(5):399–412.

10. Tait RC, Ferguson M, Herndon CM. Chronic orofacial pain: burning mouth syndrome and other neuropathic disorders. J Pain Manag Med 2017;3(1):120.

11. Gandolfi B, Rusbridge C, R M, Lyons L. You're Getting On My Nerves! The Feline Orofacial Pain Syndrome. Paper presented at: Tufts' Canine and Feline Breeding and Genetics Conference; Boston, MA, September 27–29, 2013.

12. Nakajima C, Kulik A, Frotscher M, et al. Low density lipoprotein receptor-related protein 1 (LRP1) modulates N-methyl-D-aspartate (NMDA) receptor-dependent intracellular signaling and NMDA-induced regulation of postsynaptic protein complexes. J Biol Chem 2013;288(30):21909–23.

13. May P, Herz J. LDL receptor-related proteins in neurodevelopment. Traffic 2003; 4(5):291–301.

14. Khan SA, Keaser ML, Meiller TF, et al. Altered structure and function in the hippocampus and medial prefrontal cortex in patients with burning mouth syndrome. Pain 2014;155(8):1472–80.

15. Watanabe R, Doodnaught G, Proulx C, et al. A multidisciplinary study of pain in cats undergoing dental extractions: a prospective, blinded, clinical trial. PLoS One 2019;14(3):e0213195.

16. Freeman LM, Rodenberg C, Narayanan A, et al. Development and initial validation of the Cat HEalth and Wellbeing (CHEW) Questionnaire: a generic health-related quality of life instrument for cats. J Feline Med Surg 2016;18(9):689–701.

17. Ellis SLH, Rodan I, Carney HC, et al. AAFP and ISFM feline environmental needs guidelines. J Feline Med Surg 2013;15(3):219–30.

18. Elzerman AL, DePorter TL, Beck A, et al. Conflict and affiliative behavior frequency between cats in multi-cat households: a survey-based study. J Feline Med Surg 2019. https://doi.org/10.1177/1098612X19877988. 1098612X19877988.

19. Niemiec B, Gawor J, Nemec A, et al. World small animal veterinary association global dental guidelines 2019. World Small Animal Veterinary Association Global Guidelines. Available at: https://wsava.org/global-guidelines/global-dental-guidelines/. Accessed March 24, 2020.

20. Niemiec BA. Feline dental radiography and radiology: a primer. J Feline Med Surg 2014;16(11):887–99.

21. Shenoda Y, Ward MP, McKeegan D, et al. "The cone of shame": welfare implications of Elizabethan collar use on dogs and cats as reported by their owners. Animals (Basel) 2020;10(2):333.

22. Kehlet H, Jensen TS, Woolf CJ. Persistent postsurgical pain: risk factors and prevention. Lancet 2006;367(9522):1618–25.

23. Aguiar J, Chebroux A, Martinez-Taboada F, et al. Analgesic effects of maxillary and inferior alveolar nerve blocks in cats undergoing dental extractions. J Feline Med Surg 2015;17(2):110–6.

24. Guedes AGP, Meadows JM, Pypendop BH, et al. Assessment of the effects of gabapentin on activity levels and owner-perceived mobility impairment and quality of life in osteoarthritic geriatric cats. J Am Vet Med Assoc 2018;253(5):579–85.

25. Cheshire WP. Trigeminal neuralgia : a guide to drug choice. CNS Drugs 1997; 7(2):98–110.

26. Loscher W, Rogawski MA. How theories evolved concerning the mechanism of action of barbiturates. Epilepsia 2012;53(Suppl 8):12–25.

27. Zhang Z, Gadotti VM, Chen L, et al. Role of prelimbic GABAergic circuits in sensory and emotional aspects of neuropathic pain. Cell Rep 2015;12(5):752–9.

28. Amengual Batle P, Rusbridge C, Nuttall T, et al. Feline hyperaesthesia syndrome with self-trauma to the tail: retrospective study of seven cases and proposal for an

integrated multidisciplinary diagnostic approach. J Feline Med Surg 2019;21(2):
178–85.

29. Naldaiz-Gastesi N, Bahri OA, López de Munain A, et al. The panniculus carnosus muscle: an evolutionary enigma at the intersection of distinct research fields. J Anat 2018;233(3):275–88.

30. Kidd W. Scratch reflex of the cat. In: Initative in evolution. Holborn (London): H.F. & G Witherby; 1920. p. 254–6.

31. Ellis SLH. Recognising and assessing feline emotions during the consultation: History, body language and behaviour. J Feline Med Surg 2018;20(5):445–56.

32. Boers J, Kirkwood PA, de Weerd H, et al. Ultrastructural evidence for direct excitatory retroambiguous projections to cutaneous trunci and abdominal external oblique muscle motoneurons in the cat. Brain Res Bull 2006;68(4):249–56.

33. Titeux E, Gilbert C, Briand A, et al. From feline idiopathic ulcerative dermatitis to feline behavioral ulcerative dermatitis: grooming repetitive behaviors indicators of poor welfare in cats. Front Vet Sci 2018;5:81.

34. Favrot C, Steffan J, Seewald W, et al. Establishment of diagnostic criteria for feline nonflea-induced hypersensitivity dermatitis. Vet Dermatol 2012;23(1):45.e11.

35. Pakozdy A, Gruber A, Kneissl S, et al. Complex partial cluster seizures in cats with orofacial involvement. J Feline Med Surg 2011;13(10):687–93.

36. Kitz S, Thalhammer JG, Glantschnigg U, et al. Feline temporal lobe epilepsy: review of the experimental literature. J Vet Intern Med 2017;31(3):633–40.

37. Leypoldt F, Armangue T, Dalmau J. Autoimmune encephalopathies. Ann N Y Acad Sci 2015;1338:94–114.

38. Alexopoulos H, Dalakas MC. The immunobiology of autoimmune encephalitides. J Autoimmun 2019;104:102339.

39. McQuillan RF, Bargman JM. Hyponatraemia caused by LGI1-associated limbic encephalitis. NDT Plus 2011;4(6):424–6.

40. Tröscher AR, Klang A, French M, et al. Selective limbic blood-brain barrier breakdown in a feline model of limbic encephalitis with LGI1 antibodies. Front Immunol 2017;8:1364.

41. Balducci F, De Risio L, Shea A, et al. Neurogenic urinary retention in cats following severe cluster seizures. J Feline Med Surg 2015;19(2):246–50.

42. Pakozdy A, Halasz P, Klang A, et al. Suspected limbic encephalitis and seizure in cats associated with voltage-gated potassium channel (VGKC) complex antibody. J Vet Intern Med 2013;27(1):212–4.

43. Petit-Pedrol M, Sell J, Planagumà J, et al. LGI1 antibodies alter Kv1.1 and AMPA receptors changing synaptic excitability, plasticity and memory. Brain 2018; 141(11):3144–59.

44. Hasegawa D, Ohnishi Y, Koyama E, et al. Deleted in colorectal cancer (netrin-1 receptor) antibodies and limbic encephalitis in a cat with hippocampal necrosis. J Vet Intern Med 2019;33(3):1440–5.

45. Baastrup C, Jensen TS, Finnerup NB. Pregabalin attenuates place escape/avoidance behavior in a rat model of spinal cord injury. Brain Res 2011;1370:129–35.

46. Klang A, Schmidt P, Kneissl S, et al. IgG and complement deposition and neuronal loss in cats and humans with epilepsy and voltage-gated potassium channel complex antibodies. J Neuropathol Exp Neurol 2014;73(5):403–13.

47. Budhram A, Leung A, Nicolle MW, et al. Diagnosing autoimmune limbic encephalitis. CMAJ 2019;191(19):E529–34.

48. Graus F, Titulaer MJ, Balu R, et al. A clinical approach to diagnosis of autoimmune encephalitis. Lancet Neurol 2016;15(4):391–404.

49. Pakozdy A, Glantschnigg U, Leschnik M, et al. EEG-confirmed epileptic activity in a cat with VGKC-complex/LGI1 antibody-associated limbic encephalitis. Epileptic Disord 2014;16(1):116–20.

50. Rusbridge C, Long S, Jovanovik J, et al. International Veterinary Epilepsy Task Force recommendations for a veterinary epilepsy-specific MRI protocol. BMC Vet Res 2015;11(1):194.

51. Wahle AM, Brühschwein A, Matiasek K, et al. Clinical characterization of epilepsy of unknown cause in cats. J Vet Intern Med 2014;28(1):182–8.

52. Klang A, Hogler S, Nedorost N, et al. Hippocampal necrosis and sclerosis in cats: a retrospective study of 35 cases. Acta Vet Hung 2018;66(2):269–80.

53. Claßen AC, Kneissl S, Lang J, et al. Magnetic resonance features of the feline hippocampus in epileptic and non-epileptic cats: a blinded, retrospective, multi-observer study. BMC Vet Res 2016;12(1):165.

54. da Rocha AJ, Nunes RH, Maia ACM, et al. Recognizing autoimmune-mediated encephalitis in the differential diagnosis of limbic disorders. Am J Neuroradiol 2015;36(12):2196–205.

55. Nosadini M, Mohammad SS, Ramanathan S, et al. Immune therapy in autoimmune encephalitis: a systematic review. Expert Rev Neurother 2015;15(12): 1391–419.

56. Blades Golubovic S, Rossmeisl JH Jr. Status epilepticus in dogs and cats, part 2: treatment, monitoring, and prognosis. J Vet Emerg Crit Care 2017;27(3):288–300.

57. Rusbridge C. Diagnosis and control of epilepsy in the cat. Practice 2005;27(4): 208–14.

Moving?

Make sure your subscription moves with you!

To notify us of your new address, find your **Clinics Account Number** (located on your mailing label above your name), and contact customer service at:

Email: journalscustomerservice-usa@elsevier.com

800-654-2452 (subscribers in the U.S. & Canada)
314-447-8871 (subscribers outside of the U.S. & Canada)

Fax number: 314-447-8029

Elsevier Health Sciences Division
Subscription Customer Service
3251 Riverport Lane
Maryland Heights, MO 63043

*To ensure uninterrupted delivery of your subscription, please notify us at least 4 weeks in advance of move.

Printed and bound by CPI Group (UK) Ltd, Croydon, CR0 4YY

03/10/2024

01040408-0008